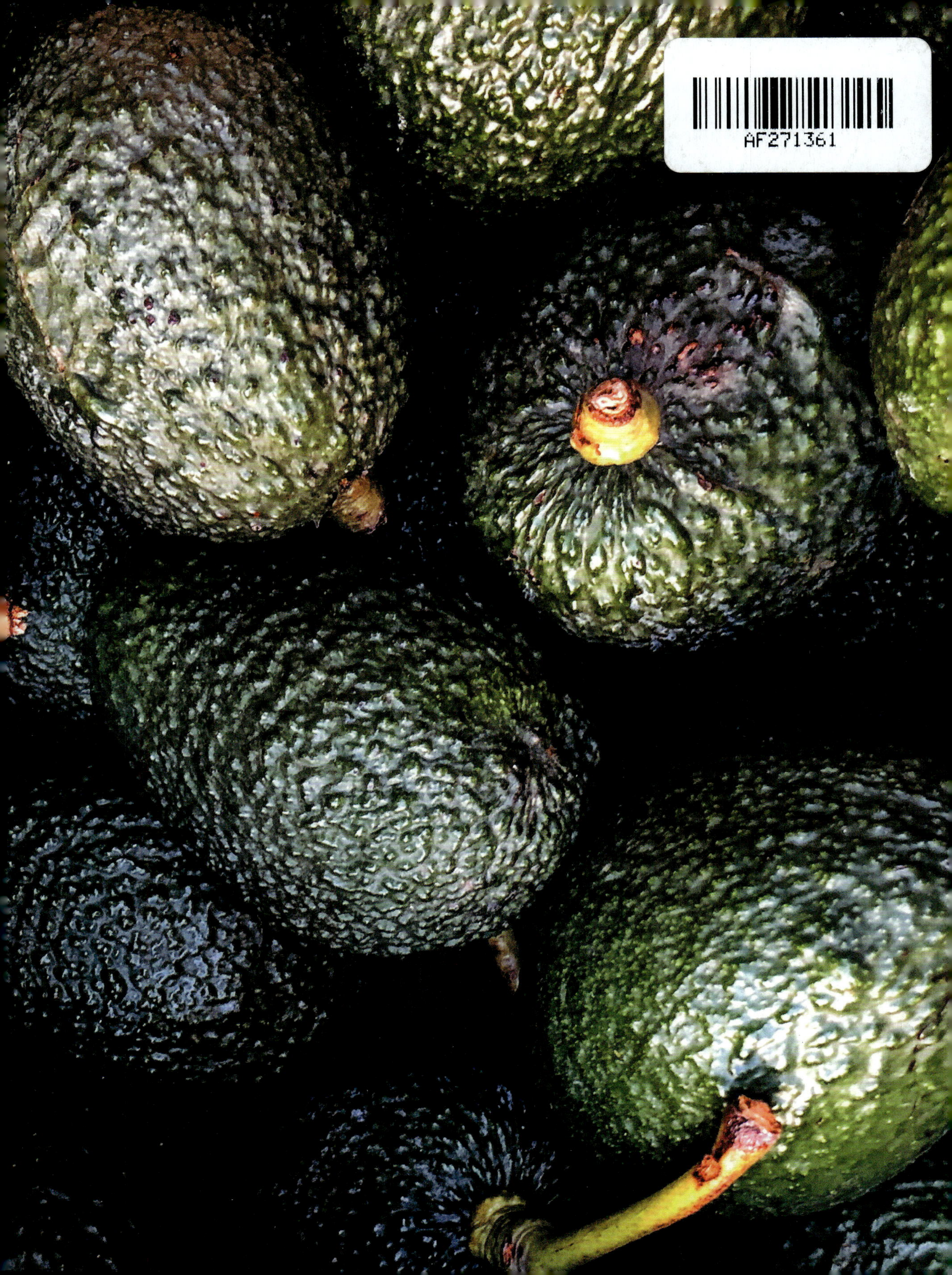
AF271361

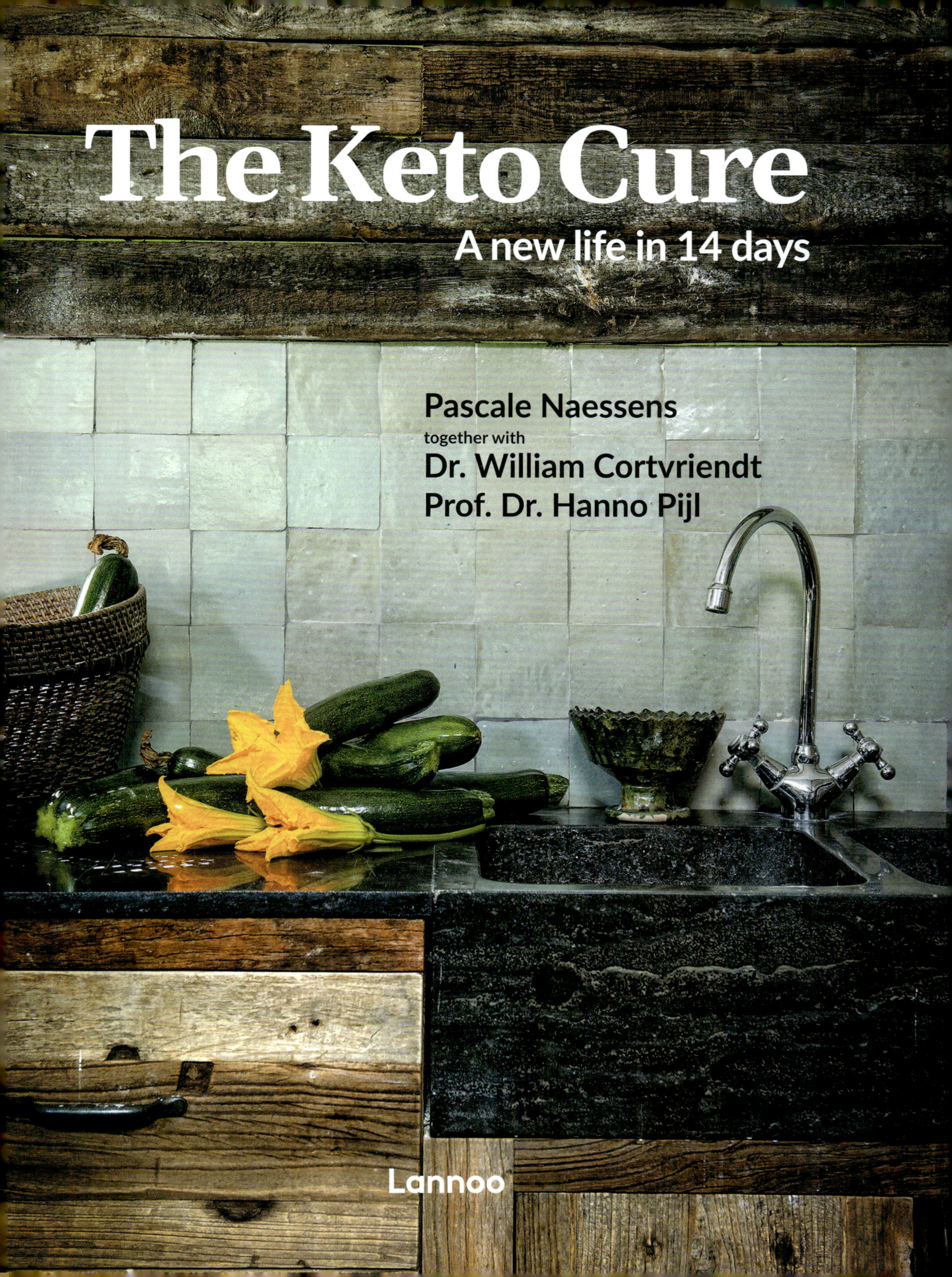

The Keto Cure

A new life in 14 days

Pascale Naessens
together with
Dr. William Cortvriendt
Prof. Dr. Hanno Pijl

Lannoo

Contents

For a more extensive index and other extras, download the free app: Pascale Naessens

The recipes in this book are for two people unless otherwise indicated.

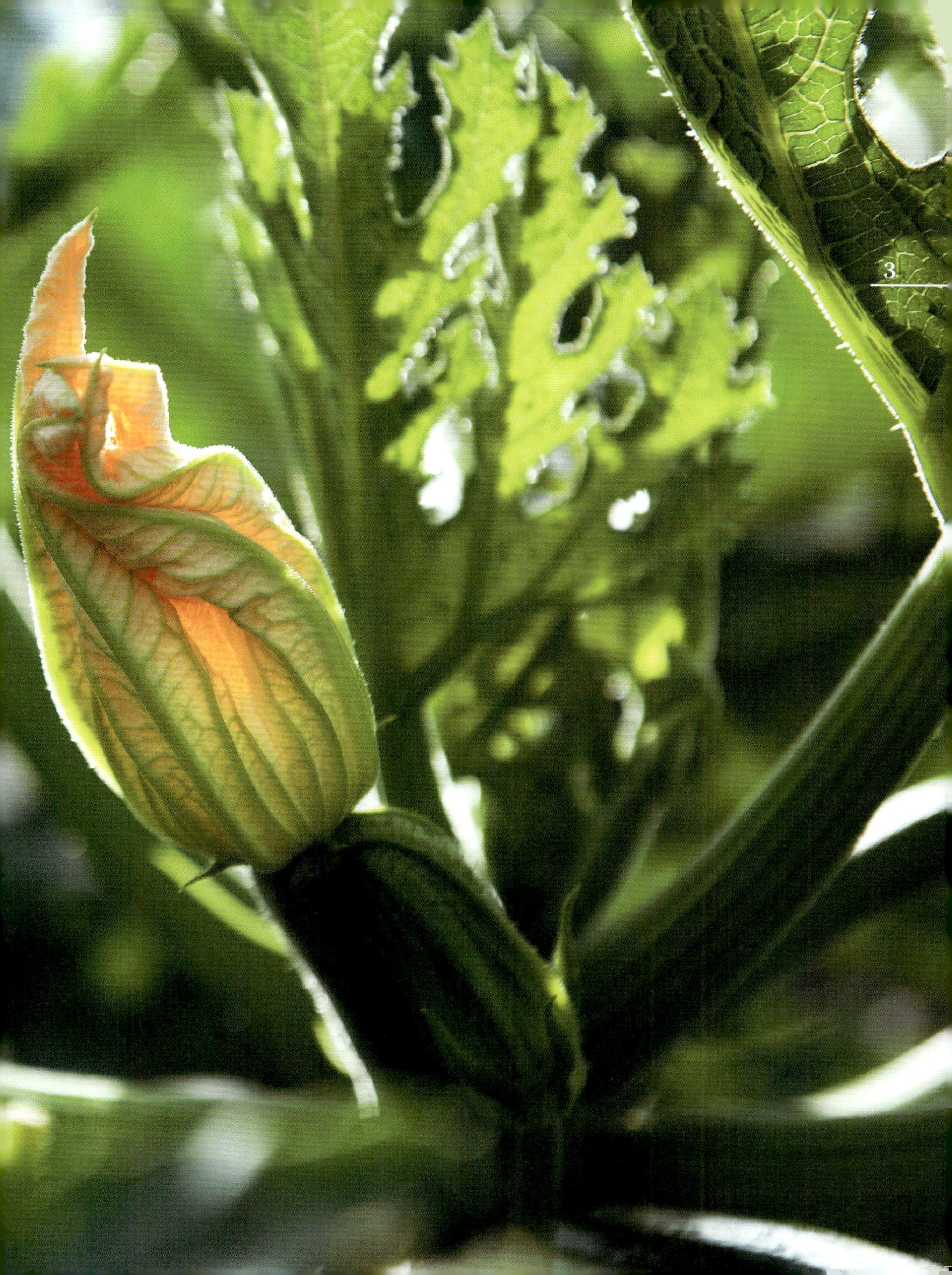
3

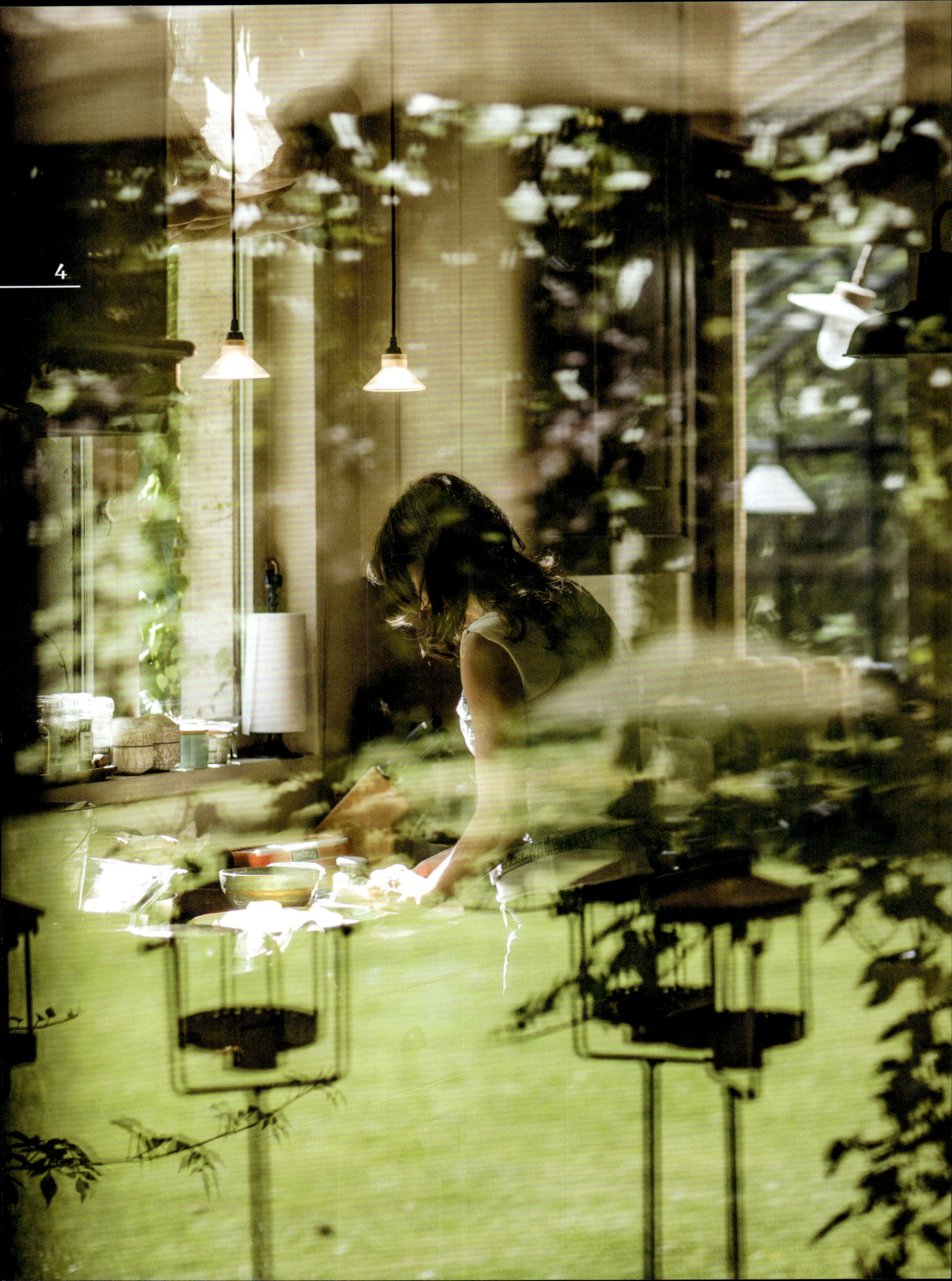

Why have I written The Keto Cure?

"I'm on a ketogenic diet." How often have I heard people telling me that? "So, what do you eat then?" I reply, intrigued. When I find out what they actually do eat, I often have to conclude that they're not following a ketogenic diet, but are eating low-carb, the same way of eating that I've been promoting in my books.

"Keto" has become a popular term, but there is a lot of confusion about it. What exactly does keto mean? With this book, I hope to provide insight into what a ketogenic (keto for short) diet is and how it differs from my way of eating, which I call "moderately low-carbohydrate" and promote in all my other books. This will help you understand what the difference is and decide if this diet will work for you.

Why would anyone want to follow a ketogenic diet in the first place? It is, after all, restrictive and relatively extreme: extremely few carbohydrates (carbs for short) and extreme amounts of fat. This is why it's important to be well-informed so you can make the right choices.

My faithful readers will know that my passion lies with the moderately low-carb way of eating. Most people achieve the desired result with this way of eating: staying slim and healthy while enjoying delicious food. But I understand that some people need to take that extra step to achieve the same results, particularly in terms of weight loss. That may be the most popular reason for following a ketogenic diet, especially when losing weight cannot be achieved by simply eating low-carb foods. A ketogenic diet can also be used as a treatment for conditions such as epilepsy, type 2 diabetes, and cancer. When it comes to the medical side of things, I believe it's important to get professionals involved. That's why I have asked Professor Hanno Pijl, lecturer in diabetology at the University of Utrecht and someone who has plenty of experience with the ketogenic diet, to contribute to my book. I have also asked Doctor William Cortvriendt, with whom I wrote *Pure & Lighter*, to help me with *The Keto Cure*. William Cortvriendt has just authored a book about cancer in which he recommends the ketogenic diet as a form of treatment. And don't forget that keto is a diet that is still in its early stages. That's why I feel that the scientific research behind it is so important. Because keto is becoming increasingly important in many aspects of life, that's what makes it so fascinating. There are currently 83 studies being conducted worldwide regarding the ketogenic diet as it relates to certain medical conditions, including two in Belgium and two in the Netherlands. (https://clinicaltrials.gov/ct2/results?term=%22ketogenic+diet%22&recrs=abdf)

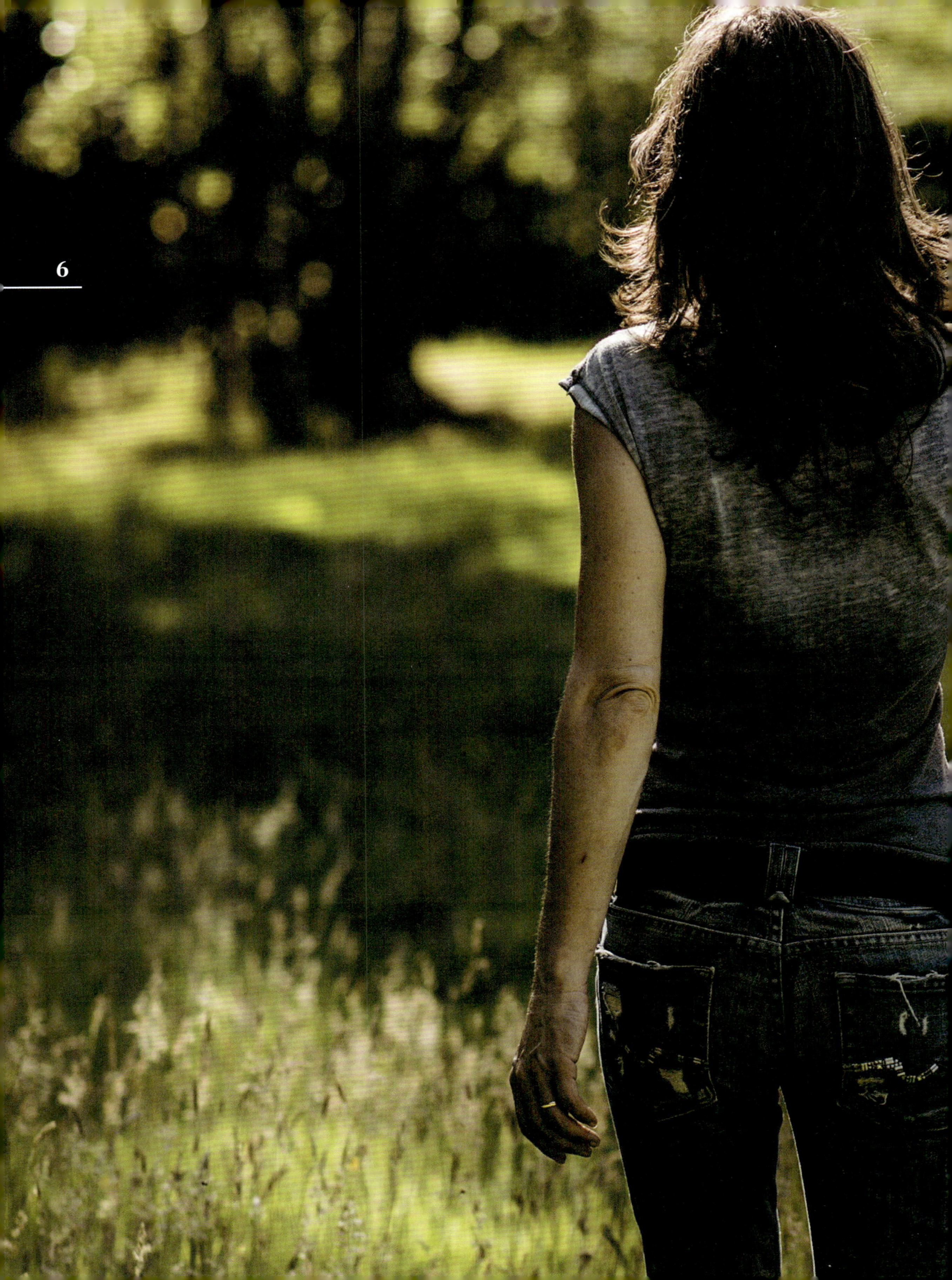

With this book, I hope to give you a thorough understanding of what a ketogenic diet is, so you can decide for yourself whether this diet is the right fit for you. If you decide to follow the diet, you can start straight away with a 14-day keto plan. You can extend this to three weeks with the extra recipes in the back of this book. These are recipes from my other books, supplemented by new recipes, but I have adapted them all to contain the correct proportions of carbs, protein and fats you need to help you reach ketosis fast and keep you there so you can instantly get to where you want to be and hopefully see some quick results. The weekly menus have been carefully planned, taking into consideration amounts of fiber, the presence of certain nutrients and sufficient intake of fluids to make the transition from burning sugar to burning fat as effortless as possible. If you decide to try them out, I wish you luck!

If you decide that the ketogenic diet is not for you, you can still use these recipes. Don't eat these dishes one after the other but alternate with a breakfast of fruit or a dish with lentils or root vegetables. That way you're eating low-carb, the way of eating I promote in my other books. I can promise you it will be a fascinating experience!

I wish you all the best on this exciting and insightful journey!
Pascale

How does the ketogenic diet relate to other ways of eating?

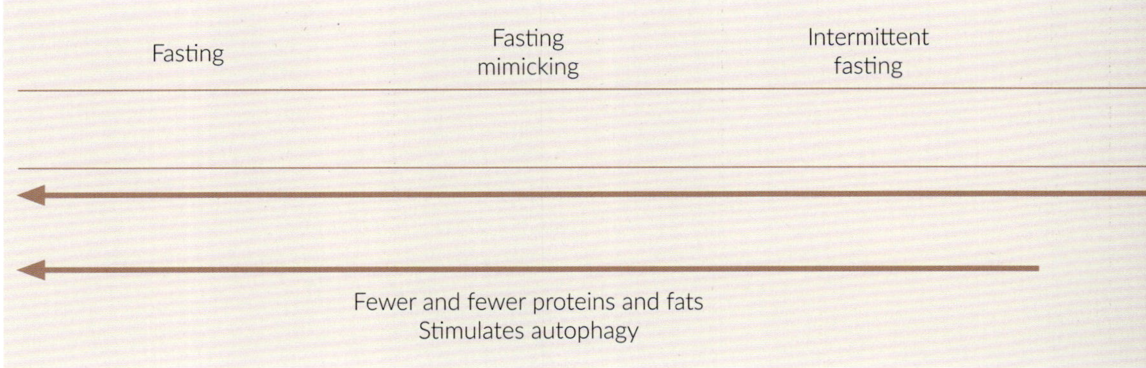

Percentage of energy from carbs = the daily energy we receive from carbs

Low-carb keto, intermittent fasting ... they're all up-and-coming diets that you should really see as a reaction to the extravagant western way of eating. They differ mostly in how few carbs, proteins and fats they contain.

There was a time when we approached health from the viewpoint of undernutrition: how can we best feed the body? In a world where more than half the population is struggling with being overweight, this approach has completely changed - the question is now: how can we get an overweight body back into its healthy state? That's why these relatively new diets are more focused on fewer carbs and fewer proteins. You will see that the low-carb, ketogenic diet is the opposite of traditional western nutrition patterns, which are rich in fast carbs, just like intermittent fasting is the opposite of the constant snacking and eating we do in the western world. The longer you follow a typically western eating pattern and the more extreme the body's reaction is to that eating pattern, for example obesity or type 2 diabetes, the more extreme the solution. Extremes lead to extremes.

But this time the extreme is overnutrition instead of undernutrition. This requires a completely different approach, one which involves fewer instead of more carbs, fewer instead of more proteins (the only thing that we should be eating more of is high-quality food).
I believe that is the reason why traditional nutritionists have trouble with these new up-and-coming diets. Their training has taught them to think from an approach of feeding the body and giving it the nutrients it needs. But what if the body has too many nutrients? In that case, less is more. The one thing these diets all have in common is that they involve some form of fasting.

Keto	Low-carb	traditional western diet
< 50 g from carbs	20 to 40 percent of energy from carbs	55 to 70 percent of energy from carbs

Fewer and fewer carbs

The many health benefits of fasting have been proven time and time again, especially in a world where food is overabundant.

The only diet you can follow effortlessly year in, year out is the moderately low-carb diet. Because it is moderate. If you think longevity is important, and if your mind and body can handle fasting, then you can also integrate intermittent fasting, fasting mimicking or even full fasting into your life.

Another important note: there are many other healthy and balanced ways of eating out there, such as the Mediterranean diet, and variations on that diet, as well as the eating habits of people in certain areas in Japan, or in the so-called blue zones (the places on Earth where people become remarkably old and age well).

Depending on where you live, your history, your culture, your genes, how your body reacts to food, and your health, you need to look for a way of eating that fits you. In the long term, this will always be a way of eating that strikes the right balance for you. We should let go of the idea that we all must eat the same way.

Fasting: No solids, only water or juices. Follow this only under the guidance of a health professional.

Fasting mimicking: A diet launched by longevity researcher Valter Longo. As the name implies, fasting is mimicked using this method. In other words: you can still eat something (1100 calories on the first day and 800 calories the four days after that) and nevertheless experience the health benefits of fasting. Consuming fewer carbs and fewer proteins are key here. For more information, see www.valterlongo.com.

Intermittent fasting: Fasting from time to time. That could be anything from skipping a meal to eating nothing or little for a few days.

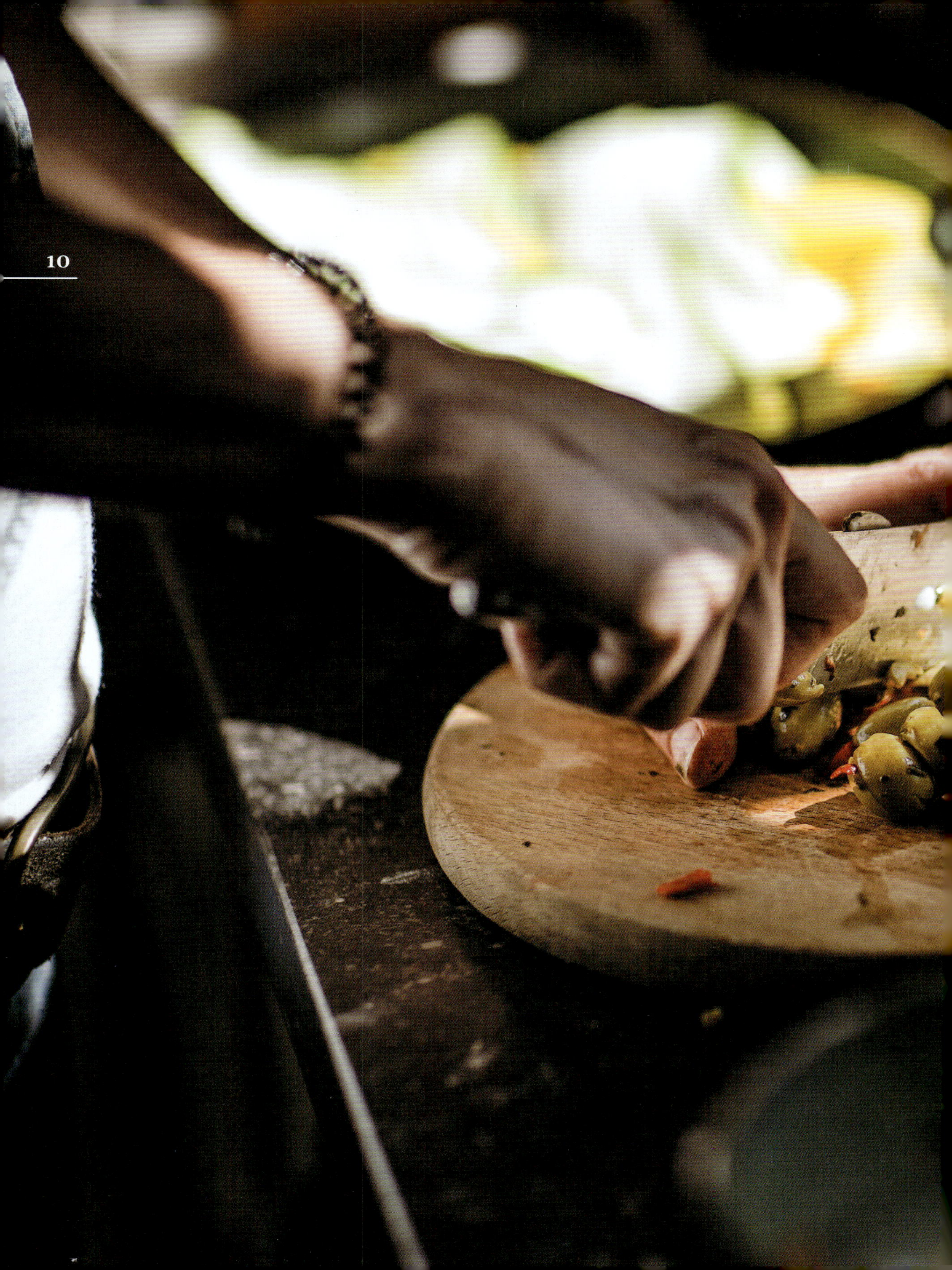

What is a ketogenic diet?

A ketogenic diet fits into the whole low-carb movement and is the strictest version of eating low-carb.

You will find ketogenic recipes in my other books—even in my very first book—but eating a keto meal from time to time is completely different to being in ketosis. To achieve ketosis, you need to eat very few carbs (sugars and starches), moderate amounts of protein and plenty of fats, day in, day out, for breakfast, lunch, dinner and whenever you consider putting something in your mouth. Your body is then forced to switch from burning sugars to burning fats. Ketones are produced during this process, a new fuel for your body. Hence the name "ketosis", also known as nutritional ketosis. People following a strict ketogenic diet only have one aim: to achieve ketosis and remain there.

Because your body starts burning fats during ketosis (both the fats obtained from the food you eat and the fats already stored in your body), this is an effective diet for people with trouble managing their weight. The ketones produced during this diet also have unique metabolic benefits for your general health, neurodegenerative conditions and in the treatment of cancer.[1]

If you want to remain in ketosis, it is important to eat as few carbs as possible every single day. One carb-rich meal is enough to kick you out of ketosis, defeating the purpose of the diet. So that's the main challenge for the beginning ketoer: reaching ketosis and staying there!

As soon as you and your body are familiar with ketosis, in other words, once your body has become a fat-burning machine, you will see that you may be able to eat slightly more carbs, but that varies from person to person. During the first few weeks, the recommended amount is fewer than 30 grams (less than an ounce) of carbs per day. Do you have trouble visualizing how much that is? To give you an idea: two slices of bread (and that includes whole-wheat bread) contain enough carbs for you to reach your daily limit. So if you're used to eating according to traditional western eating patterns, this will be a major change. For people used to eating low-carb the change will be less drastic, but it's still a major adjustment.

One thing is for certain: anyone who wants to reach ketosis will need to devote time and attention to their nutrition and be willing to make the effort to keep track of their macronutrient levels (fat, protein and carbs). This may be difficult in the beginning, but it is fascinating and insightful to see how your body reacts, and it makes you conscious of what you eat. We have given you the amount of carbs, proteins and fats per serving for every recipe in this book, making it easy to keep track of your macronutrient intake.

WHY WOULD YOU WANT TO FOLLOW A KETOGENIC DIET?

A ketogenic diet has very few carbs and extreme amounts of fats, making it quite a controversial way of eating. Moreover, few if any long-term studies have yet been published on this diet and its effects. But I think most researchers will agree that if you follow a ketogenic diet for the right reasons and for a limited time, it can be a powerful way of getting your health back on track.

- **Overweight:** Losing weight or breaking through a weight-loss plateau is the most important reason why people switch to a ketogenic diet. It has been proven that you can lose weight quickly and effectively with a ketogenic or low-carb diet. I want to point out that for people wishing to lose weight, a ketogenic diet is not the only solution. You can also lose quite a bit of weight with low-carb nutrition. I would recommend following a ketogenic diet only when a moderately low-carb way of eating is not enough to help you lose weight.
  Perhaps one of the main reasons why you lose weight is the fact that your hunger and desire for food decreases with a ketogenic diet, causing you to eat less despite the fact that you eat a lot of fat.
- **Energy levels:** Many people feel more energized and say it helps them clear their minds. I want to add that I personally don't feel any difference at all. I have been experimenting for years with a light state of ketosis and I was in ketosis for quite a while as I was writing this book. That may be because I have been eating moderately low-carb for years, keeping my blood sugar levels on an even keel and gaining many benefits in terms of my energy levels and mental well-being. Anyone eating low-carb can regularly reach a state of light ketosis.
- **Type 2 diabetes:** A diet with few carbs has a positive effect on blood sugar levels. Many people have been able to put their type 2 diabetes into remission with a ketogenic diet. Depending on how far the condition has progressed, this can also be achieved with a moderately low-carb diet.
- **Cancer:** There are currently many promising studies into the link between the ketogenic diet and cancer. A ketogenic diet doesn't cure cancer, but it does help increase the effectiveness of traditional cancer treatments. To put it simply: cancer cells need plenty of glucose to survive and they can't handle ketones. With no glucose to feed them, they become weak and more vulnerable to classic treatments such as chemotherapy. For more information, read the article written by Dr. William Cortvriendt (see page 47). He has also written a book about cancer titled *Kankervrij* (Cancer-Free), in which he discusses the positive effects of a ketogenic diet on certain types of cancer.
- **Neurological conditions:** The ketones released during a ketogenic diet are believed to positively influence Alzheimer's disease and other neurological conditions. Ketones are a premium fuel for our brains, so to speak.

- **Epilepsy:** This condition lies at the heart of how the ketogenic diet came about. The diet was developed in the 1920s for epilepsy patients. It was discovered that epilepsy patients who fasted had fewer seizures or no seizures at all. But because we cannot keep fasting forever, researchers started to look for a diet that mimicked the effects of fasting. And so, the ketogenic diet was born. This diet works better than some other epilepsy medications, especially with children, who experience a significant decrease in seizures as a result.
  (https://www.epilepsy.com/learn/treating-seizures-and-epilepsy/dietary-therapies/ketogenic-diet)

- **Ketones as super fuel for our bodies:** Athletes who not only train to burn glucose but also to burn fats, benefit from this approach. This is particularly true for endurance athletes.
  Burning fat occurs when you train and have eaten few or no carbs. When that happens, your body draws its energy from body fat.
  There has been a lot of commotion recently around the use of exogenous ketones as a super fuel. A research team from KU Leuven has shown that the use of exogenous ketones can increase physical performance by up to 15 percent. Professor Hespel, who led the research team, described the results as unprecedented. It should be noted that they are referring to ketones as a supplement. That is completely different from when your body creates its own ketones via nutritional ketosis.

There are currently many studies being conducted into the health benefits of a ketogenic diet on various conditions, including brain tumors in children, PCOS (polycystic ovary syndrome) in women, alcoholism, type 2 diabetes, breast cancer, bipolar disorders, Alzheimer's disease, Parkinson's disease, multiple sclerosis, and the effect of a ketogenic diet on gut bacteria.
You can find the full list here: https://clinicaltrials.gov/ct2/
results?term=%22ketogenic+diet%22&Search=Apply&recrs=b&recrs=a&recrs=f&recrs=d&age_
v=&gndr=&type=&rslt=
U.S. National Library of Medicine, Clinical Trials.gov

WHO SHOULD BE CAREFUL WITH A KETOGENIC DIET?

If you take medication and would like to follow a ketogenic diet, guidance from a health professional is an absolute must. Although patients with type 2 diabetes can benefit from a ketogenic diet, this must be done under the guidance of your physician. He will guide you in the gradual cutting down of your medication and/or insulin dosage as your body reacts to your new eating habits. This is very important, because if you take medication aimed at reducing glucose production, you run the risk of going into ketoacidosis (see page 18). In any case, I strongly recommend anyone taking hypertension and other forms of medication to only follow the ketogenic diet under the guidance of a professional with knowledge of the ketogenic diet.

PREGNANCY, BREASTFEEDING AND KETOSIS

If you're pregnant or breastfeeding, this is not a good time to go on a diet or start fasting, but it is essential to have a healthy and varied diet. A moderately low-carb way of eating would be a better option in this case.

However, for anyone trying to get pregnant, having a healthy body weight is essential. It is generally acknowledged that women who are overweight have more trouble getting pregnant. In this case, a ketogenic diet to lose weight first could be a possible solution but not during the pregnancy itself. Women with PCOS (polycystic ovary syndrome) who wish to get pregnant may also benefit from a ketogenic diet[2]. With a moderately low-carb way of eating, most women can also achieve weight loss and experience positive effects on their PCOS.

WHAT ARE THE DISADVANTAGES OF A KETOGENIC DIET?

- It is a very strict diet, and you have to devote a lot of time and attention to your new way of eating, especially in the beginning. It requires commitment.
- During the transition phase, you may experience side effects such as:
    - muscle cramps: taking magnesium supplements before going to bed can alleviate this.
    - keto flu, particularly headache (see page 62): drink plenty of fluids and consume more salt and minerals to combat this.
- When following a ketogenic diet, you may experience issues with your bowel movements. You can reduce this by eating more fiber from fruits and nuts and exercising more. My keto meal plan contains plenty of fiber, so you shouldn't normally experience any problems with this.
- People start off enthusiastically with a ketogenic diet, especially when it is accompanied by effective weight loss, but many people experience the diet as tedious and limiting. That's why I recommend switching over to a moderately low-carb way of eating after following a keto diet, which you can then alternate with a ketogenic diet a couple of days a week or a couple of weeks per month. You can do this depending on what you want to achieve and how easy or difficult you find following a ketogenic diet. Moreover, many experts recommend regularly going into and out of ketosis instead of staying in ketosis for long periods of time. This is also known as cycling. You cycle between a ketogenic diet and a moderately low-carb way of eating that follows a more natural eating pattern. Even the hunter-gatherers of old probably weren't in a constant state of ketosis (see page 25).

  However, there is no doubt that anyone returning to their old eating habits with plenty of fast carbs after following a ketogenic diet will see the pounds and medical conditions piling back up in no time. That is why I'm an absolute proponent of a moderately low-carb way of eating. That is not a diet but a way of life that is easy to keep up in the long term and that genuinely makes you happy. I would never want to go back to the way things were before.
- The controversy surrounding the health benefits of following a long-term ketogenic diet makes it difficult for some people to give it a try.

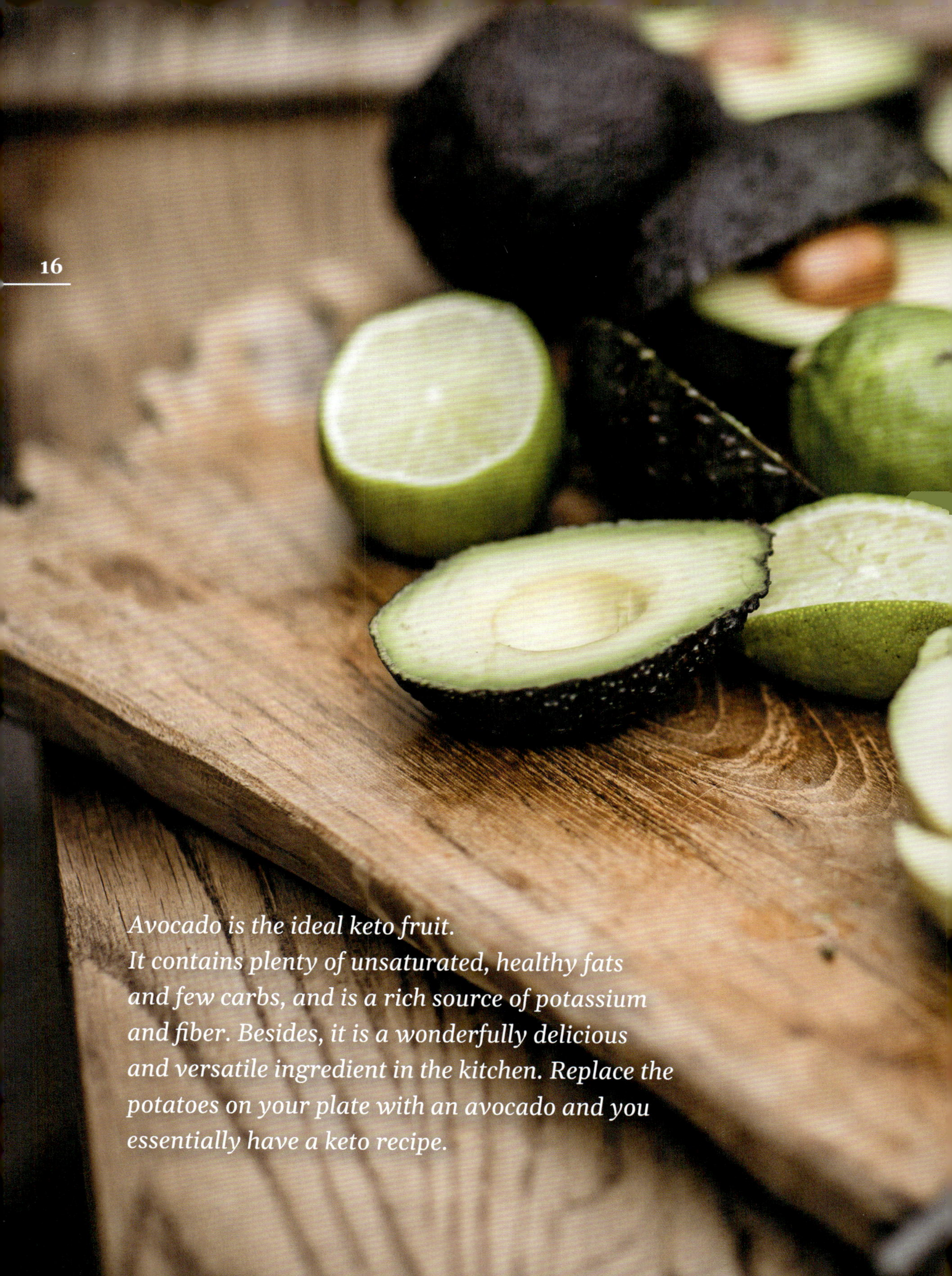

*Avocado is the ideal keto fruit.
It contains plenty of unsaturated, healthy fats
and few carbs, and is a rich source of potassium
and fiber. Besides, it is a wonderfully delicious
and versatile ingredient in the kitchen. Replace the
potatoes on your plate with an avocado and you
essentially have a keto recipe.*

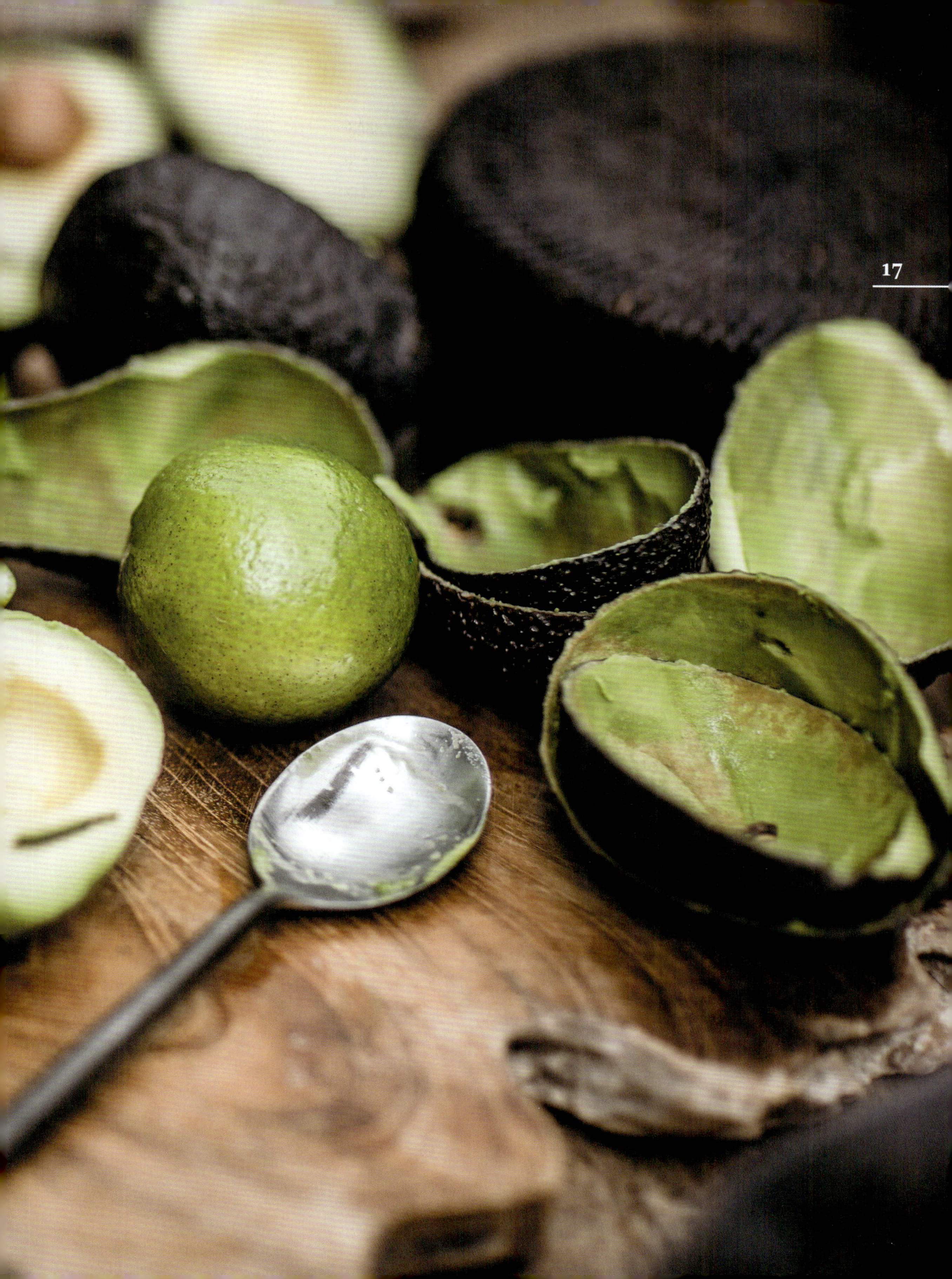

THE CONTROVERSY AROUND THE KETOGENIC DIET

Although the ketogenic diet has been shown to have many health benefits, it remains controversial, in particular because there are, as of yet, few published long-term studies. But there is good news. Because of its popularity, the ketogenic diet is currently perhaps the most researched diet out there, so we simply need to be patient a little longer.

One important bone of contention is the saturated fats and cholesterol levels. While following a ketogenic diet, a lot of foods rich in saturated fats are consumed: eggs, cheese, coconut oil, meat, butter... Saturated fats have been a source of controversy for years because some studies indicate that they contribute to cardiovascular disease. More recent studies, such as the PURE study, dispute that claim (https://www.ncbi.nlm.nih.gov/pubmed/30391990). There are also studies that show that a diet rich in fats and poor in carbs has a positive effect on the fats in the body, despite high levels of saturated fat. (https://www.ncbi.nlm.nih.gov/pubmed/20713651) https://academic.oup.com/jn/advance-article/doi/10.1093/jn/nxz308/5673196?guestAccessKey=3d f1e4fa-2899-4bd9-8625-9f45fa522d3b

Moreover, many experts suggest that we should not lump all saturated fats together. What you combine these fats with on your plate is just as important: with unhealthy carbs such as fries or with healthy vegetables?

Some experts are alarmed by the idea of keto because when they think of a ketogenic diet they immediately think of ketoacidosis. But nutritional ketosis should not be confused with ketoacidosis. Nutritional ketosis is a natural metabolic state that, over the course of history, gave people the flexibility to deal with both changes in food supply and times of hunger. Ketoacidosis, on the other hand, is an unstable and dangerous condition that only occurs with improperly treated type 1 diabetes or (in extreme cases) advanced-stage type 2 diabetes, in which both the ketone levels and the blood sugar levels reach alarming, life-threatening levels. Unfortunately, sometimes people are still confused about these two different metabolic states, which makes being informed about them all the more important.

Any diabetes patients who wish to switch to a ketogenic diet must follow the guidance of a professional. To prevent the risk of ketoacidosis, anyone taking medication to regulate their glucose levels should never start a ketogenic diet of their own accord.

WHY DOES A KETOGENIC DIET SUCCEED WHERE CLASSIC WEIGHT-LOSS DIETS FAIL?

The success stories on social media about low-carb and keto are numerous. You often see before-and-after images: on the left, a depressing-looking obese version of someone, and on the right, a slim version of that same person having lost 40, 60, 80, 100 or even more pounds. It's striking how the people in the slim photo always have a huge smile on their faces and are dressed in sexy clothes. This also goes for men, by the way. Even the staunchest critic of the ketogenic diet has to admit that these are wonderful results. It is infectious. How can you not agree that this works?

They don't look sick in the pictures, on the contrary! And we have to admit, we seldom see these kinds of results being achieved—and maintained—with a classic diet. Where are the success stories? Where are the pictures?

The most important reason why keto succeeds where all else fails, is that you don't feel hungry when you're following a ketogenic diet, because you are allowed to eat delicious and wholesome food and because fat is not off-limits. It's a completely different experience from many classic diets, where everything revolves around reducing your calorie intake. This means going hungry and, above all: having enough willpower to stick to it.

Because you don't experience that nagging sense of hunger during a ketogenic diet, you will ultimately end up eating less, and that's one of the reasons why you lose weight. That typical constant craving for sweetness also disappears. The absence of carbs stabilizes your blood sugar levels, decreasing your cravings and feelings of hunger and making you feel a lot better. According to studies by several researchers, among them Professor David Ludwig (https://www.ncbi.nlm.nih.gov/pubmed/30429127), you burn more calories with a diet that contains few carbs and plenty of fats than with a diet with plenty of carbs and little fat. You have more energy and burn more calories which, in turn, will help you lose weight.

I want to add that most people also experience these benefits by eating moderately low-carb as described in my other books. Thankfully, most people don't have to go so far as to follow a ketogenic diet. They can achieve the same results by eating low-carb. But, as I noted earlier, some people need to go the extra mile to achieve that same goal. Because everyone is different.

IS IT EASY TO KEEP UP?

For some, it is. For others, it isn't. Of course it also depends on your situation and what you want to achieve. Some people, such as those suffering from epilepsy, see it as a long-term lifestyle change while others, like those who want to lose plenty of weight fast, see it more as a short-term diet plan lasting anywhere from a few months to a few years. It seems that most people temporarily follow a keto diet to tackle overweight or other health problems, after which they switch over to low-carb nutrition.

The ketogenic diet is quite strict and that works well for some people. The boundaries of what is and isn't allowed are clearly defined. The diet offers little freedom and your menu is determined by calculations rather than "what do I feel like today?" or "what tastes good?", shifting the focus from emotional eating to functional eating. You start to see food more in chemical terms: a compound composed of fuel, vitamins and minerals. I believe that is also the reason why you see so many powders appearing in the increasingly popular ketogenic diet. The internet is rife with keto shakes (powders that you supplement with the necessary nutrients), MCT oils, protein powders, instant coffee with additives, keto supplements, collagen powders ...

When I was following a strict ketogenic diet for a while, I noticed the shift in focus myself. My nutritional needs were more functional, but I don't believe I'll ever be seduced by the functionality of powders. I am convinced that they will only make you unhappy in the long term. I am someone who loves pure, wholesome food along with the romance and allure that comes with good food. A healthy lifestyle starts with pure ingredients that have been processed as little as possible. This is the kind of food that will keep us healthy and make us happy. That's why a moderately low-carb way of eating, and all the freedom that comes with it, feels so right to me. I experience that freedom as a benefit rather than a burden. It allows me to get creative in the kitchen. And, to be really honest … keto ends up being more of the same after a while. But if I had a good reason, such as battling obesity, epilepsy, type 2 diabetes or certainly cancer, I would be able to appreciate the ketogenic diet more. The recipes in this book will show you that you can still eat delicious food even while following a ketogenic diet.

It is up to each person individually to decide whether they find it difficult to follow a ketogenic diet. The time to patronize is over. At best, we can offer ideas and try to provide as much honest information as we can so people can make their own decisions.

KETO AND VEGAN

Eating keto and being a vegan is certainly not impossible. Danielle Belardo, a vegan cardiologist, tried the ketogenic diet for two weeks and was very enthusiastic. But—as I mentioned earlier—she only did this for fourteen days. There are quite a few people who follow a vegan keto diet; you can find them on social media. Dr. Carrie Diulus, for example, has been following a vegan keto diet for years as a type 1 diabetes patient, and she writes openly and honestly about her experiences. But you often see that many vegan keto followers aren't too strict with the rules and actually eat low-carb instead of keto. There is absolutely nothing wrong with that, but I like to present you with the whole picture, so you know what you're getting yourself into. People who follow a ketogenic diet have good reasons for doing so. People who follow a vegan keto diet have excellent reasons for doing so. It's not something you do for fun.
If you combine keto and vegan, you won't be making things easy for yourself because the list of ingredients to choose from becomes severely limited. Moreover, this combination is not without its contradictions. A vegan diet tends to focus on more carbs, such as sweet potatoes, turnips, squash, red beets, lentils, chickpeas, beans and quinoa; all ingredients that don't fit into a ketogenic diet. It's not surprising that some vegans, perhaps because of the limited nature of what they can eat, are forced to look for alternatives and often end up using processed foods. That in itself is a contradiction, because healthy nutrition starts with wholesome, natural ingredients that have been processed as little as possible.
In other words, eating keto and vegan is not impossible, but you need to be exceptionally motivated and creative to keep it up. Furthermore, you'll want to keep a bit of variation in your diet. In this keto meal plan, you'll find a number of vegan recipes. You will also find several delicious vegetarian keto recipes in Julie van den Kerckhove's books.

KETO AND MEAT

When describing a ketogenic diet, people often think of eating bacon, meat, eggs and mounds of butter and coconut oil. But you can also choose to use more olive oil, fish, vegetables, nuts, seeds, olives … to add variation to your diet, as I do in the recipes in this book.

DO I CONSUME ENOUGH FIBER WITH A KETOGENIC DIET?

That also depends on the choices you make. If you follow the meal plan in this book, you certainly will, because I believe that getting enough fiber and keeping your bowels healthy is essential. Whole-wheat products are not the only place you will find fiber, as some would have you believe, it's also in vegetables, leafy green vegetables, nuts, seeds such as chia seed, flaxseed and pumpkin seeds, avocado, coconut, pecans, kale, broccoli, cauliflower, other types of cabbage, spinach, mushrooms, eggplant, asparagus, zucchini, tomatoes …
The variety or boredom of eating keto depends mostly on how much effort you're willing to put into it.

THE TECHNICAL SIDE OF KETO

When you always combine large amounts of carbs with fats and proteins in your diet, as is customary in the west, your body will use the glucose from carbs as your most important source of energy; sugars are easily converted by the body. But your body can also use fats and even proteins as a source of energy. In fact, at this very moment, your heart cells are using their favorite fuel, ketones, as a source of energy. So even when you're not in ketosis, your body does produce ketones, albeit in small quantities. So the body uses a mixture of all these potential fuel sources.

But when the body gets too few carbs (i.e. glucose) due to fasting, strenuous exercise or a ketogenic diet, for example, the body will switch to fats as its primary source of energy, either from body fat or the fats found in your food. During this process, the liver converts fatty acids into ketones that can be used by most of the cells in our bodies, such as the cells in our muscles, brain and most organs. In this case, the brain switches largely from glucose to ketones as a source of energy—a more efficient source producing fewer free radicals. This is part of the reason why this process has neurological benefits, and also explains the many studies being carried out on the effects of a ketogenic diet on Alzheimer's, Parkinson's and epilepsy.

The longer you stay in ketosis, the more efficient your body becomes in using ketones as a source of energy. Fewer ketones will be passed in the urine. That's why urine strips are a less effective measure of whether you're in ketosis.
It's not that your entire body starts using ketones as a fuel source. Some cells don't have the right enzymes or energy cells to use ketones. These include red blood cells and certain cells in the brain and liver which continue to use glucose as a source of fuel. This doesn't mean that you should continue to eat carbs. Your liver can produce glucose from amino acids (the building blocks from which proteins are made) and glycerol (one of the compounds found in fats) with a process called gluconeogenesis. This allows your blood sugar levels to remain well within acceptable levels during ketosis. Ketogenesis (ketone production) and gluconeogenesis (glucose production) work side by side in your body.

The transition from burning sugars to burning fats in your body is a relatively slow process and goes through different stages. After two days, enough ketones are produced to start ketosis (although this process may take longer in some people). With nutritional ketosis, the body receives enough energy and glucose from fats and protein without having to break down muscle tissue, which is what happens when the fat reserves are used up. At that point, the body will break down the muscles to produce the glucose needed by those cells which can only function with glucose as an energy source. This occurs during long-term fasting, for example during hunger strikes and with anorexia patients.

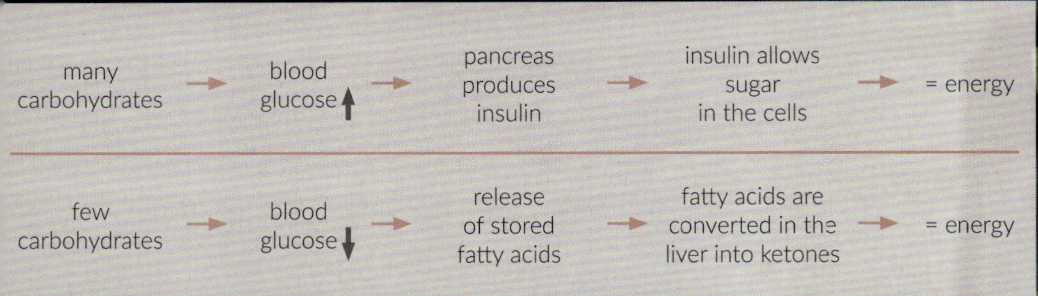

EATING PLENTY OF FAT AND FEW CARBS IS NOT THE ONLY WAY TO REACH KETOSIS

There are other ways to reach ketosis:

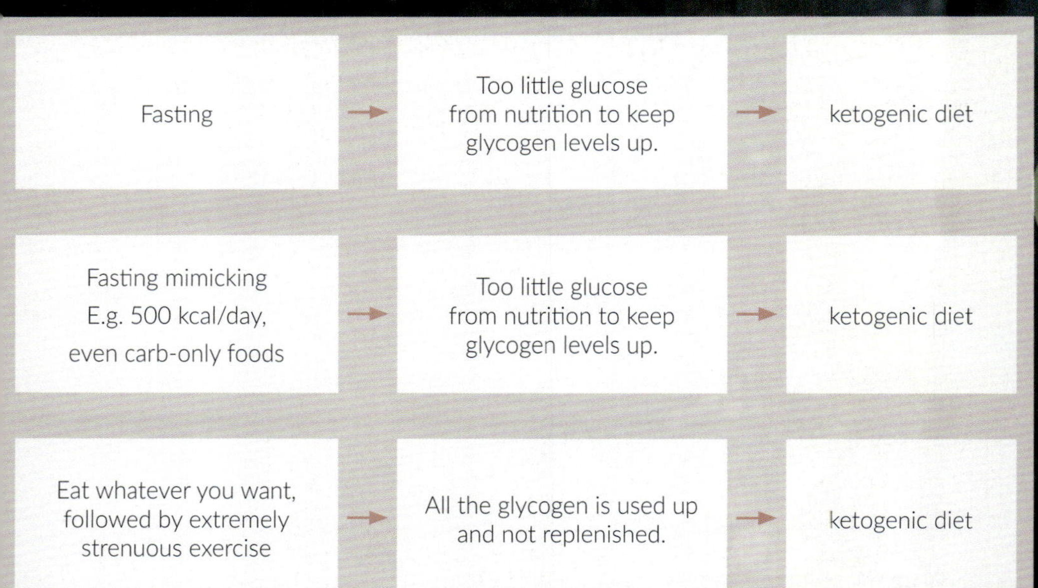

Marathon runners will always have reached ketosis by the end of a marathon, even after eating an excessive amount of rice porridge beforehand, for example. This is because they will have used up all their glycogen reserves (glucose) without being able to replenish them in time. So it's not so much the consumption of large amounts of fat that puts you in ketosis, you just need to make sure that your glycogen reserves are not replenished, causing your insulin levels to drop.

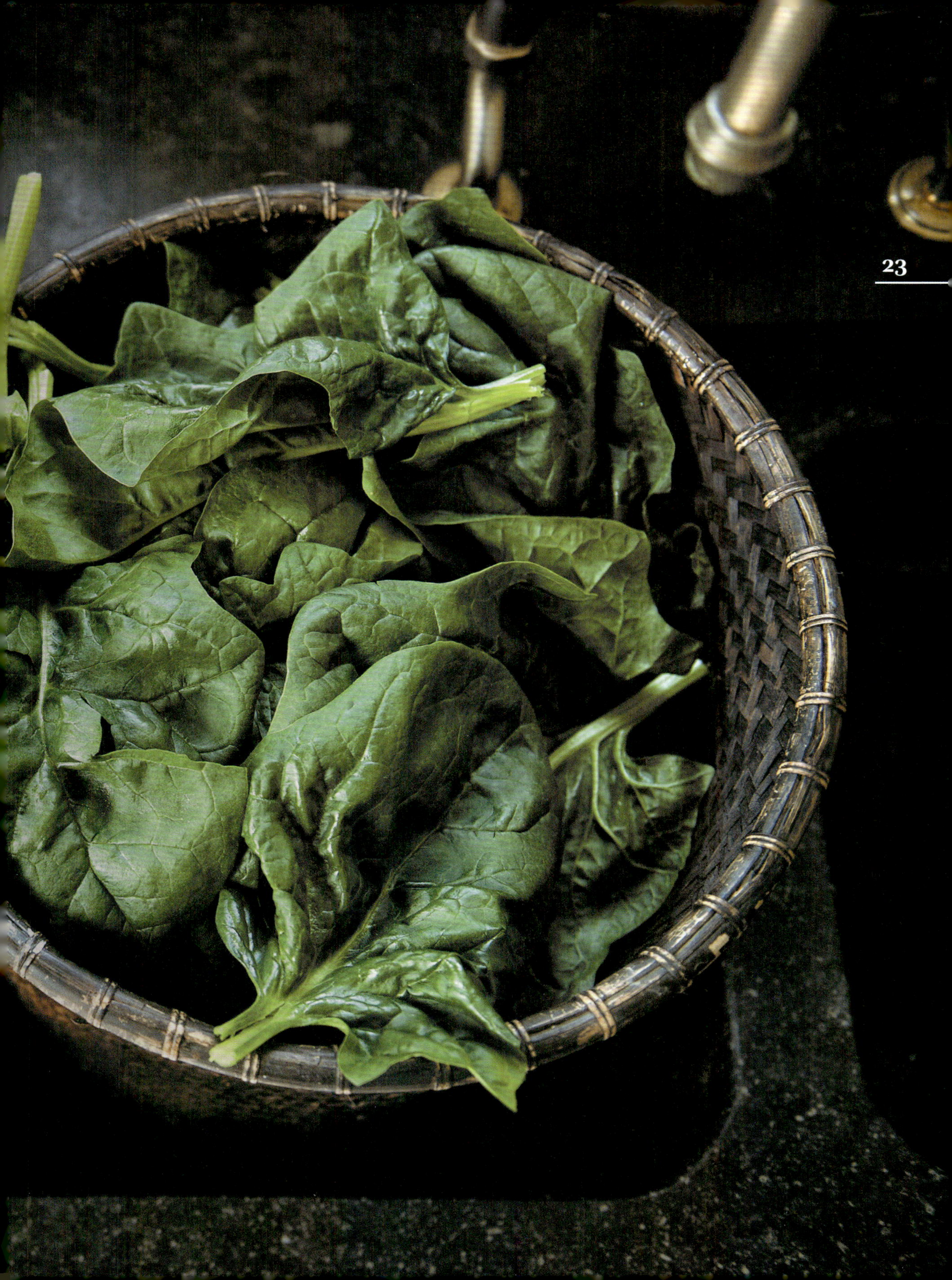

The reason why we eat so much fat during a standard keto diet is that you need to eat something and fats have the least effect on your insulin and glucose levels. No one wants to go hungry. To be able to keep this up and still feel great, you must eat enough. The art lies in finding that balance: if you eat too little fat, you'll start to go hungry and your body will go into stand-by mode after a while, making you tired and less likely to lose weight. If you eat too much fat, you will not lose weight or even gain weight.

The recipes in this book are well-balanced in terms of the proportions of carbs, fats and proteins. Most people will therefore reach ketosis fairly quickly if they stick to the recipes. Some people may need to look further for the right balance, especially those who are insulin resistant. They would do well to decrease their carb intake even further.

HOW DO YOU KNOW WHEN YOU'RE IN KETOSIS?
The best way to know whether you're in ketosis is to measure your ketone levels.
People who follow a ketogenic diet have one goal: to reach ketosis because they want their bodies to produce ketones in order to benefit from all the health advantages they offer. For those who are serious about going keto, the only way to go is to purchase a ketone meter. You can measure ketones through your breath, your urine, or your blood.

When the body burns fat, it produces three types of ketones, each of which can be detected in a different way:
- Acetone is more of a byproduct and is released through the breath (which explains why your breath sometimes smells funny, something that doesn't happen to everyone). You can use a special breath analyzer to test whether you're in ketosis. This is a fairly accurate measurement method. I personally use this test the most. It's easy to use, you can test yourself anytime and anywhere and it's fun to do. The downside is that this test is quite expensive, and it's not universally available. The easiest way is to purchase one online. There are several models on the market.
- Acetoacetate (AcAc) is measured in the urine using strips that change color. It is a simple and cheap testing method. After a while, however, your body becomes more efficient in using up ketones and therefore fewer ketones will be passed in the urine. That's why this test is not accurate in the long term.
- Beta-hydroxybutyrate (BHB) is measured with a blood test similar to the blood tests used by diabetes patients. You can often measure both your blood glucose and ketone levels using the same device. Measuring your blood is the most accurate testing method. The disadvantage is that this device is not readily available everywhere, and constantly pricking your fingertips can get very irritating after a while.

Ketone concentration in the blood (millimolar)	State
< 0,2	not in ketosis
0,2 – 0,5	light ketosis
0,5 – 3,0	nutritional ketosis
2,5 – 3,5	ketosis from training or strenuous exercise
3,0 – 6,0	ketosis from fasting
15 – 25	ketoacidosis

Note: So, the more ketones your body produces, the better? No. The important thing is whether
or not you are in ketosis.

WHY IS IT IMPORTANT TO MEASURE YOUR KETONE LEVELS?

If you really want to follow a ketogenic diet, it's important that your body produces ketones so you
can achieve your goal. It doesn't help if you follow a strict diet and don't reach ketosis. The only thing
that leads to is frustration. If reaching ketosis is not your goal but you do feel better eating fewer
carbohydrates, then follow a low-carbohydrate diet as described in my other books. That saves you
a lot of counting and measuring.

IS KETOSIS A NATURAL STATE FOR HUMANS?

At this very moment, your body is making ketones that can be used as a source of energy,
albeit in small quantities. When you fast, and even at night, your body produces more ketones.
It is also interesting to note that breastfed babies are often in a light state of ketosis. Ketones are
therefore no stranger to us.

We currently live in a world of abundance, but for our ancestors, such as the hunter-gatherers,
it wasn't always certain that they could find enough food to sustain themselves. Their nutritional
intake was dependent on the hunt, the seasons, the weather ... Most of their carb consumption
came from berries, roots and honey, but these were all seasonal products and therefore not always
available. To be able to deal with this food scarcity (and lack of carbs), nature provided humans with
a way to draw energy from their own fat reserves. When fat is burned, ketones are created which
serve as fuel for our ever-hungry brains. As soon as the summer arrived or there were enough carbs
available, the body could go back to burning glucose instead of fat. Switching between these two
metabolic states of burning sugars and burning fats is a very natural situation for the human body.
It's the one thing that all scientists can agree on. However the question that remains is, were our
hunter-gatherer ancestors generally in a state of ketosis or in a state of burning sugars? The verdict
is definitely still out on this subject.

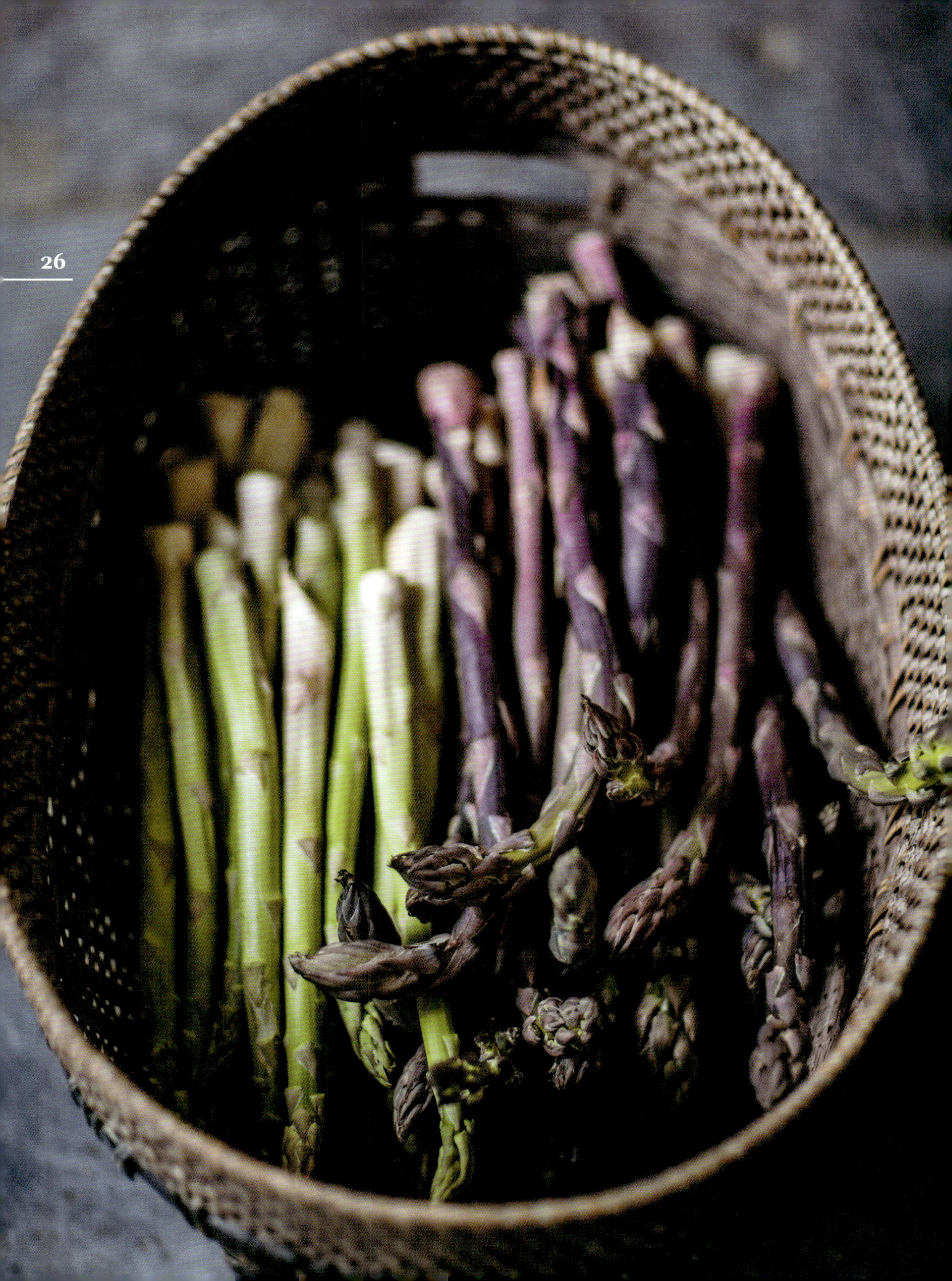

We can't go back in time, but we can learn from the indigenous communities who continue to live in tribes today. How they eat largely depends on where they live. Communities in northern regions devoid of berries and roots, such as the Inuit, are more dependent on meat and fat (note: they consume more carbs than you'd think from the glycogen found in muscle tissue). They most probably find themselves in ketosis for longer periods. The Tsimani in Bolivia and the Hadza in Tanzania might like to eat more meat but may often come back from a hunt emptyhanded, obliging them to eat readily available plant-based foods, perhaps even fruit and honey when in season. They will more often be in a metabolic state where they burn sugars. What both groups have in common is that neither suffers from typical western conditions such as overweight, type 2 diabetes, high blood pressure or cardiovascular disease that plague many of us today and which would be the case if they were to switch to a typically western way of eating. So, whether we are typically in a state of ketosis or burning sugars most of the time doesn't seem to play a role in the development of these conditions.

Conclusion: Nutritional ketosis is a natural metabolic state that, over the course of history, gave people the flexibility both to deal with changes in the food supply and to cope with times of hunger. Perhaps it's this ability to switch between the two metabolic states (burning sugars and burning fats) that will ultimately benefit our health, with the current ketogenic diet mimicking the natural scarcity of food and a moderately low-carb diet mimicking the summer seasons with their berries and roots. We have also learned that many forms of fasting have health benefits.

THE KETOGENIC DIET AND ENDURANCE SPORTS

Athletes who not only train to burn glucose but also to burn fats benefit from this approach. This is especially true for endurance athletes. You can only store a certain amount of glucose/energy in the form of glycogen. Once that supply is used up, often described by athletes as hitting a brick wall, you no longer have any energy. The storage capacity of fat is far greater in comparison to that of glycogen. In other words, if you train your body to burn fat, you give your body access to a tremendous store of energy.

You can condition your body to switch from burning sugars to burning fat by training at moments when you have eaten few or no carbs, forcing your body to draw their energy reserves from body fat. The best way to do this is with the guidance of a sports professional who has expertise in the field of metabolism.

Since a study published by KU Leuven in Belgium showed that endurance athletes benefitted from the use of exogenous ketones, online sales of exogenous ketones have increased significantly. It should be noted that they are referring to using ketones as a supplement, which is an entirely different situation from that described in this book, which refers to nutritional ketosis for people who do not engage in strenuous activity. Consuming exogenous ketones inhibits the production of internal ketones.

WHAT ARE MCT OILS AND HOW DO THEY FIT INTO A KETOGENIC DIET?

Fatty acids are classified by their chain lengths: short-chain, medium-chain and long-chain fatty acids.

SCT: *short-chain triglycerides*. Quite rare in food, these fatty acids are produced primarily by gut bacteria in our intestines. One example is butyrate, a compound containing four carbon atoms.
MCT: *medium-chain triglycerides*. These fatty acids contain six to twelve carbon atoms. They are primarily found in coconut oil and palm oil and, to a lesser degree, in butter.
LCT: *long-chain triglycerides*. These contain 13 to 21 carbon atoms per fatty acid chain. They are most prevalent in foods such as meats, fish, olive oil, nuts, and avocados.
VLC: *very long-chain triglycerides*. These fatty acid chains contain more than 22 carbon atoms.

Medium-chain fatty acids behave differently in the body to the other fatty acids—much like glucose. First, they reach the liver faster because they don't have to go through the whole digestion process like long-chain fatty acids. Second, they are able to oxidize quickly. This can lead to ketone formation, where they are used as an energy source rather than stored as fat.

Because of these benefits, MCT oils used to be particularly recommended for people who had trouble digesting fats. As more and more studies illustrated the benefits of ketones, the popularity of MCT oils increased greatly, especially with people looking to follow a ketogenic diet, where everything revolves around the production of ketones. That's why pure MCT oil is now available as a supplement. These products are mostly manufactured from coconut oil with its MCT content of 50 to 60 percent.

You may often read that one to four tablespoons of pure MCT oil per day will cause you to burn fat and give your brain a boost. But the big question is whether you achieve the same results with the ketones from MCT supplements as you do with the ketones produced by your own body fat.

Studies looking at the role of MCT oil in weight management showed that MCT oils had a slight edge when it comes to losing weight. The researchers themselves, however, stress that more research needs to be carried out to be able to draw solid conclusions.

MCTs are also supposed to give your brain a boost, but the studies linked to these findings were conducted with Alzheimer's patients whose brains were no longer functioning well on glucose due to old age or lifestyle choices and who respond better to ketones. The question is whether this conclusion applies to healthy people as well.

According to the experts, it is important to first define what exactly you mean by "being in ketosis." If being in ketosis means that you have ketones circulating in your blood, then MCTs and exogenous ketones can help you reach ketosis. But that is not the same as nutritional ketosis, where you find yourself in a state of burning fat and your body makes ketones by burning its own body fat.

Jeff Volek and Stephen Phinney, two authorities in the field of the ketogenic diet, discourage using MCT oil as a supplement because it detracts from the benefits you would enjoy with a nutritional ketogenic diet.

MCT oils are certainly beneficial in specific situations, for example for patients suffering from epilepsy. They allow these patients to eat slightly more carbohydrates while remaining in ketosis. They can also be beneficial to people wishing to reach or remain in ketosis. But, as Dr. Bill Wilson says, it's the cheater's way.

The ketogenic diet is fascinating, and we regularly see promising studies being conducted into its health benefits for different conditions, even as an anti-aging treatment. MCT oils can certainly play a role in these treatments. MCTs can help you stay in ketosis more easily, but don't think that you can achieve the same results with four tablespoonfuls of MCT oil per day as you would with nutritional ketosis. If you're not willing to change your eating habits, you won't see huge results, especially when you're looking to lose weight.

You can find a handy summary of the various studies into the benefits MCT oils at https://healthybutsmart.com/mct-oil-benefits.

INTERMITTENT FASTING AND A KETOGENIC DIET

I have already written at length about intermittent fasting in my book *Low carb cookbook 2*. In theory, intermittent fasting can go hand in hand with a ketogenic diet, but I advise you not to move too quickly. First, try to familiarize yourself with a ketogenic diet, find out how it feels for you, and only then take it to the next level. Some people start a ketogenic diet full of enthusiasm, skip breakfast, and restrict their calorie intake to boot. The result is usually that they feel miserable, don't lose weight, and give up very quickly. Take it one step at a time, feel how your body reacts, and don't take the next step until it feels right to do so.

WHAT IS THE DIFFERENCE BETWEEN EATING LOW-CARB AND A KETOGENIC DIET?

For me, eating low-carb means plenty of vegetables, nuts, seeds, fish, meat and fruit on the menu. And I am not afraid to use fat. But I do limit my intake of bread, pasta, potatoes, rice ...
When you describe what a ketogenic diet involves, you're talking about ... right, how much carbs, fats and proteins you eat. We don't talk about nutrition, but about macronutrients. We don't talk about meal plans, but we do talk about metabolism. The term ketogenic refers to the metabolic state that your body finds itself in. You need to weigh your food, calculate your macros, and measure your ketone levels. In other words, we're definitely talking about a diet. That is not the case with the moderately low-carb way of eating that I promote in my other books and that I live by. That is a way of life, a way of eating that gives you plenty of freedom. Forget weighing, measuring or counting. Nonetheless, with these eating habits you also sometimes find yourself in a mild form of ketosis. But as I have often said, some people need to take things one step further to achieve what others can achieve by simply eating low-carb. For those people, a ketogenic diet can make a world of difference.

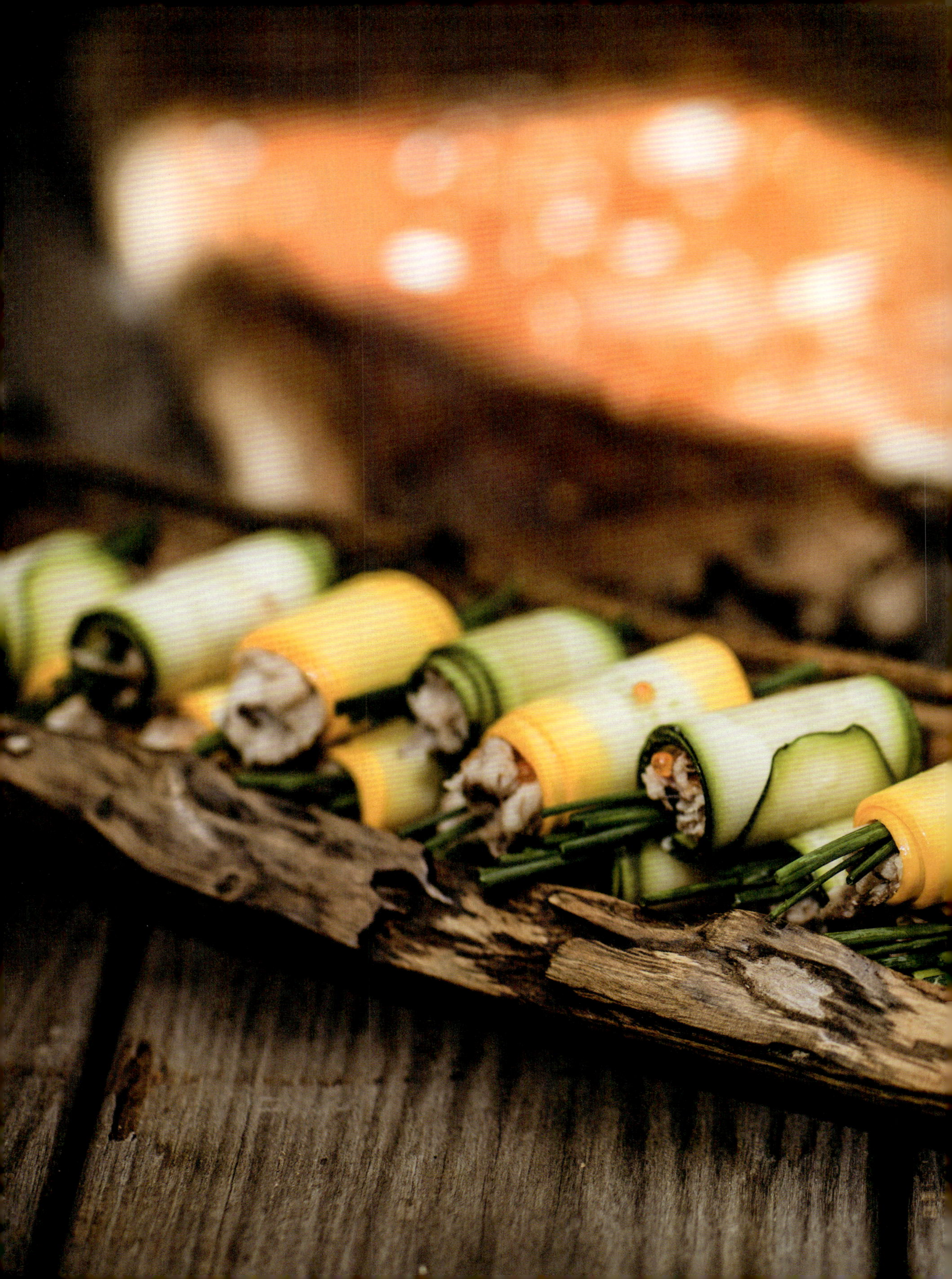

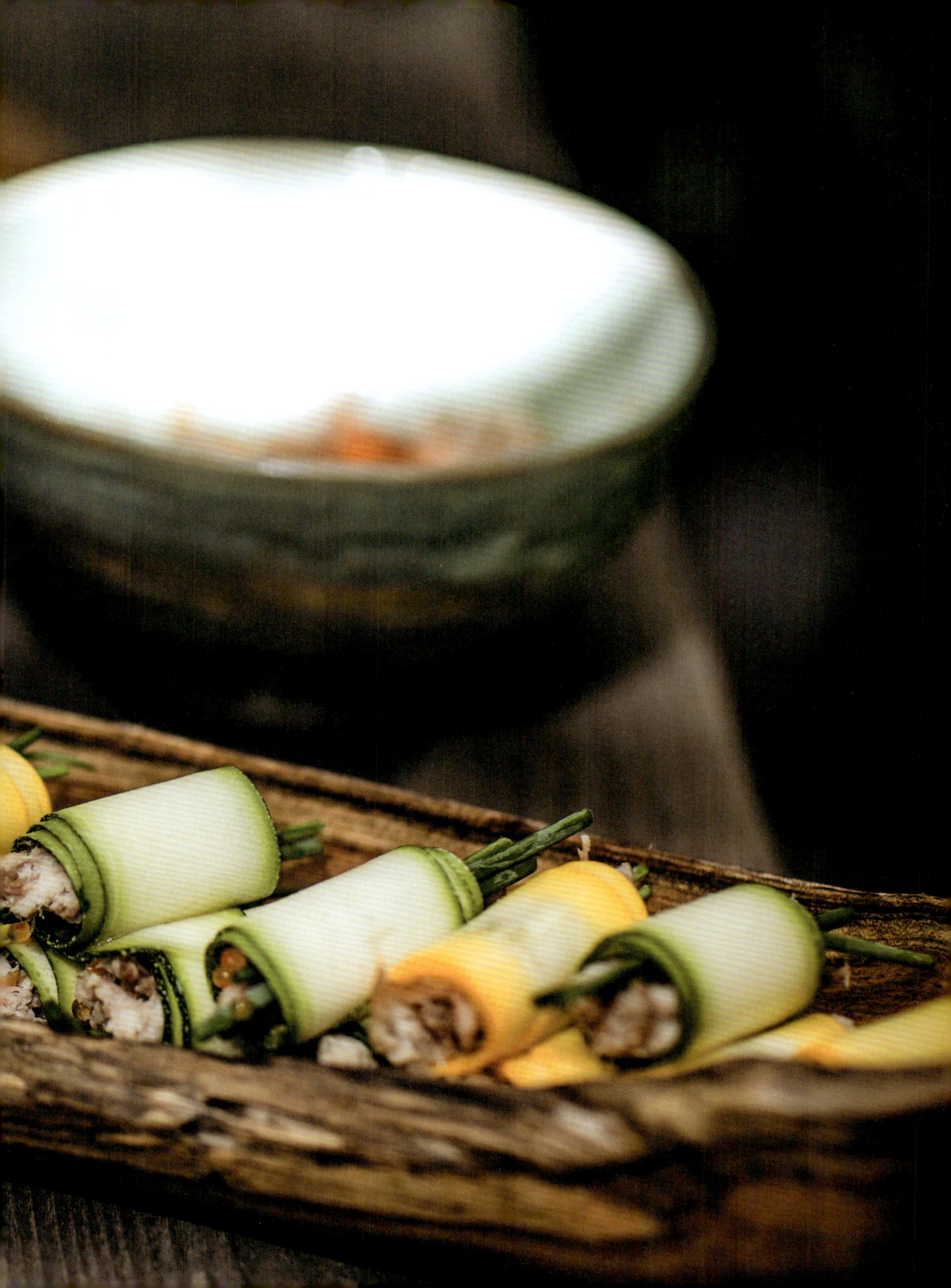

MY PERSONAL VISION ON A LOW-CARB WAY OF EATING AND MY EXPERIENCES WITH THE KETOGENIC DIET

I personally feel at my best with a moderately low-carb way of eating. What this basically comes down to is that I don't eat any bread, pasta, potatoes, rice, etc. And what this means is that I automatically use keto recipes and recipes that contain healthy carbs such as fruit and vegetables rich in carbs on a regular basis. I sense that I tend to keep to the natural nutritional rhythm of our forefathers as much as possible and switch between the two metabolic states.

As described in my earlier section *Is ketosis a natural state for humans?* humans would naturally and regularly switch between their two main sources of energy: fat and glucose. It was the availability of food that determined which system the body would use to store energy. But, because of the constant abundance of carbs today, there is no longer any need for the body to switch over to burning fat.

I eat carbs mostly in the morning with my breakfast fruit. On average 400 grams (14 ounces) of fruit with a low and moderate carb content such as strawberries, blueberries, blackberries, raspberries (most berries have a low carb content), peaches, nectarines, apricots, oranges, kiwi, papaya—and no bananas, grapes or dried fruit, which tend to contain a lot of carbs. During the rest of the day I often eat the way I describe in this book, mostly dishes with few carbs and plenty of healthy fats.
This means that my body is not in a permanent keto state, but because I eat few carbs—especially on days when I have eggs for breakfast—my body automatically switches from burning sugars to burning fats. And to me, that seems like a natural state where I have the best of both worlds. This allows me to enjoy the benefits of carb-rich fruits and vegetables with all their fiber and polyphenols and my body knows how to easily switch to burning fat on days that I eat less carb-rich fruits or vegetables. This transition takes place in a natural, effortless manner. Without counting and calculating. Switching from one metabolic state to the other is also called cycling, a method promoted by researchers in favor of a long-term keto diet. This method also fits in with what humans were experiencing naturally; the hunter-gatherer also went in and out of ketosis depending on the food that was available at the time.

In other words, eating low-carb and a ketogenic diet have a lot in common, also in terms of their health benefits, but there is still a huge difference. The ketogenic diet is the strict version. The health benefits such as weight loss, putting type 2 diabetes into remission, better blood values, increased energy levels, a general decrease in ailments in and fewer issues with the gut and digestive system are mostly similar. There are a variety of testimonials from people who have lost 40, 60, or even 80 pounds with a moderately low-carb way of eating.

But you will undoubtedly lose weight faster with a ketogenic diet. I am aware that there are also people who, despite the fact that they eat low-carb, don't lose their excess weight and have more success with a ketogenic diet.

With a moderately low-carb way of eating, you don't have the metabolic advantages of ketosis, the state in which your body constantly burns fat to produce ketones. These can play an important role in combatting various conditions such as neurodegenerative diseases, certain forms of cancer or epilepsy.
It is therefore important to find out which way of eating fits you and your body. The more knowledgeable you are about the options available, the clearer that choice will be.

WHAT IS THE DIFFERENCE BETWEEN EATING THE OCCASIONAL KETO DISH AND BEING IN KETOSIS?

A keto recipe is a recipe that has very few carbs, moderate amounts of protein and large amounts of fat. All my books contain plenty of keto recipes; even my very first book contains many keto recipes. But this doesn't mean that when you eat the occasional keto dish, you're in ketosis or are following a ketogenic diet. If you sometimes alternate keto dishes with dishes that contain healthy carbs, such as dishes containing carrots, lentils or quinoa or a breakfast with fruit, then you will end up eating relatively few carbs but too many to reach ketosis. In that case, you're following a low-carb diet and your body will first draw its energy reserves from glucose before reverting to burning fat once the glucose supply runs out. On the other hand, when you eat exclusively keto recipes—morning, noon and night—that contain very few carbs and plenty of fats, your body will be forced to switch to fat as its primary source of energy. When these fats are broken down, the liver produces ketones which serve as fuel for your body. When your liver is constantly producing ketones, you're in ketosis. If you regularly eat keto dishes combined with dishes that do contain some carbs (fruit, lentils, carb-rich vegetables ...), you're not following a ketogenic diet, but a diet low in carbs, the way of eating I personally subscribe to and promote in my other books.

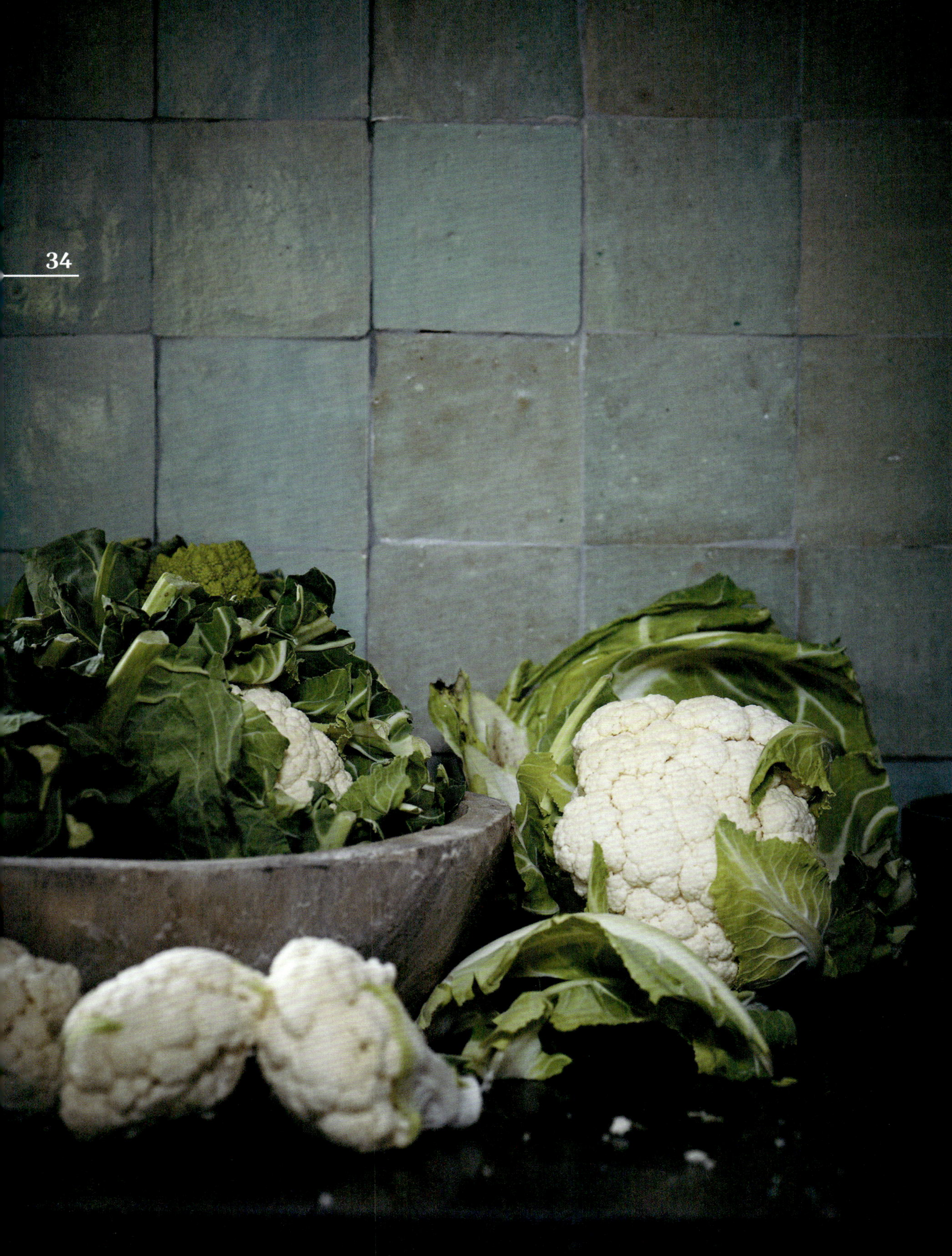

What do the experts say?

I am no stranger to the ketogenic diet, but when I started to write this book, I immediately realized how delicate the subject is. The ketogenic diet is not only a relatively technical diet, but it is a diet still in the early stages of being discovered, which gives rise to quite a bit of controversy. Especially when it comes to its effects on medical conditions such as diabetes or cancer, I believe it's important to get professionals involved. That is why I have invited two medical professionals intimately involved with the ketogenic diet to share their insights and give us their in-depth analysis of the ketogenic diet in relation to their field of expertise.

My co-authors and I have read all the texts in this book.
We felt it was important that we all shared the same vision.

Professor Hanno Pijl is an endocrinologist who will give us an even more in-depth look into the ketogenic diet as it relates to diabetes. Read his article on page 37.

Doctor William Cortvriendt has just completed his book, *Kankervrij* (Cancer-free), in which he recommends the ketogenic diet as a form of treatment.
Read his article on page 47.

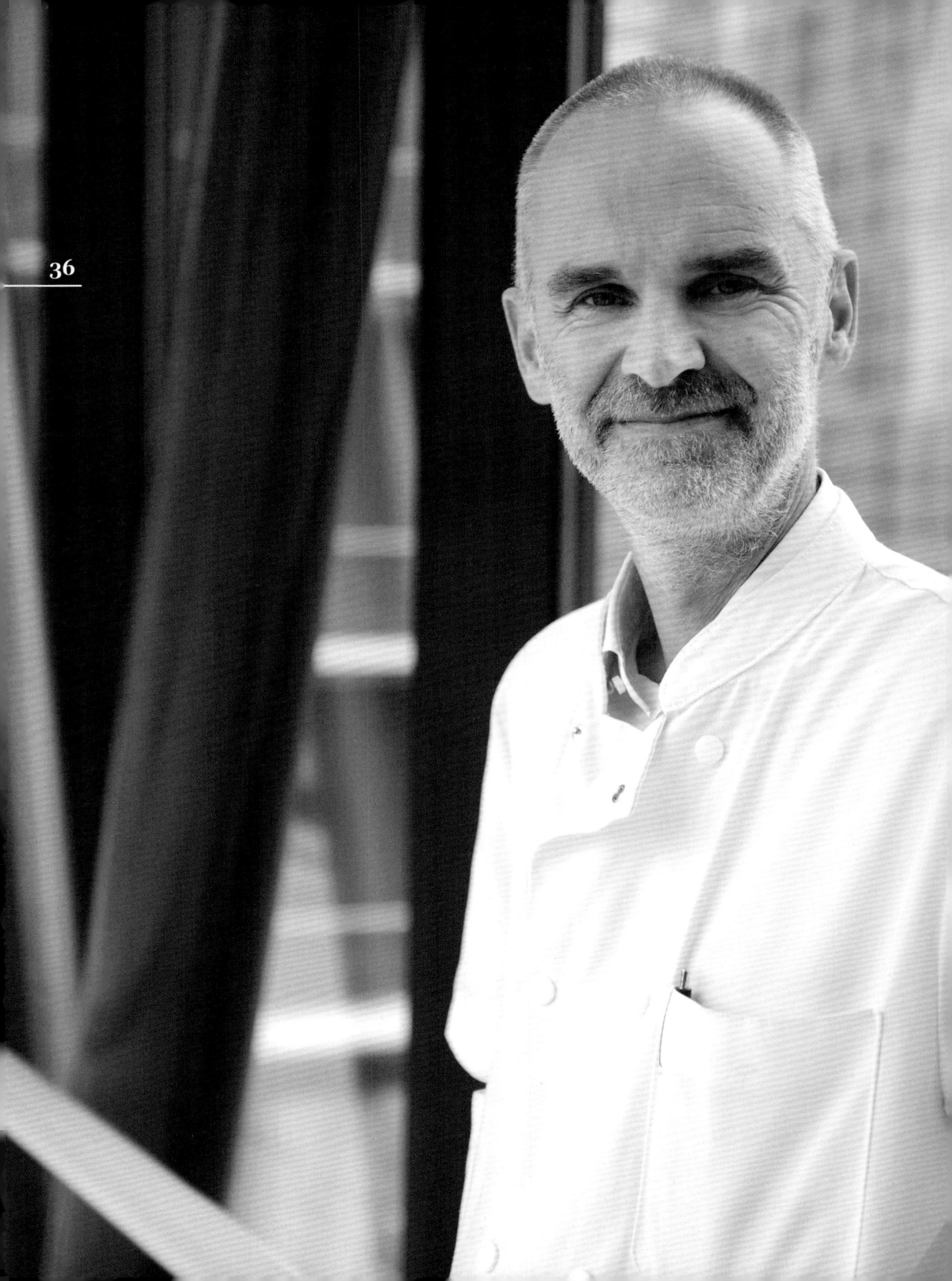

PROFESSOR HANNO PIJL

*I first met Professor Hanno Pijl when I interviewed
him about healthy nutrition. He is an endocrinologist
whose work includes counseling people with diabetes.
He also conducts scientific research, working together
with world-renowned experts such as Valter Longo
and Professor Dariush Mozaffarian. He is one of those
physicians who realize that nutrition and lifestyle are
critical elements of treatment and that you first need
to work with nutrition before resorting to medicine.
Together with Karine Hoenderdos, he wrote the book*
Diabetes Type 2? Maak jezelf beter *(Type 2 Diabetes?
The cure is in your hands). At the University Medical
Center in Leiden, where he works, he counsels diabetic
patients and others on changing their eating habits
to a low-carb or even ketogenic way of eating.*

Ketogenic nutrition: what does the science say?

By Prof. Dr. Hanno Pijl

WHAT IS A KETOGENIC DIET?

Ketosis is a biological phenomenon dating back to prehistoric times that helped us survive in times of food scarcity. Keto acids are the byproducts of the breaking down of fats. When there is little food, our bodies draw energy from our fat reserves. We use that fat as a source of fuel, which is then converted in the liver to keto acids. These are then released into the bloodstream by the liver. We can start talking about ketosis when the concentration of keto acids in the blood is high. These keto acids can, in turn, be used as a fuel source. And that is, of course, useful when there is nothing to eat. Moreover, the metabolism of keto acids has been shown to cause less cell damage and inflammation than the conversion of glucose. You can imagine how all that helps us survive periods of food scarcity.

But does that mean you have to eat very little to reach ketosis? No, you don't have to, as long as you are careful about what you eat. Carbs, particularly the most common carbs in our diet, starch and sugar, are in fact nothing more than long chains of glucose molecules (although there are many different types of sugars that all have a slightly different structure). Starch and sugar are converted in the gut to glucose molecules. The glucose is absorbed by the gut lining and transported to the bloodstream. The blood flows past the pancreas, which is responsible for making insulin. The level of glucose in the blood is the main trigger for insulin production. Protein triggers this production less, and fat very little or not at all. Insulin slows down the burning of fat and the resulting production of keto acids. Which makes sense, when you consider the fact that insulin is primarily produced when there is a lot of glucose present in the blood. That glucose can then be used as a source of fuel, making the burning of fat unnecessary. When you eat very little starch and sugars (typically less than 50 grams a day, or less than 20 grams a day if you're being really strict), the insulin concentration in your blood remains low and you end up burning primarily fats and producing keto acids. Proteins also stimulate insulin production, which means that you also have to limit your protein intake if you really want to eat keto. At the same time, you can continue to eat fat as this doesn't stimulate insulin production in your body. That fat then serves as a source of energy in the absence of glucose. A happy coincidence is that the keto acids produced during the conversion of fats in the liver can also be used as a fuel. That is especially important for the brain. The brain cannot burn fats, which makes it entirely dependent on ketones in the absence of glucose. A ketogenic diet contains very little starch and sugar, and limited amounts of protein. To be able to keep this up for more than a couple of weeks, you need to make sure that you're getting enough fuel in your body. You can do this and remain in your state of ketosis by eating lots and lots of fat (at least 70 percent of your nutrition).

FOLLOWING A KETOGENIC DIET, HOW DO YOU DO IT?

I am happy to leave the answer to that question to Pascale, and you will find plenty of tips on how to do so elsewhere in this book. However, I would like to address one common misconception: that ketogenic nutrition, by definition, consists of many animal products. This misconception stems from the idea that starches and sugars are found almost exclusively in plant-based foods. That does not automatically mean, however, that all plants contain starches and sugars: there are plenty of plant-based foods that contain neither. You can also eat keto and be a (lacto)vegetarian (with full-fat dairy products and eggs) or even vegan (with plant-based fats, vegetables that contain plenty of fiber and little starch, and fruits that are relatively low in sugars). A vegan ketogenic diet is hard to maintain. You'll need to do your best to find enough variety to keep your food interesting and to make sure you're getting all the right nutrients.

HOW QUICKLY DO YOU REACH KETOSIS?

It generally takes a day or two before you reach ketosis when you consume 50 grams of starch per day. The process is quicker if you consume less starch. Times may vary per individual and are dependent on your own metabolic rate and state once you decide to eat keto. As soon as you eat more starch or sugar, you will immediately get kicked out of ketosis: the insulin produced as a reaction to the increase in the blood glucose levels inhibits the production of keto acids very quickly. But the ketosis will return just as quickly once you start eating keto again.

IS A KETOGENIC DIET HEALTHY?

There are an increasing number of scientific indications that a ketogenic diet, at least when followed for shorter periods of time, is good for us. However, we still lack thorough research on the effects of ketogenic nutrition compared to, for example, Mediterranean nutrition patterns or vegetarian diets with more carbs. Moreover, there are not enough long-term research studies (lasting more than two years) into how safe the diet is (although no major issues have been reported with children who follow a long-term ketogenic diet to combat epilepsy). So, what do we know about ketogenic diets?

HEALTHY PEOPLE WITHOUT OVERWEIGHT

There are very few studies that have evaluated the effects of ketogenic nutrition on healthy people who are not overweight. There are, however, a couple of points I would like to share here.

Before agriculture arrived on the scene some ten thousand years ago, a mild state of ketosis was probably the norm for most people. People had far less to eat than they do now, in particular far less starch and sugar, the main sources of glucose in our diet. Although carbs have always been part of our diet, our ancestors ate mostly fats and proteins before the rise of agriculture. Since farming was introduced, some 60 to 70 percent of our food has consisted of high-carb crops. But early farmers, just like the hunter-gatherers before them, were regularly faced with food shortages. It is only since the Industrial Revolution that large parts of the world's population have had an abundance of food at their disposal and never been forced into a state of ketosis.

When the starch and sugar in our diet is replaced by fat, we experience far fewer glucose and insulin spikes in the blood. That leads to more fat burning and less glucose burning, a decreased production of unhealthy free radicals and inflammation after meals, an improved sensitivity to various hormones and a healthier metabolic profile.

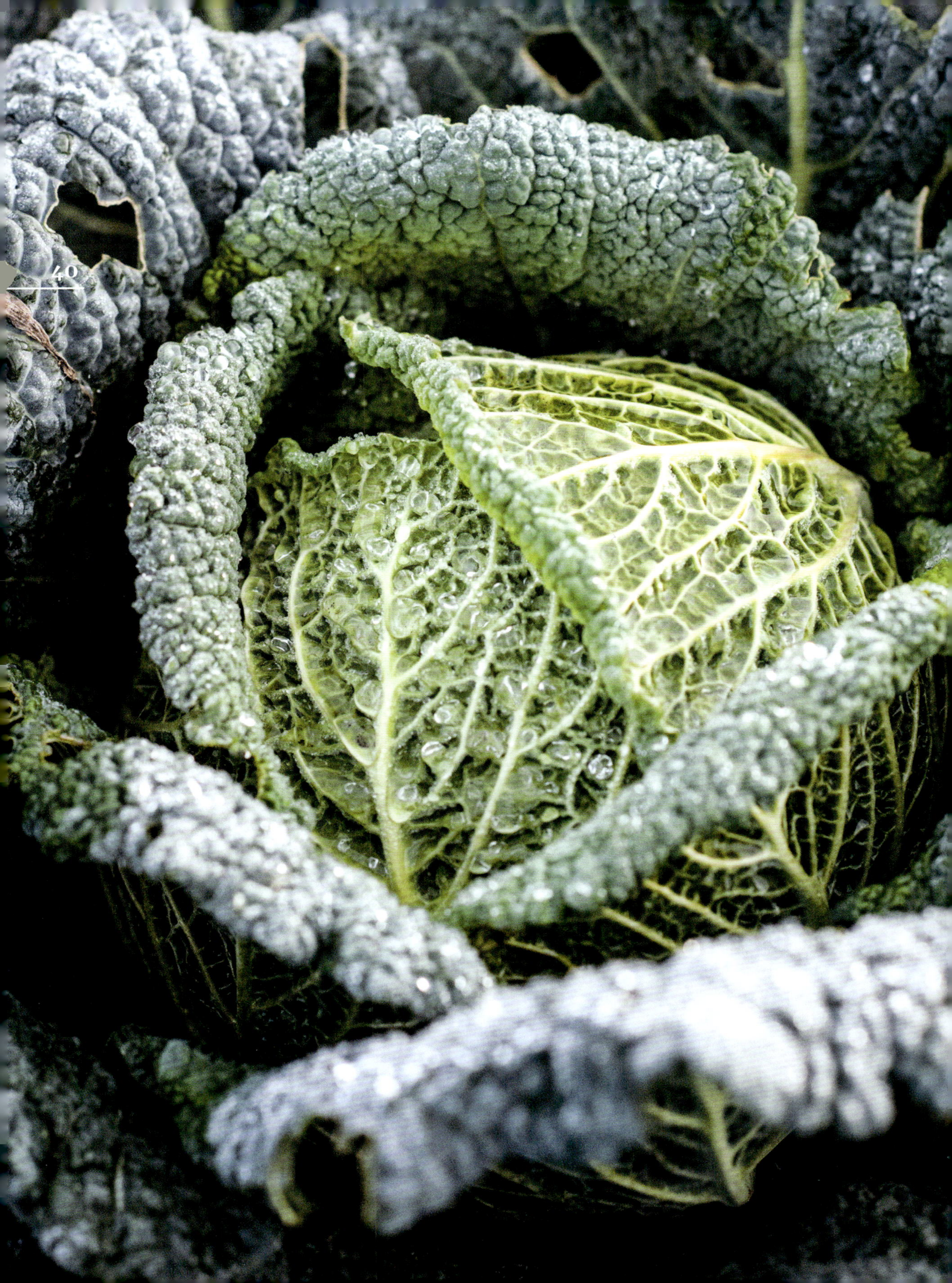
40

Ketogenic food contains, by definition, a lot of fat. This fat can be saturated or unsaturated. Saturated fat has been given a bad rap since food health guidelines in the 1960s indicated that too many saturated fats were believed to increase the risk of cardiovascular disease. In recent years, there has been much heated discussion about saturated fats. It seems that the truth is less clear-cut than we initially thought. Until recently, we viewed saturated fat as a single type of fat (animal fat), whereas in fact it's a collective term for many different types of saturated fatty acids. And each of those fatty acids has its own impact on our health. Some saturated fatty acids increase our cholesterol levels and give rise to inflammation, while others are very beneficial. Moreover, data exists suggesting that replacing saturated fats with carbs does not necessarily decrease the risk of developing certain conditions. Finally, ketogenic nutrition, even when it does contain large amounts of saturated fats, has other effects on fats in the blood that decrease the risk of cardiovascular disease. This has to do with the fact that too much glucose can be converted by the liver into unhealthy (saturated) fatty acids. When you limit your consumption of starch and sugar, the production of these unhealthy fatty acids decreases. In short, there is little evidence to support the idea that ketogenic nutrition increases the risk of cardiovascular disease. In fact, there is more evidence to indicate that the risk will actually decrease. Because no long-term studies into this phenomenon have been carried out as of yet, it is always wise to test the level of fat in your blood after a while when following a ketogenic diet.

PEOPLE WITH OVERWEIGHT AND METABOLIC SYNDROME

People with overweight are often, but not always, more resistant to insulin. That is why their blood glucose levels are usually elevated and they are at a higher risk of developing diabetes. But an increased resistance to insulin can also lead to a complex series of changes in the body's metabolism, a condition collectively called metabolic syndrome. Metabolic syndrome increases the risk of cardiovascular disease and cancer. Weight loss increases your sensitivity to insulin, causing the metabolic syndrome to disappear.

If you want to lose weight, limiting your starch and sugar intake is more effective than limiting your fat intake, at least in the short term. This is especially true for ketogenic nutrition with people who are resistant to insulin and suffer from metabolic syndrome. In the long term (more than a year), this advantage over foods containing fewer fats disappears. Why that is the case remains a mystery. The most probable explanation is that people find it difficult to maintain changes in their eating patterns over the long term, especially when they're constantly being enticed to make the wrong choices.

PEOPLE WITH DIABETES

An increasing number of studies indicate that ketogenic nutrition is beneficial for people with overweight and type 2 diabetes. A century ago, when diabetes couldn't be treated with medicine, a ketogenic diet was the only way to improve the condition of people with diabetes. With the advent of insulin and other medications, we developed the optimistic idea that medication could easily neutralize the effect of carbs on our nutrition. But the reality turns out to be quite different. By far the most glucose in our bodies comes from what we eat. Starch and sugar are the main sources. If you consume less glucose, you don't have to work so hard to get it out of your system, which means you require far less medication to manage your blood glucose levels. Therefore, people with overweight and type 2 diabetes almost always suffer from metabolic syndrome. Less starch and sugar can also help put a stop to that. Recent research shows that a ketogenic diet is highly effective in putting type 2 diabetes into remission. That means people often require less medication, have healthier blood glucose levels and feel much better overall. The following case study helps illustrate this:

Wim was 41 years old when he was diagnosed with type 2 diabetes in 2001. He was treated with medication according to standard protocol, and although his blood glucose levels improved, they never really stabilized. Over the course of several years, his medication was increased to keep his blood glucose level stable. He also had to take pills to manage his blood pressure and cholesterol levels. Meanwhile, he continued to gain weight. In 2014, he was advised by his physician to start injecting insulin because his blood glucose level was still not under control despite the medication he was taking. A year later he was injecting 200 units of insulin per day (a high dose) and had gained another 20 pounds—and his blood glucose levels were still too high. Then his son said to him: "Dad, if you keep going like this, you're not going to live to see me graduate." From that moment onwards, Wim decided to take a different approach. He had seen a program on television about the harmful effects of sugar. After doing some research of his own, he banned starch and sugar from his diet and started eating unprocessed foods with plenty of fish, full-fat dairy products, nuts and vegetables. Within two days (!) he had to stop his insulin injections because his blood sugar levels were dropping at an alarming rate. If you don't consume glucose, you don't have to inject it out of your system. Moreover, he soon started feeling better and found he was able to exercise more. Within a month, Wim was able to stop taking his blood glucose, blood pressure and cholesterol medications. He lost 80 pounds within six months. He felt like a completely new human being. Since 2015, he has been doing sports intensively. Today, he consumes slightly higher levels of whole-grain starch (but not nearly at the levels before his turnaround!) without raising his blood glucose levels too much. As of 2020, he is still off the medication, both for his blood glucose and for his blood pressure and cholesterol. He does notice that during stressful periods or when he eats more starch or sugar, his blood glucose levels tend to rise. The predisposition to develop diabetes, regardless of lifestyle, never goes away!

This story is certainly not unique, but it is special for two reasons. First, on paper it sounds easy to turn your eating habits around and start exercising regularly, but it is much harder for many people to put it into practice. Wim often compares it to training to be a top-class athlete. We as human beings simply have the tendency to eat whatever people put in front of us, and to sit down whenever we have had enough to eat. Starchy and sugary foods are abundantly available everywhere, all the time, and we can do practically everything without having to get up from our chairs. Secondly, not everyone with type 2 diabetes can live without medication, even with optimal nutrition and exercise. This has to do with the amount of insulin these persons can still produce themselves.

For many people with type 2 diabetes, insulin production decreases over time. We don't know exactly why this happens but, without insulin, you can never stabilize your blood glucose levels. Eating less starch and sugar certainly helps a lot, but you will still need pills or even insulin injections to keep your blood glucose levels acceptable.

It is important to realize that contacting your physician is essential before starting with ketogenic nutrition to treat your diabetes. The reason for this is that, in the beginning, you will very quickly need to adjust your medication levels to make sure your blood glucose levels don't crash. You should also be aware that, ultimately, some people will still be dependent on medication to manage their blood glucose, blood pressure and cholesterol levels. This primarily concerns people with overweight who have chronic diabetes (for more than ten years), or people who continue to suffer from diabetes despite having a relatively normal weight. With both these groups there is often, but not always, something else going on with the production of insulin.

In most cases, you don't have to eat keto the rest of your life to keep your diabetes in remission. As soon as the blood levels have stabilized for a while and your weight is at an acceptable level, the intake of carbohydrates can often be increased somewhat (but certainly not back to pre-diabetes levels!) without increasing your blood glucose levels. Then you can resort to a moderately low-carb way of eating such as the one Pascale promotes in her other books.

Little research has been conducted into the effects of ketogenic nutrition on type 1 diabetes. In theory, it should be effective, but with type 1 diabetes—more so than with type 2 diabetes— the risk of developing dangerously low sugar levels is far greater. That is why people with type 1 diabetes must always inject themselves with long-acting insulin. If you eat few carbs, your blood sugar concentration could drop if you are not careful about how much insulin you inject. On the other hand, just like with people with type 2 diabetes, you need less insulin if you eat less starch and sugar. A recent study conducted with 273 children who ate an average of 36 grams of carbs per day showed that it had a positive effect on their metabolism.

PEOPLE WITH CANCER
Experiments with animals have shown that ketogenic nutrition has a positive effect on the treatment of cancer. But there is little data on how safe and effective a ketogenic diet is for humans with cancer.

Periodic bouts of eating keto have been shown to protect mice from the side effects of chemotherapy, while at the same time inhibiting the growth of cancer cells. This is how it works. When you remove sugars, starches, and (to a degree) proteins from the diet of a mouse with cancer, the glucose and protein concentrations in their blood decrease. Healthy cells notice that they are not getting the energy and materials they need to grow. They react to this stressful situation by changing their metabolism. They stop growing and multiplying.

Instead, they defend themselves against all other potential forms of stress (such as heat, radiation, harmful substances, and chemotherapy). Moreover, they start using their energy for regeneration and maintenance. In other words, healthy cells react by protecting themselves against the side effects of chemotherapy. Cancer cells are not able to make this switch, however, because they are genetically damaged. They continue to focus on growing and multiplying without restraint. Furthermore, they have a unique form of metabolism: they can only burn glucose or one specific type of protein. No fats or keto acids. Cancer cells therefore become very vulnerable when less fuel becomes available. Moreover, ketogenic nutrition lowers the concentration of insulin in the blood, and insulin stimulates the growth of cancer cells. Less fuel, fewer substances to thrive on and less stimulus for growth inhibits the growth of cancer cells, particularly when combined with chemotherapy.

As we have said, there is still not much research into how safe and effective ketogenic nutrition is for people with cancer. Although the results found in mice look promising, all too often we find that medication or nutrition works differently with humans. That's why more research is necessary to find out whether eating keto has the same effect on humans as it does on mice and if we can use ketogenic nutrition as an effective cancer treatment.

HOW SAFE IS A KETOGENIC DIET?

Some people doubt whether eating keto is safe. There are two main reasons for that. The first reason is the fear of eating too much saturated fat. As described earlier, there are some important things to note regarding this fear. The second potential problem with ketogenic nutrition is the lack of nutritional fiber. Fiber is non-digestible carbohydrate. Some types of fiber are converted by bacteria in the gut into healthy saturated (!) fats, others remain in the intestines and make bowel movements easier. So, fiber is truly important to our health. Some nutritional scientists fear that the primary source of ketogenic nutrition comes from animal products (because they do not contain any sugars and starches). Were that the case, you would consume very little fiber. But there are perfectly good ways to combine keto and lactovegetarian and even vegan foods. The question remains: is ketogenic nutrition, when used as the basis for your eating habits, the optimal choice for the long term? I happen to doubt that. People are omnivores and generally eat as varied a diet as possible to achieve optimal health. Periodically eating keto for limited periods of time, however, such as for one week every month, or for a couple of weeks to help keep your diabetes in remission, seems to be a healthy, safe option.

Finally: make sure that you consume enough salt and drink enough water when eating keto. One of the side effects of ketogenic nutrition is that your kidneys release a lot of sodium and magnesium and with it a lot of water. This is often a good sign for people with diabetes because it helps lower their blood pressure, but on the other hand, you run the risk of having too few minerals in your blood (especially sodium and magnesium) when you are following a sodium-reduced diet at the same time. This can lead to cramps, but also to more serious conditions if the shortage becomes too great or lasts too long. So, make sure that you consume enough salt and eat enough vegetables (to keep your mineral levels up).

IS A KETOGENIC DIET SUITABLE FOR EVERYONE?

A ketogenic diet is not for everyone. Some people become weak, dizzy or tired. This sometimes passes with a little perseverance, but for other people it is a reason to stop. Try it for yourself to see if it is the right fit for you.

People suffering from any health conditions should first consult their health professional to find out whether it is a good idea to start eating keto. This is particularly true for people with diabetes (who often have to reduce their medication fairly quickly) and cancer (who are not allowed to lose too much weight), but this is also good advice for people with other conditions. Health professionals should know when you are undertaking something that may have an impact on your health.

(INTERMITTENT) FASTING, IS THAT THE SAME AS EATING KETO?

Fasting is also a ketogenic process. With most people, the ketones are produced after a day of fasting, but this period may vary from person to person. From what we know so far, the effects of fasting on our health are primarily caused by the lack of glucose and proteins. Fat plays a smaller role. This does not mean that less fat, or no fat at all as is the case in full fasting, doesn't have its benefits. You could see ketogenic nutrition (also known as fat fasting) as a modified form of fasting. It mimics the effects of fasting, but they are less pronounced because large amounts of fat are consumed to replace the missing starch and protein. On the other hand, it is easier to stick to a ketogenic diet than it is to keep up a full fast, simply because you can still eat quite a lot.

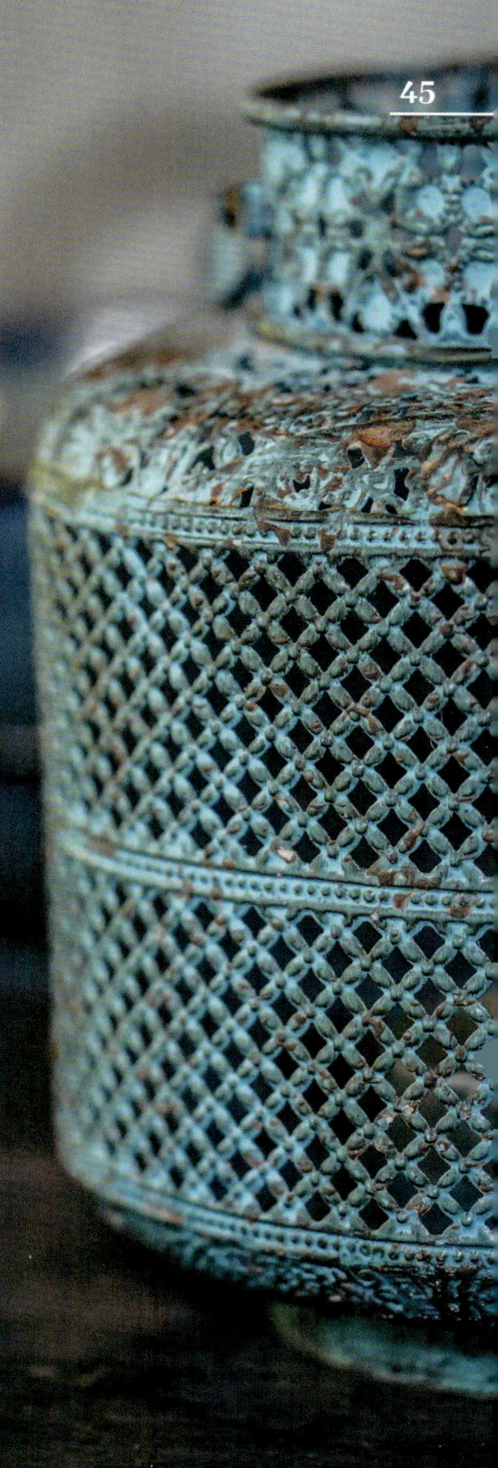

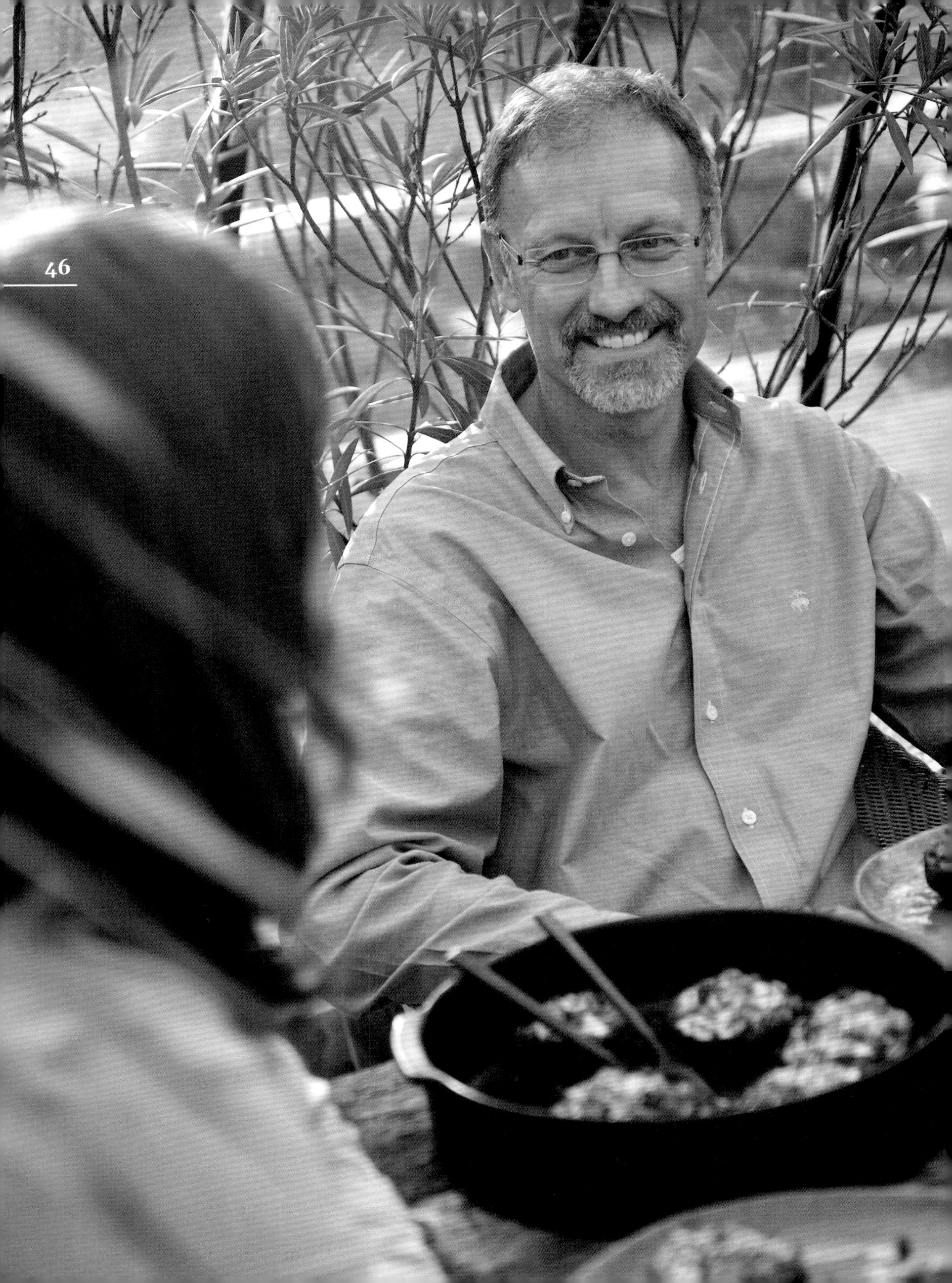

DOCTOR WILLIAM CORTVRIENDT

I wrote my book Pure & Lighter together with William Cortvriendt. He has authored various books, including Lichter *(Lighter) and* Living a Century or More, *in which he recommends a low-carb way of eating. His book* Living a Century or More *was adapted into a television program in the Netherlands, providing advice to people on leading a healthier life. He authored the book* Kankervrij *(Cancer-free), in which he recommends the ketogenic diet. I have asked him to explain why a ketogenic diet is recommended for people with cancer.*

The ketogenic diet as a supplemental treatment for conditions such as cancer

By Dr. William Cortvriendt

In recent years, the ketogenic diet has seen a huge surge in popularity. And, if current developments in the US and now also in Belgium and the Netherlands continue, this popularity is set to grow. In the US, ketogenic nutrition has rapidly become the country's most popular diet.

We have known for over a century that a ketogenic diet is an effective form of therapy for epilepsy. But as various effective medicines became available over the course of the last century, the ketogenic diet slowly faded into the background. All that has changed in the last five years. Many people have discovered that they feel much healthier after following a ketogenic diet for a short or longer period. Moreover, the ketogenic diet has been shown to be a powerful means to lose weight quickly and effectively in serious cases of obesity, and to put type 2 diabetes into remission in many instances. There are also indications that it can inhibit the progression of diseases such as Parkinson's disease and Alzheimer's disease. For cancer patients, the ketogenic diet may also make traditional cancer treatments more effective, as I shall discuss later on.

OUR ENERGY SUPPLY, NOW AND THEN

From an evolutionary standpoint, our energy metabolism is geared towards burning glucose and fatty acids. And when food is scarce, the liver produces ketones by breaking down fatty acids. History has shown that regular intervals of ketone production were, until very recently, the rule rather than the exception. During our evolutionary process, eating food every day, let alone three meals a day, was anything but normal. If the hunting was poor or the weather bad, little to no food would be available for days. When we no longer receive nutrition for two days or longer, the glucose reserves in our bodies quickly run out and we are forced to burn fatty acids instead. Our fat tissue contains far greater reserves of fatty acids and can provide us with months' worth of energy without us having to eat anything. In addition, the liver converts some of those fatty acids into ketones, that are used to fuel our brains instead of glucose. In contrast to ketones and glucose, fatty acids are not able to access our brains as easily. Furthermore, ketones have proven to be a clean and healthy fuel alternative for the cells in our bodies, releasing fewer harmful free radicals in the process when compared to burning glucose.

Not only do we eat and snack more often than our ancestors did and no longer have to go for very long without food, but what we eat has also changed drastically over the last few decades. In particular our consumption of fats has decreased, while our consumption of carbs has increased significantly. This has also changed our metabolism. Thanks to our high-carb, western way of eating, our bodies are completely geared toward burning glucose and we never really reach ketosis. The following figure illustrates the relationship between what we eat and to what extent we use glucose, fatty acids and ketones as a source of energy.

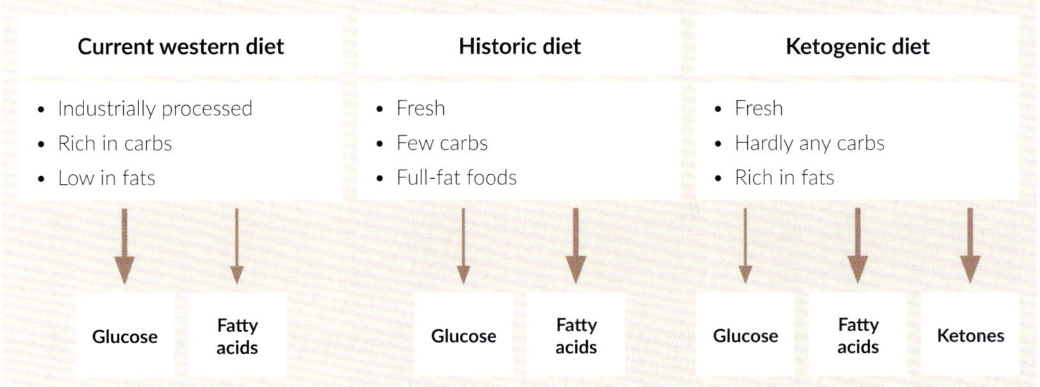

The consequences of dietary choices on the nature of the foodstuffs we use for our energy metabolism.

The ketogenic diet comes closest to the situation that arises when too little food is temporarily consumed, either as a result of food scarcity or voluntarily fasting for a period of time. In contrast to fasting, a ketogenic diet can be kept up for a longer period.

Because of this change in eating behavior, a large part of the world's population is, in fact, constantly living with raised blood sugar levels. The health consequences of this have become more than clear to us by now. The excessive consumption of fast carbs and the subsequent saturation of our cells with glucose has dangerous implications for our health. First of all, the glucose that comes from sugars and other carbs is not a substance that our bodies can use for anything other than a source of energy. When we consume too much of it, there is only one thing our bodies can do with this surplus and that is store it, usually in the form of fat. In addition, we suffer from a chronically high blood sugar level from hormones such as insulin and the growth hormone IGF-1 (insulin-like growth factor 1). All this results in not only overweight, but also a fatty liver, chronic inflammation in the body, increased ageing, type 2 diabetes, cardiovascular disease, dementia—and cancer. It's no coincidence that many of these conditions are positively affected by replacing our modern western nutrition with a low-carb eating pattern. Especially in a number of conditions such as serious obesity, type 2 diabetes, or even cancer, it has been shown that an even further reduction in carbohydrate intake via a ketogenic diet can play an important role in the treatment and even cure of these conditions.

WHAT DO WE TRY TO ACHIEVE WITH A KETOGENIC DIET?

The aim of every ketogenic diet is to lower the blood sugar level (in other words, the amount of glucose in your blood) enough to allow the liver to convert fatty acids into ketones. These ketones then replace glucose to a great extent as a source of fuel. When that happens, we say that you have reached ketosis. Moreover, the often elevated blood levels of certain hormones such as insulin and IGF-1 also decreases. That has several important positive consequences such as an increase in fat metabolism, a rapid decrease in overweight and a decrease in what is called insulin resistance. This is one way to deal with serious obesity and can potentially put type 2 diabetes into remission.

Moreover, it improves the metabolism of the brain cells, providing an effective treatment of epilepsy and inhibiting the progression of degenerative diseases such as Alzheimer's and Parkinson's.

Various proponents of this diet also claim that they feel healthier, have more energy, and can think more clearly. Some endurance athletes also swear by a ketogenic diet because the conversion from glucose to fatty acids and ketones gives them a far more stable source of energy for their muscles to draw from. Other studies, where participants followed the ketogenic diet for over a year, have shown that it is safe.

HOW OFTEN AND FOR HOW LONG SHOULD YOU FOLLOW A KETOGENIC DIET?

With all this positive news about the ketogenic diet, it has grown to be quite a fashionable trend in many countries. The logical next question then is whether it's something you should do every day and whether it's suitable for everyone. My answer to this depends on the duration and the reason that you want to adopt the ketogenic diet.

Contrary to a low-carb way of eating, following a ketogenic diet is not easy. To effectively reach ketosis with a ketogenic diet, you must follow a very strict, almost carb-free eating regimen. You are barely allowed fruit, you need to be careful with your vegetables, and you even have to keep your protein amounts in check. The amino acids that you consume when you eat too many proteins are converted by your liver into glucose, so if you eat too many proteins, you will be kicked out of the ketosis that you're striving to achieve with a ketogenic diet. Moreover, naturally occurring ketosis is meant to effectively counterbalance short periods of food scarcity. A continual state of ketosis, which is what people following a long-term ketogenic diet look to achieve, is not a natural metabolic state for our bodies. You also need to take into account that there are a number of contra-indications for a ketogenic diet such as pregnancy, type 1 diabetes, cardiac arrhythmia, surgery where large portions of the intestinal tract are removed, and certain rare genetic conditions.

So, my advice is that you should aim to achieve a state of ketosis that lasts longer than two to three weeks only if it is part of a treatment of the aforementioned conditions such as obesity, type 2 diabetes and cancer. For people who wish to adopt the ketogenic diet for their general health, it is advisable to first try a low-carb approach like the one Pascale has already promoted and illustrated in many of her earlier cookbooks.

This is an eating pattern that I would recommend to anyone any day. It is also the way of eating that Pascale Naessens, Hanno Pijl and I have enjoyed for many, many years. To supplement this, you may follow a ketogenic diet for two weeks once every six to eight weeks. An increasing amount of data suggests that this is when unhealthy or damaged cells are cleared away so that young and healthy cells can take their place.

There are reasons to assume that regularly reaching ketosis for short periods of time keeps our cells young and healthy. And, although we don't know for sure, it may even be plausible that such relatively short periods of ketosis might prevent cancer. After all, the damaged cells being cleared away could include cells which might have the potential to turn into cancerous cells.

Those familiar with eating low-carb will find that reaching ketosis is a relatively simple process. Your metabolism is already used to burning fatty acids, supplemented by the ketones already produced by the liver. This can happen as quickly as when you have a longer period between dinner and breakfast the next day. When transitioning from low-carb nutrition to a ketogenic diet, your body will be able to generate large quantities of ketones quite effortlessly, so that reaching ketosis almost happens by itself.

WHY KETOGENIC NUTRITION WORKS AGAINST CANCER

The anti-carcinogenic function of a ketogenic diet is not only relatively unknown to the general public but also to many oncologists and therefore deserves some further explanation.

With the help of a ketogenic diet as part of a cancer treatment program, the aim is to weaken the cancer cells by reducing the availability of glucose, essential for their growth. Although the fact that the metabolism of cancer cells differs from normal cells has been known for almost a century, it is surprising that this has never or rarely been considered until quite recently in evaluating how we can prevent and treat cancer more effectively.

What all cancer cells have in common is that certain parts of the cells, also known as the mitochondria, are seriously damaged. In healthy cells, these mitochondria make sure that the reaction between oxygen and glucose, fatty acids, and ketones occurs, producing ATP (adenosine triphosphate), which in turn is used by our cells as a source of energy.

In cancer cells, this normal process of generating energy is inhibited, while it is these very cells that require lots of energy for their quick and uninhibited growth. Cancer cells are therefore forced to generate energy in another way without using the mitochondria and without requiring oxygen. This process is called fermentation. But only glucose can be converted into energy through fermentation. Fats and ketones are not suited to this process.

This means that the supply of energy to cancer cells has three important differences compared to normal cells. First of all, cancer cells are far more dependent on glucose, precisely because they are not or barely able to burn fatty acids and ketones. The second difference is that fermentation produces only a sixteenth of the energy produced per molecule of glucose than when glucose is burned with the aid of oxygen. The result is that cancer cells are only able to grow and multiply when large quantities of glucose are readily available, or when plenty of proteins are available from which the liver can make its own glucose when blood sugar levels are low. This means that cancer cells are almost completely dependent on the supply of large quantities of glucose through sugar and other carbs from our food or—in a pinch—from high-protein foods.

The third difference concerns the waste products created during metabolism. When glucose reacts with oxygen, carbon dioxide and water are produced, which is easily disposed of through the lungs and the kidneys. When glucose is fermented, however, it produces lactic acid, which acidifies the environment surrounding cancer cells. When certain parts of our bodies become acidic, our bodies think that this is a result of fermentation due to a lack of oxygen. The body reacts by creating more blood vessels to supply oxygenated blood to that area, a process also known as angiogenesis. Through the excess production of lactic acid and the resulting acidification, cancer cells (through angiogenesis) indirectly increase the supply of nutrients feeding the tumor.

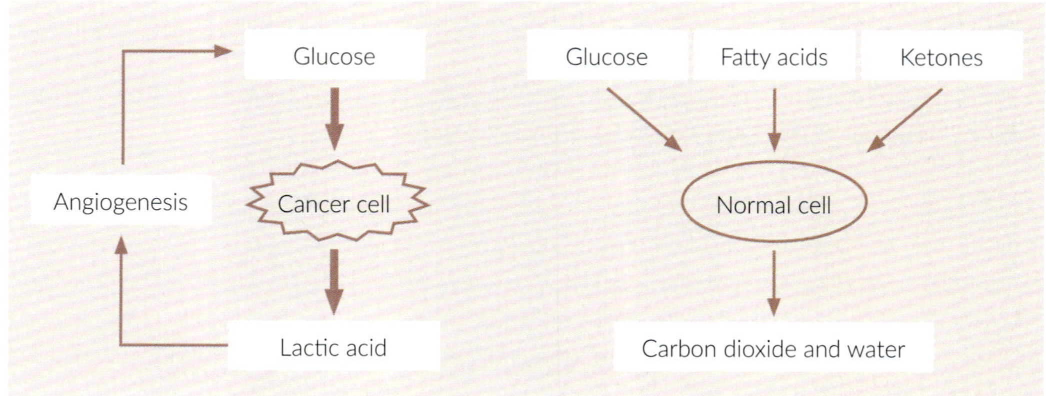

The essential difference between the supply of energy to a cancer cell and a normal cell. The cancer cell is dependent on the fermentation of large quantities of glucose from our diet. Lactic acid is formed during this process which causes an increase in the production of new blood vessels, which in turn increases the flow of glucose and other nutrients to the tumor.

This has gradually led to the insight that inhibiting the flow of glucose to cancer cells by lowering blood sugar levels may be an effective supplementary treatment for cancer. A decreased supply of energy will weaken the cancer cells and inhibit their growth.

Moreover, it also reduces the production of lactic acid. This inhibits the development of angiogenesis, which means that fewer blood vessels leading towards the tumor are created by the body. And that, in turn, decreases the flow of glucose and other nutrients feeding the tumor, decreasing the growth of cancer cells even further.

For most normal body cells, a low blood sugar level is not a problem because they can switch to burning fatty acids—with the notable exception of our brain cells, because they are not able to burn fatty acids. Our bodies solve this issue by having the liver produce ketones from fatty acids when the blood sugar level is low. They can be used as a source of energy by the brain cells and most other normal cells in the body, but not by cancer cells. In other words, if we succeed in lowering our blood sugar levels enough, we can inhibit the supply of energy to cancer cells, while other healthy cells

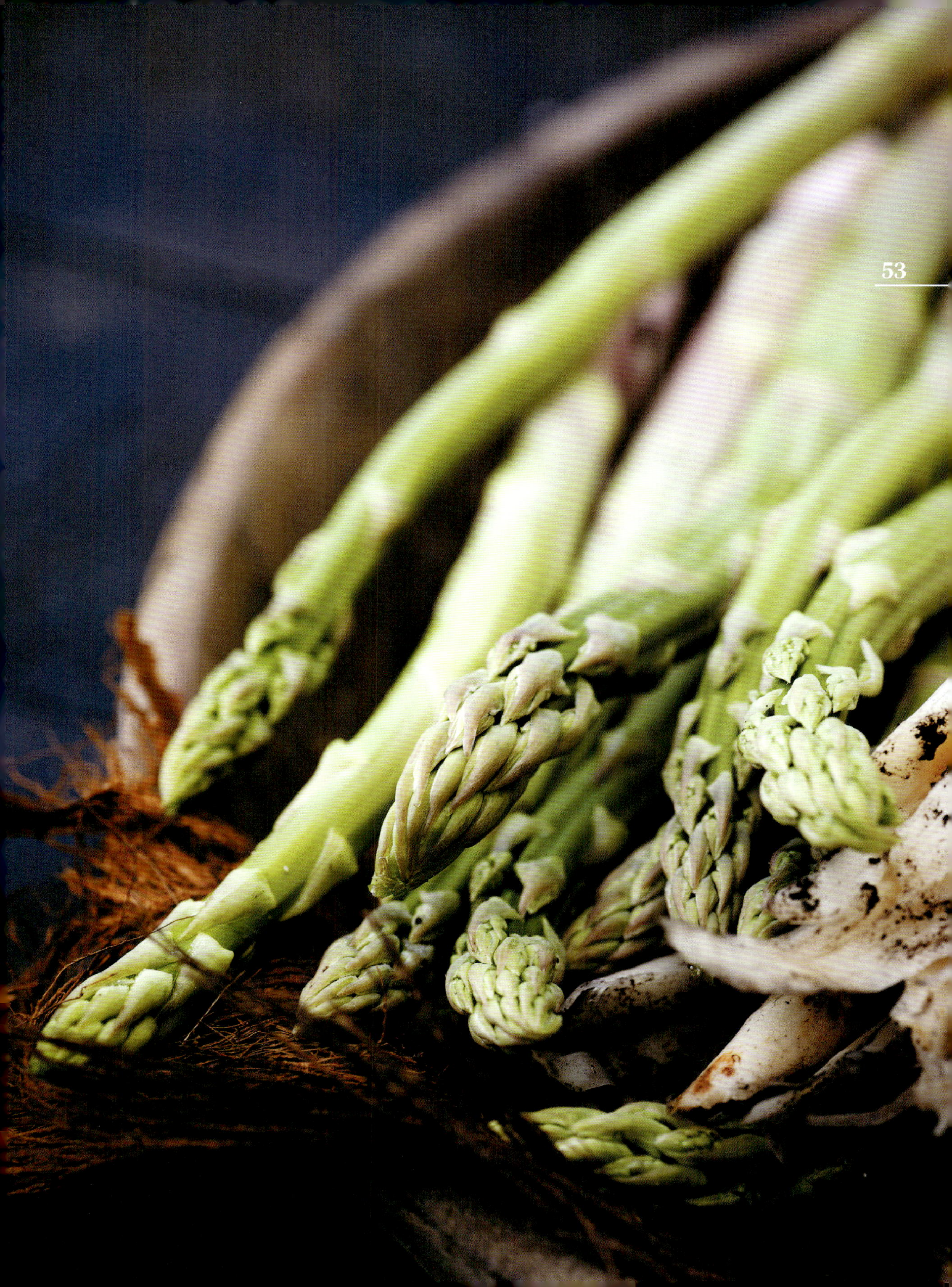

simply switch to burning fatty acids and ketones. And we can realize such a drop in our blood sugar levels and the subsequent changes in our metabolism with the help of a ketogenic diet.

WHAT TYPES OF CANCER BENEFIT FROM A KETOGENIC DIET?

In theory, all cancer cells have damaged mitochondria, which would mean that almost every cancer cell has to resort to fermentation to meet its energy needs. This also means that a ketogenic diet should, in theory, be suitable to treat any type of cancer.

There are, however, a couple of points that should be noted here.

First of all, the beneficial effects of a ketogenic diet in treating cancer have mostly been proven through testing on animals. The first tests conducted on humans are admittedly positive and promising, but they are still limited. Furthermore, that all cancer cells have damaged mitochondria is a fact, but the extent of the damage may differ. What is clear is that the more serious the damage to the cancer cells' mitochondria, the more dependent they are on fermentation for energy. They therefore require more glucose and are more vulnerable to a restriction in the supply of glucose. An oncologist can get a good idea of how dependent the type of cancer is on the supply of glucose through what we call a PET-scan. These scans are used today as a diagnostic tool to identify cancers and potential metastases. A radioactive substance is linked to glucose molecules and injected intravenously. The radioactive glucose collects in the cancer cells in the tumor. This not only (literally) highlights where the cancer cells have accumulated, but also shows how much glucose they need. And it is clear that the more glucose the cells need, the more vulnerable they will be when they lack that glucose. We also know from research studies that during a ketogenic diet, the already weakened cancer cells become more vulnerable to the effects of chemotherapy and radiation therapy treatments.

Besides the fact that some cancer cells may still be able to react glucose and fatty acids with oxygen to some degree, there are a few other factors that may reduce the effectiveness of a ketogenic diet. The first of these is the amount of glucose in our blood, also called our blood sugar level. A ketogenic diet will cause this to drop drastically, but it will never go all the way down to zero, because the liver always sets a baseline through the production of glucose from amino acids. Besides ketones, the cells in our brains are still about 30 percent dependent on glucose as their energy source. This means that you can inhibit the growth of cancer cells with a ketogenic diet, sometimes even stop it, but you can never let cancer cells go 100 percent hungry!

Another factor that can only be partially influenced by a ketogenic diet is the availability of the amino acid glutamine. This amino acid can more or less be fermented by cancer cells to supply them with part of their energy needs. Glutamine is an amino acid present in almost all proteins in our diet and can also be produced by our own bodies from other amino acids. The only thing we can do to limit the supply of glutamine through nutrition is to not consume any more proteins than strictly necessary and to avoid any supplements that contain glutamine.

In any case, a ketogenic diet can clearly play an important part in the treatment of all types of cancer. But, because cancer cells are very versatile, that diet will always need to be part of a complete treatment plan that also includes traditional treatments such as surgery, radiation therapy and chemotherapy. Additional analyses in my book *Kankervrij* show that you can make other adjustments in your lifestyle that can significantly improve your cancer prognosis.[3]

WHAT ARE SOME CONCRETE RESULTS THAT YOU MAY EXPECT FROM A KETOGENIC DIET WITH CANCER?

The use of a ketogenic diet as part of a cancer treatment is relatively new and most of the research so far has involved studies conducted on animals. In about three quarters of these animal studies, a ketogenic diet was shown to have had a clear anticarcinogenic effect.[4]

From studies carried out on the effects of a ketogenic diet on people, we know for certain that it drastically reduces blood sugar levels. There is also extensive research available showing a strong correlation between blood sugar levels and cancer prognoses. They show time and time again that the higher your blood sugar levels, the worse the prognosis, and vice versa.[5]

Based on these results, you should indirectly be able to conclude that a ketogenic diet would also improve your prognosis through a lowering of the blood sugar level. The studies measuring the effect of a ketogenic diet on cancer patients primarily concern studies where a small number of patients show significant improvements. The first recorded instances of such improvements and a decrease in tumor size date as far back as 1941 and 1942.[6]

More recent studies have shown remarkably positive clinical results in combination with data from PET-scans. These studies show that, with a ketogenic diet, the cancer cells are less able to take in glucose.[7] One study, based on a four-week ketogenic diet, indicated that there is a correlation between the subsequent decrease in insulin, the decreased rate of tumor growth and the degree to which PET-scans show that there is a reduced intake of glucose by the cancer cells.[8]

Such a result is an important indication for a causal correlation between the ketogenic diet, the subsequent reduced intake of glucose by cancer cells and the resulting anticarcinogenic effects. Another study shows that a reduced intake of glucose also leads to a reduction in the production of lactic acid. This means that, with a ketogenic diet, cancer cells can effectively ferment less glucose and convert it into energy.[9] The study also showed that, after following a ketogenic diet, the so-called HER2-expression was reduced, a general measure for the decreased activity of cancer cells in a certain type of (HER2-positive) breast cancer.

There are also various publications that report surprising and exceptionally positive results in a number of individual patients with cancer after following a ketogenic diet.[11] We also know that a ketogenic diet can make traditional radiation therapy and chemotherapy treatments more effective. From cell and animal studies, we know that cancer cells are less able to neutralize oxygen free radicals than normal cells. Because radiation therapy and chemotherapy result in the release of large numbers of oxygen free radicals, it is also an important explanation of why cancer cells are more damaged by radiation therapy and chemotherapy than normal cells.[12]

We also know that cancer cells produce large quantities of lactic acid through the fermentation of glucose, which in itself works as an antioxidant that cancer cells can use to protect themselves from radiation therapy and chemotherapy.[13]

Various studies emphasize that the reduced possibility for fermentation by cancer cells during a ketogenic diet or fasting result in a reduction in lactic acid production, and that is the reason why the cancer cells of patients who follow a ketogenic diet are more vulnerable to radiation therapy and chemotherapy treatments.[14]

It is also important to note that the ketogenic diet can help combat cachexia, the wasting away of the body that frequently occurs during advanced stages of cancer. Cachexia occurs when the insatiable hunger for energy and nutrients from the increasing numbers of cancer cells cannot be stilled by nutrition alone.

As a result, the cancer cells break down normal tissues that are rich in protein, with muscle tissue being the main victim. Some of the amino acids that are released are then directly used by the cancer cells as material for further growth and the rest is converted by the liver into glucose, which in turn serves as fuel for the cancer cells. During this stage, the cancer cells eat up all your remaining healthy tissue.

In cancer patients, it has been shown that a ketogenic diet can reduce the breaking down of proteins in the body, leading to a reduction in cachexia and sometimes even resulting in weight gain.[15]
We don't know how long a ketogenic diet should be followed with cancer patients. Theoretically, the diet should continue as long as actual cancer cells are visibly present in the body, monitored with the help of PET-scans. Because as long as the PET-scan continues to show spots with an active visible intake of glucose, cancer cells are showing that they are still taking in glucose and actively continuing to grow.

But what do you do when the cancer has gone into remission and there are no more visible cancer cells in the body? In that case, my advice would be *never* to go back to a "normal" western eating pattern with plenty of fast carbs. If during remission dormant cancer cells remain in the body, high-carb foods and the raised blood sugar levels they cause will implicitly invite those cells to grow and multiply once again. I advise you to keep eating low-carb once you are in remission, as recommended in the recipe books *Living a Century or More, The recipe book, Pure & Lighter* and all of Pascale's other cookbooks.

Moreover, I would recommend switching once every two or three months to a ketogenic diet for two weeks. You can precede these short periods of eating keto with a couple of fasting days to enable you to reach ketosis quickly and easily. With cancer, it won't matter too much whether you reach ketosis a couple of days earlier rather than later in most cases. The challenge is to stick to it for longer periods of time. Supplementing a ketogenic diet with one or more short fasting periods can be of particular benefit just before chemotherapy or radiation therapy treatment. There are studies that show that this may reduce the side effects associated with chemotherapy and radiation therapy such as nausea and inflammation.[16]

The fasting doesn't need to be a full fast. You can achieve the same positive results with what people call FMD (Fast Mimicking Diet), where you drink broth and eat small quantities of salad with perhaps a small piece of meat or chicken.

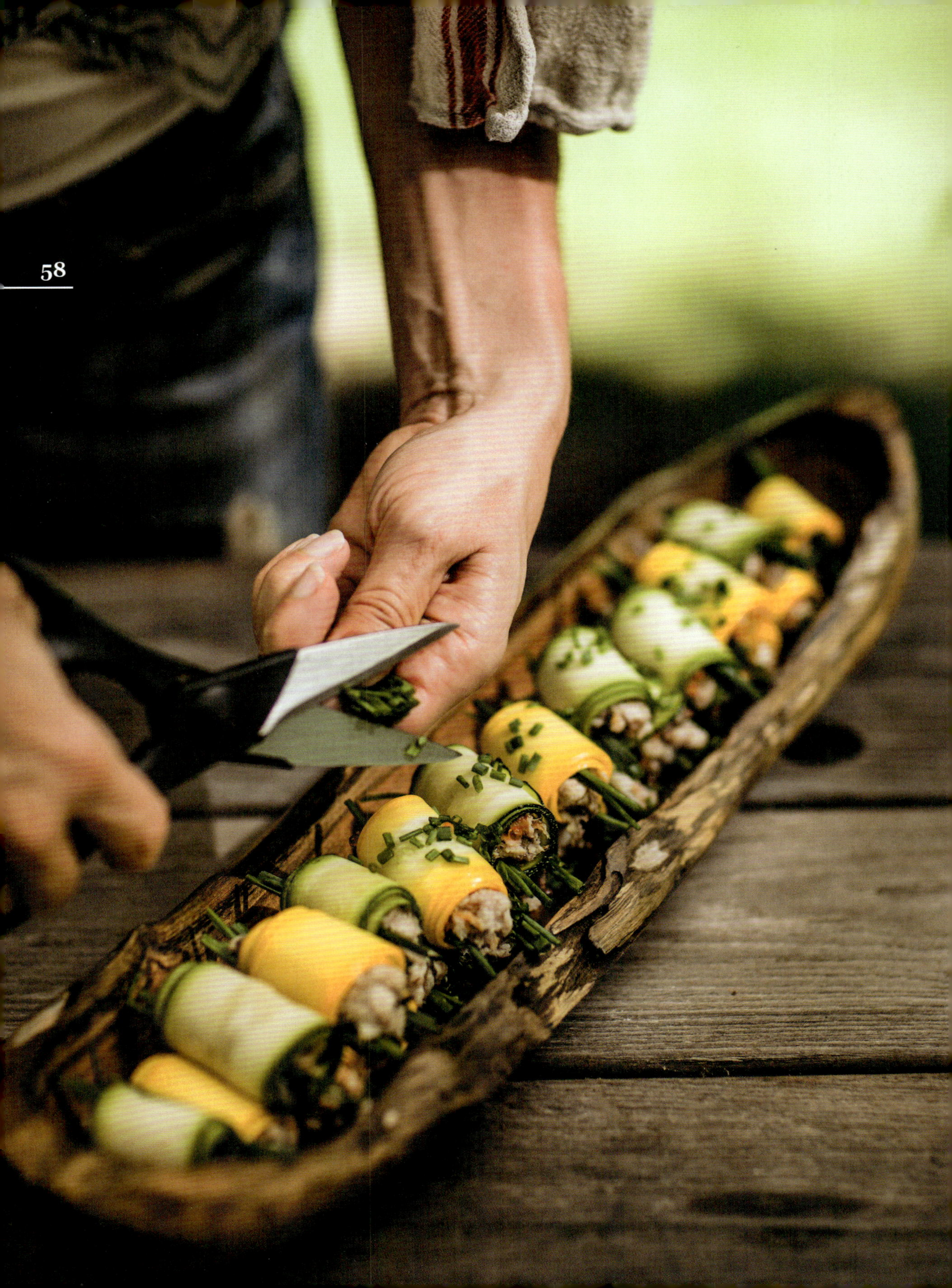

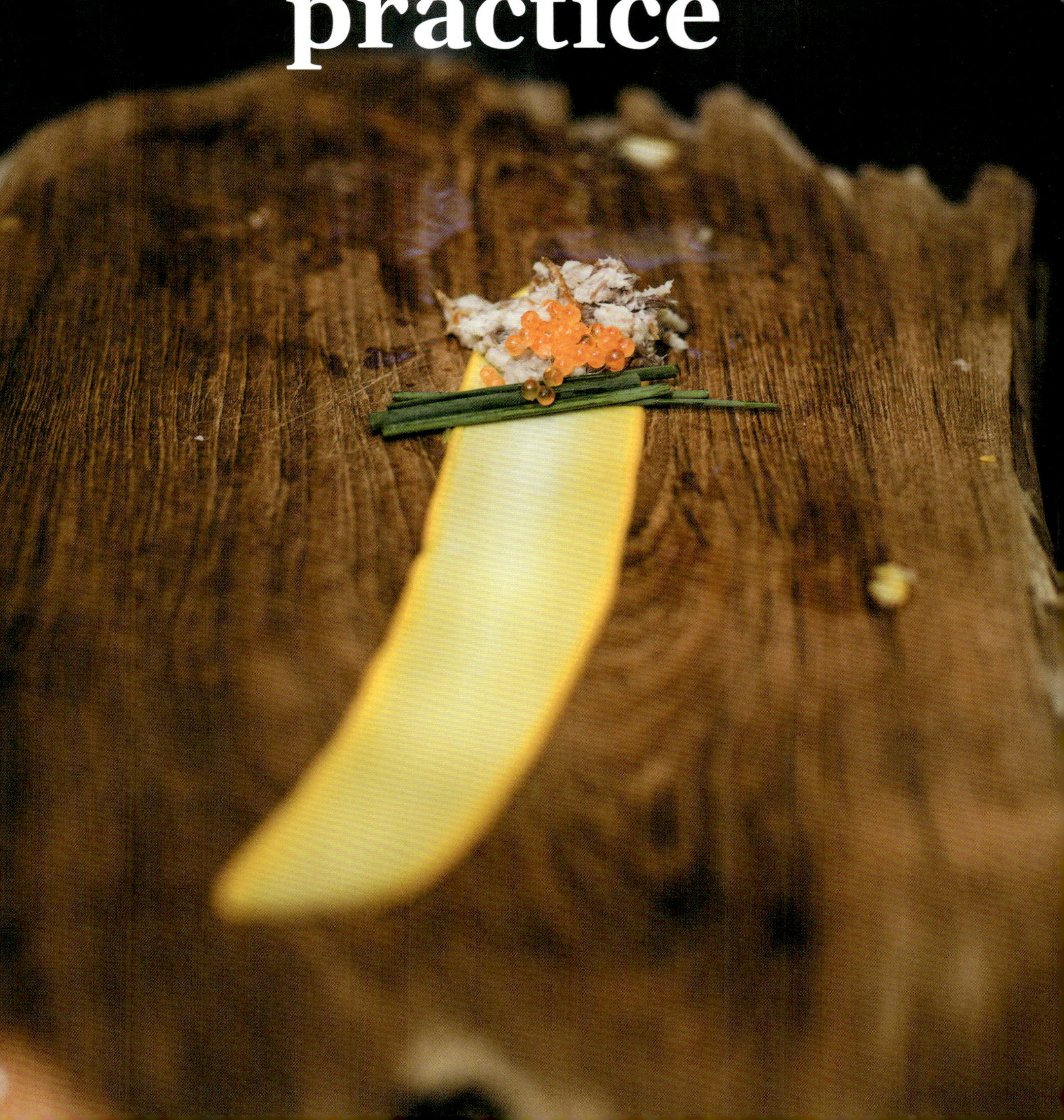

Keto in practice

Figuring out the nuts and bolts of a ketogenic diet

HOW MANY CARBS, HOW MUCH PROTEIN AND HOW MUCH FAT?

There is no such thing as a standard ketogenic diet with a specific ratio of macronutrients. The ideal ratio may vary from person to person, depending on whether you have an active lifestyle, are young or old, your metabolism rate ...

The most commonly used ratio is:
- Less than 50 to 30 grams of carbs per day (in my keto meal plan, I have managed less than 30 grams net carbs per day, except for the last day).
- about 1 gram of protein per kilogram of your ideal weight.
- Fats for the remainder.

Here's a handy practical tip: try to focus on limiting your carb intake as much as possible. That is the most important thing to remember, the rest will follow. Beware of hidden carbs. Keeping the carbs down is far more important than keeping your fat intake up. Yes, the keto diet contains plenty of fats, but they're mostly fats from healthy foods. In other words: eat the fat that comes with the food and don't avoid it—embrace it. Always use full-fat products, never light. Where you used to use just one spoonful of olive oil, use several. If you used to cut away the fat from the meat, leave it on from now on. Is your goal to lose weight? Don't go too crazy on the fat, but you're certainly not allowed to go hungry.

KEEP IT SIMPLE AND STICK TO THE RECIPES IN THIS BOOK

I have already done all the hard work for you and calculated your macronutrients: with each recipe, you will find the proportions of macronutrients in each dish. As you know, this is partly a collection of dishes from my earlier books where I have adjusted the quantities so they have the right proportions to help you reach or stay in ketosis. This 14-day keto meal plan should help you reach ketosis effortlessly. Should you decide to keep going after that, you can use the extra recipes in the back of the book and start to experiment with some of your own recipes.

HOW MUCH AM I ALLOWED TO EAT?

The recipes in this book are for two people or two servings. But if you are hungry or have an active lifestyle, eat more and adjust the amounts accordingly. The idea is: eat when you're hungry, stop when you've had enough. Feel free to skip a meal, but for the truly fanatic amongst us, it's better to keep to the meal plan and quantities outlined in this book. Some enthusiasts start a ketogenic diet and then also reduce their calorie intake because they want to lose weight fast. If you are new at this, I strongly discourage you from doing so, because it may mean that you will fall short of your goal. First try to get comfortable with a ketogenic diet. Feel how your body reacts. Once you know how it feels, you can start to experiment.

The carbs in this 14-day keto meal plan are kept low to help you reach ketosis quickly, less than 30 grams (1 ounce) of net carbohydrates per day. As soon as your body has grown accustomed to burning fats, you may want to allow more carbs. Start with 5 to 10 grams of extra carbs per day, stick to that for a week and see what it does to your ketone levels. Where the limit lies depends on the individual and how much exercise you get.

A KETOGENIC DIET OFTEN CALCULATES WITH NET CARBS. WHAT ARE THOSE?

With a keto diet, you often see things like: *20 net carbs*. Carbs include fiber (and alcohol), but fiber cannot be digested by humans. They add bulk to your feces, which is a good thing, and soluble fiber together with resistant starch (another type of fiber) are exceptionally beneficial for the bacteria in your gut. So they are important, but they don't contain any calories and don't have any effect on your blood sugar level. That's why they are left out of the equation with a ketogenic diet. We work with net carbs instead, the total carbs minus the fiber. In this book we also work with net carbs.

Be aware of the fact that, depending on which app or list you use to calculate fats, carbohydrates and proteins, there may be differences.

HOW MUCH PROTEIN ARE YOU ALLOWED TO EAT IN A KETOGENIC DIET?

This is still a point of discussion. According to some, you need to eat protein sparingly; on the one hand because your body can produce glucose from proteins and on the other hand because proteins increase your blood sugar levels, inhibiting the burning of fats in the body. But other experts believe that proteins don't play such a large role and that women, especially women during menopause, would benefit from eating slightly more protein to help them lose weight. Which leads to other people disagreeing with those other people etc.
In this book, I have stuck to the most frequently used proportions in a ketogenic diet:
20 to 30 percent protein, which means that every day, between 20 and 30 percent of your energy should come from proteins, or about 1 gram of protein per kilogram of your ideal weight.
Just to give you an idea: 100 grams of salmon contains 22 grams of protein and 100 grams of steak contains 30 grams of protein.

Admittedly it may take a while to find the right proportion because the optimal proportions for reaching ketosis may vary from person to person. In other words, these are just guidelines.

HOW LONG DOES IT TAKE TO REACH KETOSIS?

If you're used to eating fewer carbs, for example if you're already following a low-carb diet, this may happen after two or three days. If you have a longer way to go, you may need three or four days to get there. Most people aren't true fat burners until after ten days. But it takes three weeks to a month before you can really talk about a fully keto-adapted body.

If you can't reach ketosis, the first thing you have to do is reduce your carb intake even more. And then you can also increase your fat intake. Still not in ketosis? Reduce your protein intake. Eat smaller servings of meat or fish.

One important note: most people following this meal plan will reach ketosis within a few days because I have kept the amount of carbs extremely low, but it may still be hard for some people to reach ketosis, especially people who are resistant to insulin. Also, remember that if you take any medication, you must first consult your physician to find out whether a ketogenic diet is suitable for you and whether your dosage needs to be amended.

BE CAREFUL WITH HIDDEN CARBS

Just in case you didn't know it already: carbs are everywhere. Many people think they'll be fine as long as they avoid bread, pasta, rice and potatoes. Wrong.

1 apple (180 g)	19 g net carbs (what you're more or less allowed in one day)
A handful of cashews (30 g)	10 g net carbs (half of what you're allowed in one day)
1 onion (100 g)	8 g net carbs
100 g leek	6 g net carbs
1 large tomato (180 g)	5 g net carbs
cooked carrots (100 g)	5 g net carbs
celeriac (100 g)	5 g net carbs
squash (100 g)	5 g net carbs
Greek yogurt (100 g)	4.9 g net carbs
Brussels sprouts (100 g)	4 g net carbs
coconut milk (100 g)	2.5 to 4 g net carbs

KETO FLU

During the first few days, some people may experience symptoms similar to those of the flu, such as headaches and a sense of tiredness. This is most common with people for whom the ketogenic diet is a big adjustment. The body is used to consuming plenty of sugars and is to some extent dependent on them. The transition from burning sugars to burning fats requires your body to adapt and that doesn't happen all at once. Headaches may be one of the side effects. Thankfully, not everyone experiences them.

When you reduce your carb consumption the body switches from retaining water and salt to releasing them. That's why it's important to eat more salt and vegetables that contain plenty of potassium, especially during the first weeks (the keto meal plan accommodates for this). The glycogen (sugar) reserves in your body that also retain water are depleted, causing water to be released. For those reasons, you will notice that you will have to go to the bathroom more often and that you lose more weight during the first week. Don't be fooled: that's mostly body fluids. It is therefore very important to eat more salt and drink plenty of fluids.

It is better to anticipate those changes and incorporate a number of eating habits, especially in the first weeks.

- Drink more water: 1.5 to 2 liters per day
- Use more salt
- Eat foods rich in potassium: spinach, purslane, pecans, meat, flaxseed …

That's why it's ideal to drink plenty of broths and soups during the first weeks, as they contain plenty of minerals, water and salt. The keto meal plan has taken this into account as well. I have also included plenty of vegetables that contain ample potassium and fiber to reduce the risk of getting headaches or constipation. You can also choose to take magnesium supplements, especially if you're suffering from cramps.

ALCOHOL AND KETO

I would recommend not drinking any alcohol during the first weeks, or waiting until your body has completely adjusted to fat-burning mode. Alcohol with a ketogenic diet, especially in the beginning, can give you headaches. I can draw from personal experience. One glass of wine made me feel as if I had just polished off three glasses of extremely bad wine. A glass of white wine or champagne will not immediately kick you out of ketosis, but for some reason your body has more trouble breaking down alcohol when you're in ketosis. Perhaps this has to do with the fact that your liver has to work extra hard to do so: it has to make ketones and break down alcohol at the same time. Moreover, your liver will choose to break down the alcohol first at the expense of your fat metabolism and subsequent weight loss. If you want to drink a glass of wine, chase with a glass of water.

WHAT IF I'VE MESSED UP AND AM NO LONGER IN KETOSIS?

Well, we all mess up sometimes. Don't let it get you down. See it as a lesson learned and start over. You're usually back in ketosis in two or three days. The most important thing is to eat enough so you don't feel hungry.

STILL TOO HUNGRY WHILE EATING KETO? A FEW TIPS:

- Decrease your carb consumption even further, because it is generally known that carbs stimulate the feeling of hunger. The more carbs you eat, the more you will want to eat.
- Eat slightly more proteins and fats.
- Eat more vegetables with your meal with extra olive oil.
- Try to avoid or eat fewer snacks. Eat for example just a few nuts if you're really hungry.
- Eat plenty of leafy green vegetables. They are exceptionally healthy and feed the bacteria in your gut that help give you that hungry feeling.
- Regularly drink homemade meat or fish broth with sea salt.
- Make sure you get enough sleep.

CAN I USE SUGAR SUBSTITUTES?

Yes, but I advise you to do so as little as possible. And if you do use them, use xylitol or erythritol, also known as polyols or sugar alcohols. They are naturally occurring compounds and belong to the carb group. They contain few calories and have little to no influence on blood sugar and insulin levels. They won't kick you out of ketosis if you use too much. Sounds good, right? Not quite. Plenty of research has been conducted on sweeteners—natural and otherwise—and they show time and time again that they don't help you to achieve your goal, which is to lose weight. The reason for this is that they continue to stimulate your craving for sweet, so you end up eating more rather than losing weight. There is also a lot of controversy around the effects of low-calorie sugars on our brains (they may give our brains the wrong idea), the bacteria in our gut (it doesn't make them any healthier) and diabetes.

There is also something of a paradox here. Many people follow a ketogenic diet to get rid of their sugar addiction and craving for carbs. Moreover, the ketogenic diet is, by definition, a sugar-free diet. Why would you follow a ketogenic diet for your health, yet add sugars to everything you eat? We all know that it's that sweetness that's the biggest problem, so make the choice to avoid it. And remember, the less sugar and sweeteners you eat, the less you'll crave sugar. Just use it occasionally, at parties for instance, but don't make a habit of it by having it with your breakfast every morning, for example.

A KETOGENIC DIET IS ABOUT COUNTING AND CALCULATING, ESPECIALLY IN THE BEGINNING

Let me be honest. It may be fascinating, but this is definitely the least fun part of the ketogenic diet for me. Goodbye eating with your heart and gut, hello calculator. There are several useful apps out there that can help you with this. Just enter what you want to eat, and the app immediately calculates the exact amount of carbs (and net carbs), fiber, fats and proteins that food contains. Some apps are free, others you need to pay for.

EAT PLENTY OF LOW-CARB VEGETABLES:

The carbs you do eat in a ketogenic diet should come primarily from vegetables and not from fast or processed carbs.
Vegetables that grow above ground generally contain fewer carbs than vegetables or roots that grow underground.

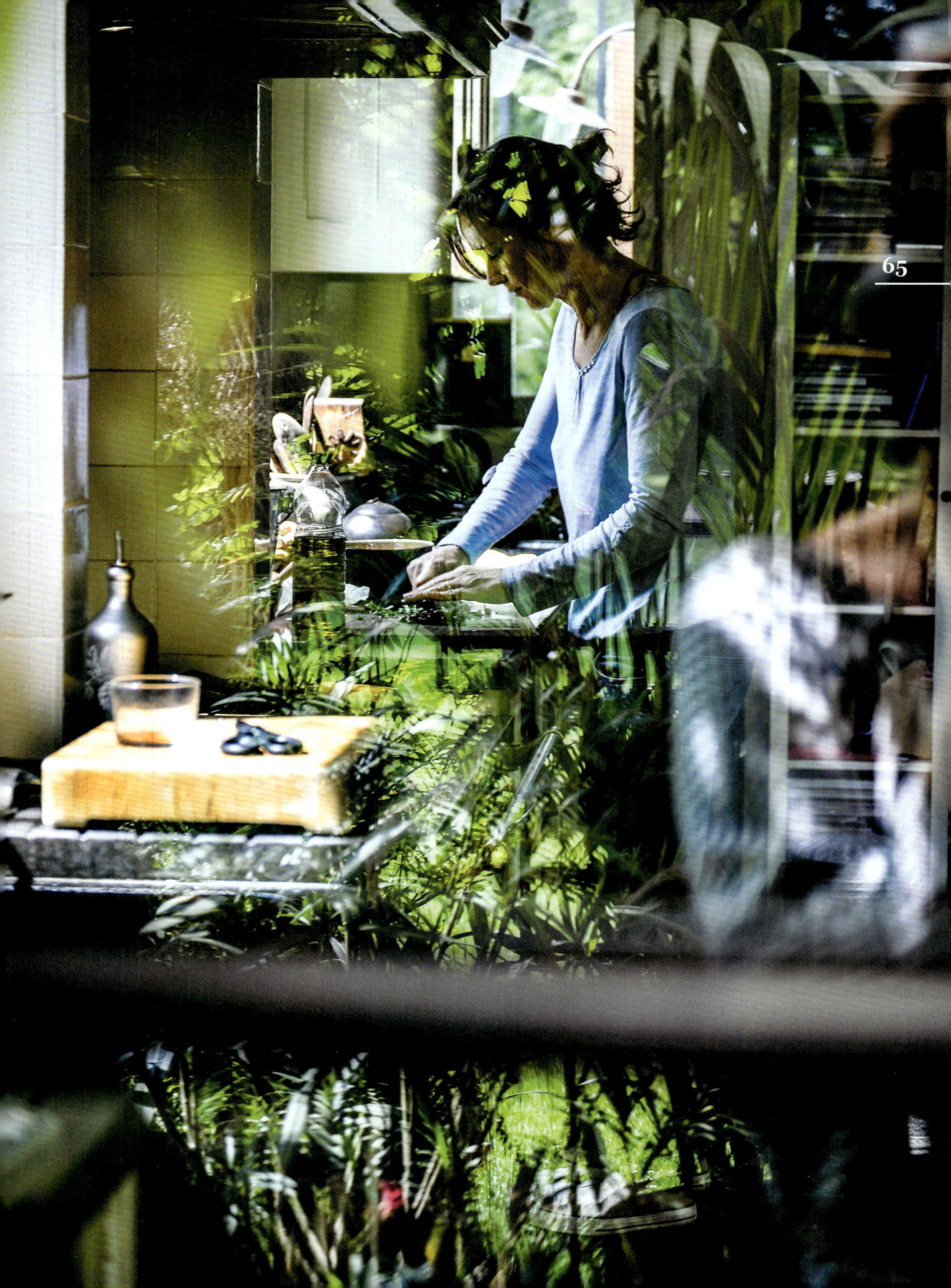

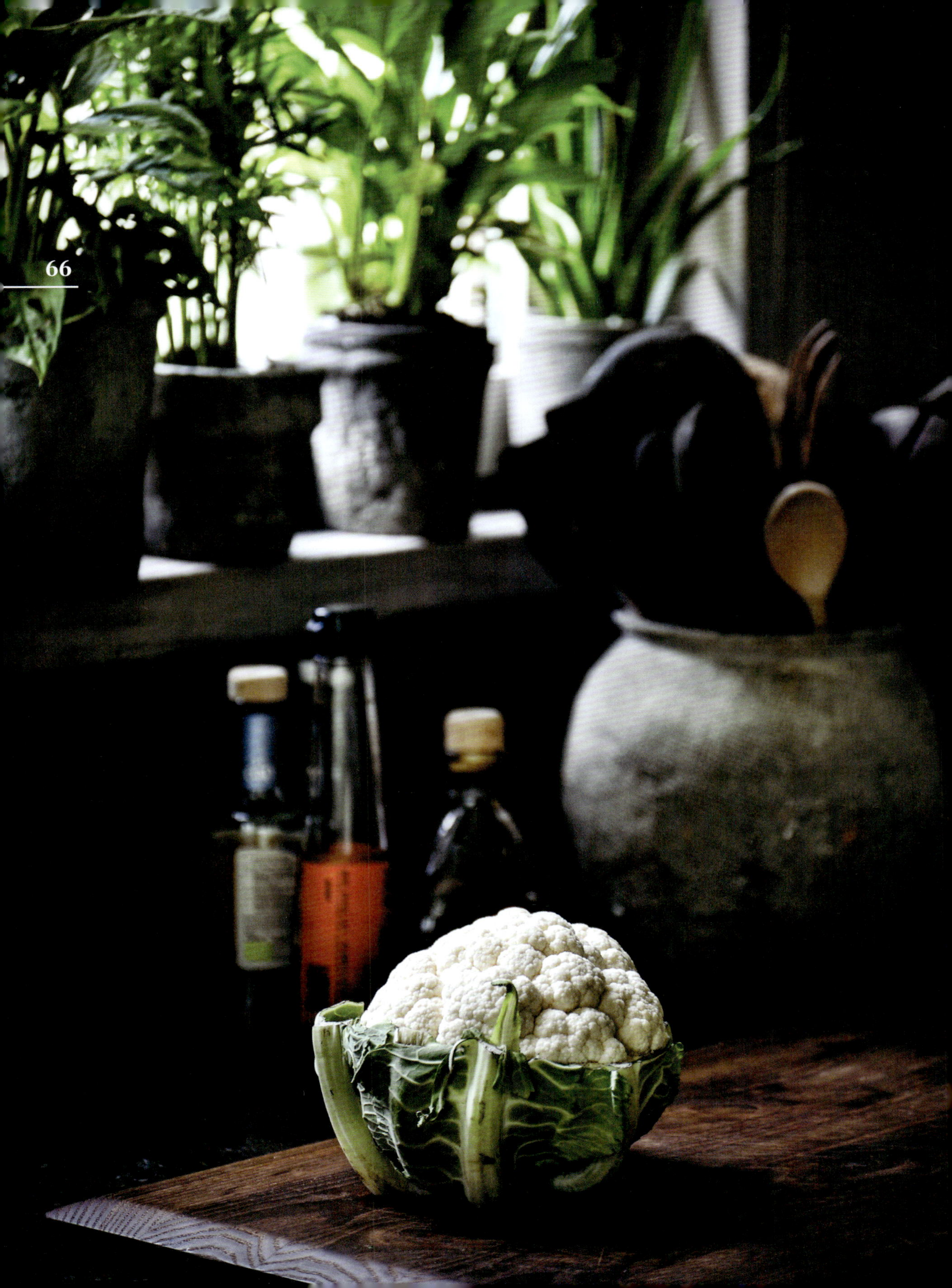

Favorite keto vegetables, per 100 g:

- chicory   1 g net carbs + good source of potassium and magnesium
- spinach   1 g net carbs + good source of potassium and magnesium
- purslane   1 g net carbs + good source of potassium
- avocado (fruit)   2 g net carbs + good source of fiber and potassium
- asparagus   2 g net carbs + good source of fiber and potassium
- zucchini   3 g net carbs + good source of potassium
- cauliflower   3 g net carbs + good source of potassium
- eggplant   3 g net carbs + good source of fiber
- kale   3 g net carbs + good source of potassium
- cabbage   4 g net carbs + good source of potassium
- broccoli   4 g net carbs + good source of fiber and potassium

WHAT TO EAT AND WHAT TO AVOID: A BRIEF OVERVIEW

During the first few weeks, it's best to keep your carb intake low. Once your body has adjusted to burning fats, you can eat more vegetables from the "eat in moderation" category.

EAT:

Leafy vegetables: spinach, lettuce, purslane, water cress, fresh herbs

Avocado, green or white celery, cauliflower, chicory, asparagus, kale, white cabbage, green cabbage, cucumber, zucchini, broccoli, mushrooms, green chilies, bok choy ...

All types of fish and meat, most dairy products (always full-fat and without added sugars)
All fats

EAT IN MODERATION:

Tomato, leek, red and yellow bell peppers
Root vegetables: beets, celeriac, carrots, onion
Pumpkin, artichoke, Brussels sprouts
Green beans, eggplant, spring onions
Nuts and seeds: the most suitable nuts are pecans

AVOID:

Vegetables: parsnip, potatoes, sweet potatoes ...
Starchy foods: bread, pasta, rice, fries ...
Most fruits (except for berries) and fruit juices
Beans, lentils, chickpeas, quinoa, whole grains

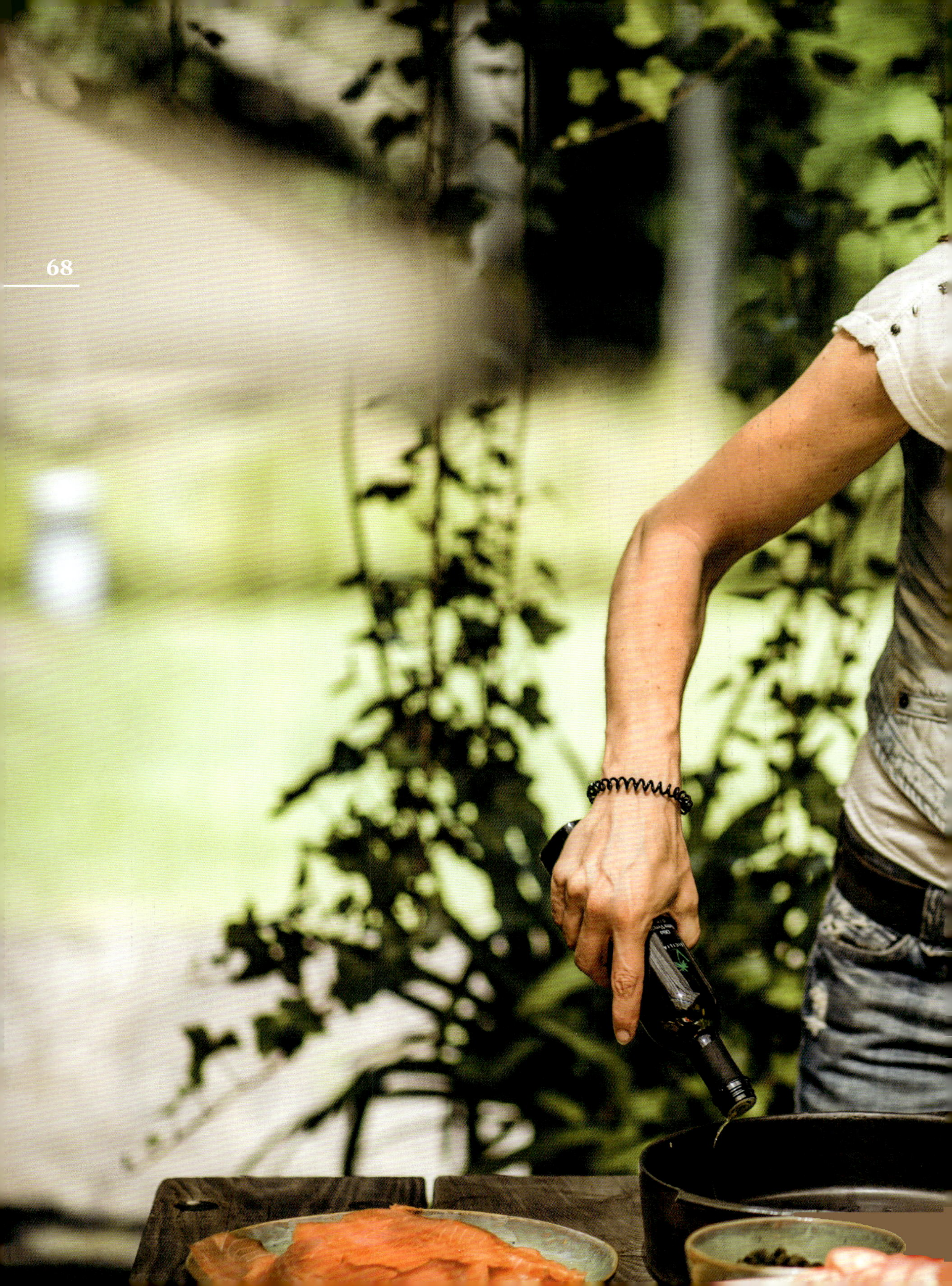

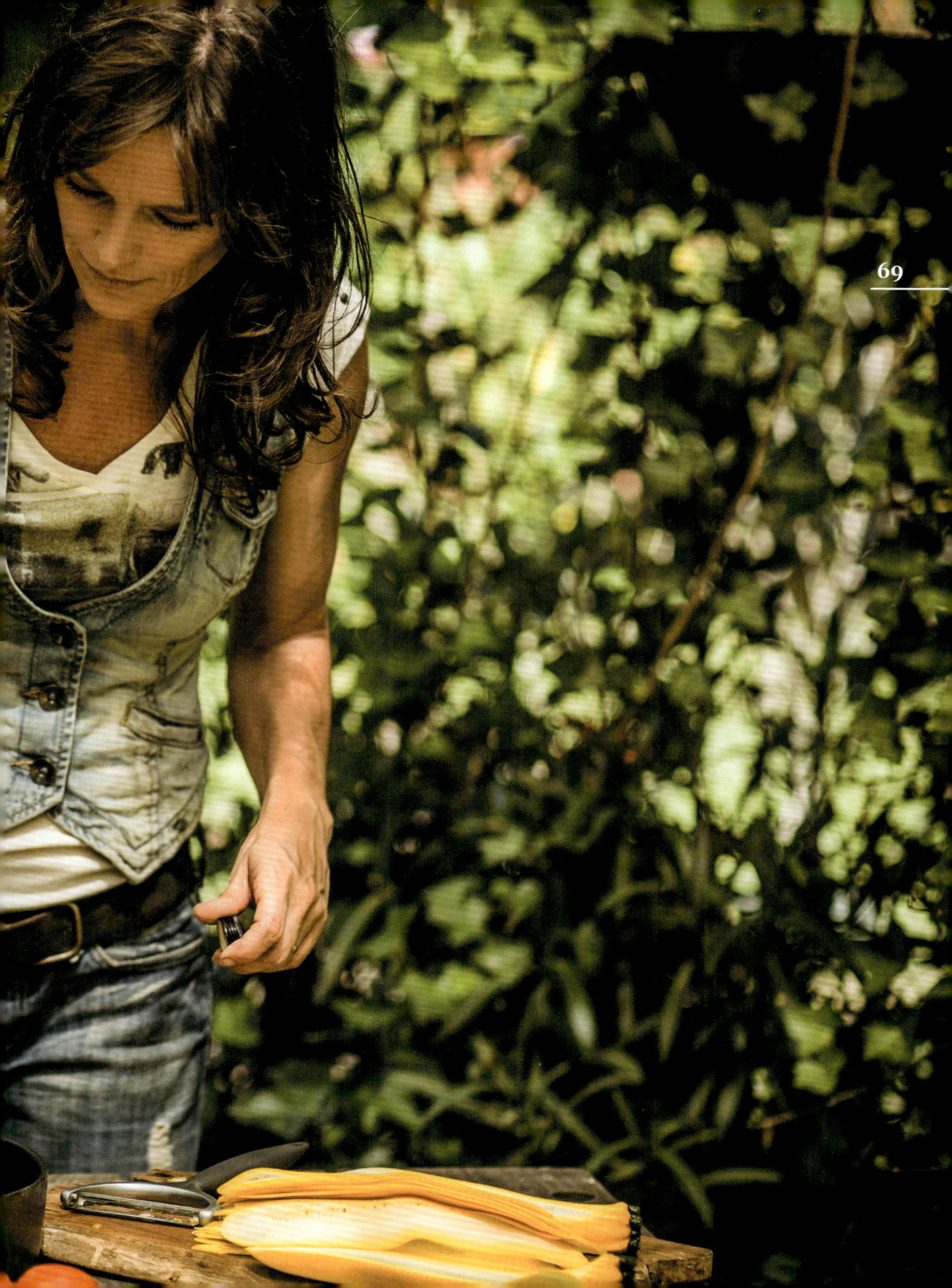

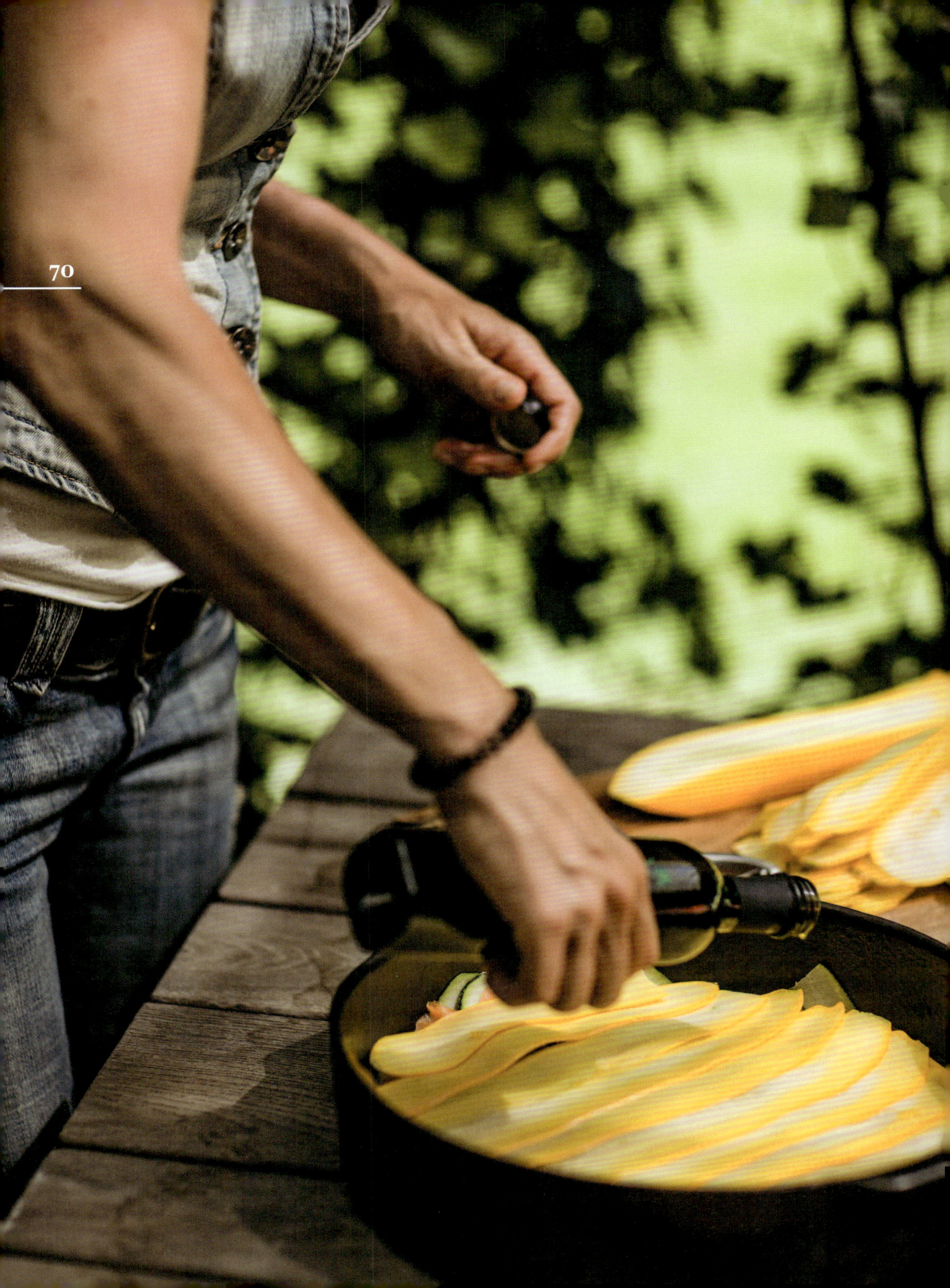

14-day meal planner

RECIPES

- Know beforehand what you are going to eat. It is very important that you have a plan, that you get organized and do your shopping on time so that you have everything you need at home and don't come across any last-minute surprises. You can follow the weekly meal plan in this book or adjust it to your own needs.
- Make a "what if" list. What if you are going out for dinner? What if you have no time and have to eat lunch on the go? What if you get hungry in between meals? Draw up a list of answers and solutions. Be proactive and be prepared.
- Drink plenty of fluids. Besides water, broths and soups are ideal, also as a source of salt and minerals.
- Stay away from the scales and savor your new way of enjoying food. See it as a journey and a great learning experience.
- Are you hungry? Eat more. Are you full? Stop eating. The idea is that you eat until you have had enough. Whatever you do, you shouldn't feel hungry.
- Make sure that you always have something on hand or in the fridge for on the go or for those unforeseen moments when you don't have time to cook a meal. Think about keeping some of my crackers or nut bread on hand.
- The recipes are for two people or two servings, but if you have an active lifestyle or need more, adjust the amounts accordingly. The idea is: eat when you're hungry, stop when you've had enough (which is not the same as eat as much as you want :-)).

IMPORTANT!
Always listen to your body. If eating keto doesn't feel good, STOP doing it.

14-day meal planner

How do you use this 14-day meal planner and the other recipes in this book?

The simplest way is to keep to the 14-day meal plan, but you can also replace recipes or use ideas from the extra recipes list. If you don't have much time, you can also make the same breakfast or lunch more often, but I want to inspire you, of course :-). Whatever you do, make sure that you don't exceed 30 grams of net carbs per day during the first week. If you are still enthusiastic after completing your first 14-day adventure into keto and would like to continue, this book contains enough recipes for a third week. After that, you're free to choose your own recipes as a full-fledged ketoer. You can find quite a few keto recipes in my other books as well.

breakfast

WEEK 1

Smoked salmon with avocado and purslane

Smoked salmon with mascarpone and fish eggs

Seeds and nuts with full-fat sour cream

Roasted nuts and seeds with sour cream

Overnight macadamia nut chocolate mousse

Philippine-style eggplant

Spinach omelet roll-up with mushrooms and cheese

WEEK 2

Mini-quiche with ham

Mini-quiche with ham

Creamy cheese with roast tomatoes and fresh herbs

Seeds and nuts with full-fat sour cream

Roasted seeds and nuts with full-fat sour cream

Brown mushrooms with poached egg and avocado sauce

Greek-style yogurt with berries and seeds

lunch

Warm feta with vegetables and pecans

Asian chicken broth

Instant cold spinach and avocado soup

Burrata with tomatoes, cream and pesto

Avocado with bacon and snow peas

Zucchini noodles with pine nuts and basil pesto

Stuffed avocado with crawfish

Brown shrimp with guacamole

Eggplant noodles

Avocado with mushrooms and dry-cured ham

Zucchini with smoked salmon,
soy sauce and capers

Spinach soup with sliced almonds

Spinach with tomato, turmeric and feta

Stuffed avocado with crawfish

dinner

Chicken broth with spinach

Pointed cabbage with shrimp

Lamb chops with cauliflower,
cream and sautéed green beans

Spiced fish with coconut milk,
lime and tomatoes

Pizza

Cod with green curry and cherry tomatoes

Chicken with olives and mushrooms

Beef broth with savoy cabbage
and marrow bones

Beef broth with tomato and cream

Zucchini with smoked salmon,
soy sauce and capers

Cod with spinach, tomato, eggplant
and pistachio pesto

Vegetables with hazelnuts

Pointed cabbage spaghetti with olives

Cooked chicken with vegetables

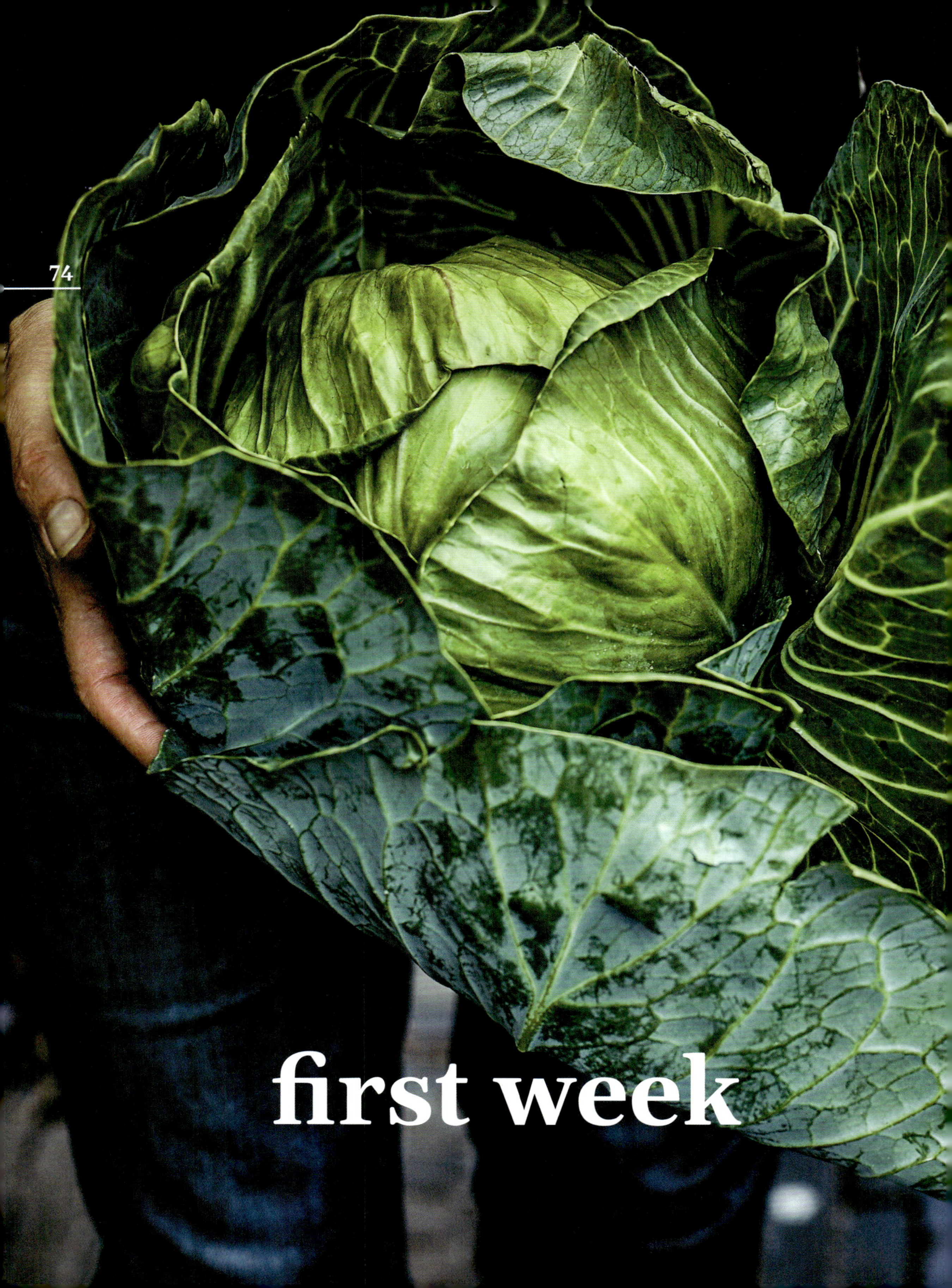

first week

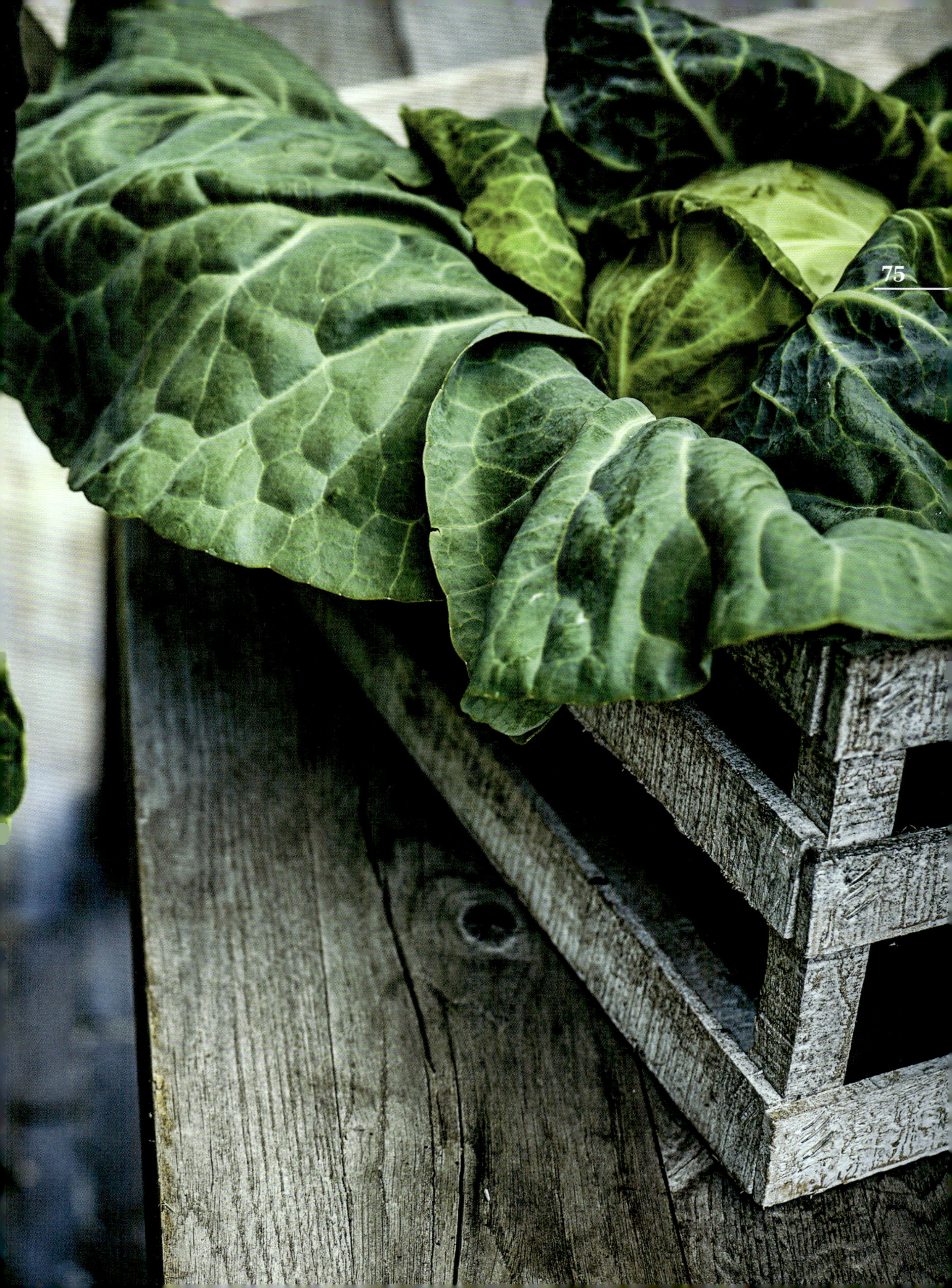

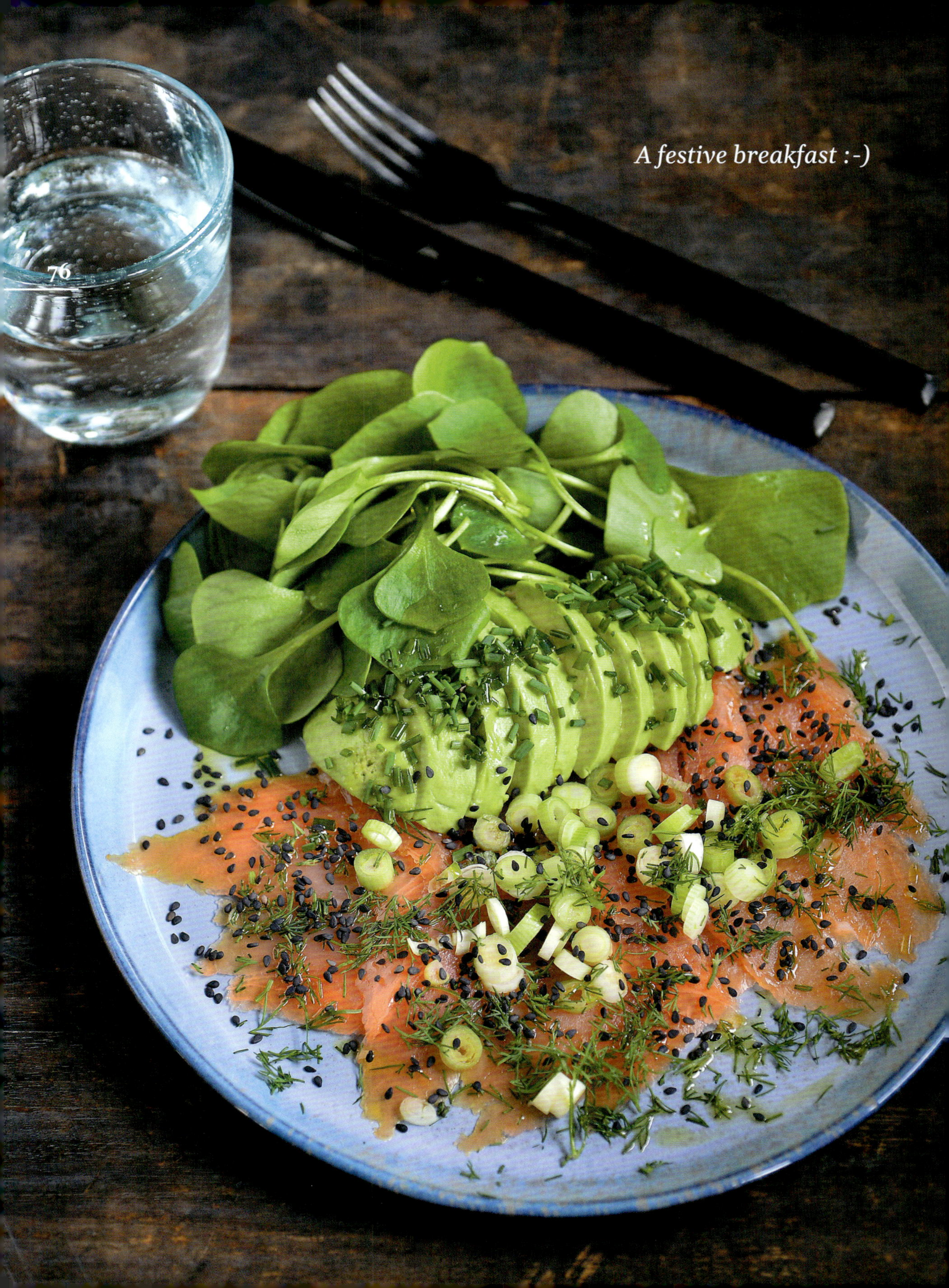

A festive breakfast :-)

Smoked salmon

WITH AVOCADO AND PURSLANE

Ready in less than 10 minutes - serves 2

10 1/2 oz (300 g) smoked salmon

2 avocados

1 bunch purslane 3 1/2 oz (100 g)

4 spring onions

1 oz (30 g) dill (optional)

black sesame seeds (optional)

1 1/2 oz (40 g) olive oil

Arrange the ingredients on a plate and top with the finely chopped spring onions, dill, and black sesame seeds. Drizzle olive oil over the salad, especially the purslane.

Tip: ketosis
If you would like to reach ketosis quickly, or if you can't reach ketosis, this is an ideal breakfast, and certainly one of the healthiest. It contains few carbs, many healthy omega-3 fats from the salmon and unsaturated fats from the avocado, and lots of potassium and fiber from the avocado and the purslane. Moreover, smoked salmon contains quite a bit of salt, which comes in handy because you lose a lot of body fluids during the first days of a ketogenic diet. That's why it's also highly recommended that you drink plenty of fluids. Enjoy your breakfast!

Tip: why is avocado such an ideal ingredient in the ketogenic diet?
Avocados are not only delicious and versatile in the kitchen, they also contain lots of healthy fats such as monounsaturated fats, and few net carbs. They do contain a lot of carbs but most of these are fiber and don't affect your blood sugar level. Avocados are also exceptionally nutritious and rich in potassium and fiber. If you leave off the carbs in a recipe and replace it with avocado, chances are that you have an ideal keto recipe. The only downside is ... as delicious as they are, even avocados can get boring after a while ;-)

Per serving: 39g P (20%) / 67.9g F (77%) / 5.2g NetC (3%)

DAY 1
BREAKFAST

Warm feta

WITH VEGETABLES AND PECANS

Ready in 25 minutes - serves 2

7 oz (200 g) feta

1 head of broccoli (14 oz/400 g)

2 spring onions

1/4 red bell pepper (2 1/2 oz/70 g)

1 oz (30 g) pecans

2 oz (60 g) olives (your favorite olives)

1 1/2 oz (40 g) olive oil

Preheat the oven to 400 °F (200 °C).
Slice the feta in two, place the slices in an ovenproof pan and bake 10 minutes in the oven or until the feta starts to color slightly on the corners.
Chop the broccoli into florets, the spring onions into thin rings and the bell pepper into cubes. Sauté the vegetables in the olive oil. Add your favorite olives; it doesn't matter if they're green or black, as long as you like them. Season with salt and black pepper.
Coarsely chop the nuts.
Place a slice of feta on each plate and arrange the vegetables next to the cheese. Garnish with the nuts.

Per serving: 23g P (15%) / 56g F (81%) / 7g NetC (4%)

DAY 1
LUNCH

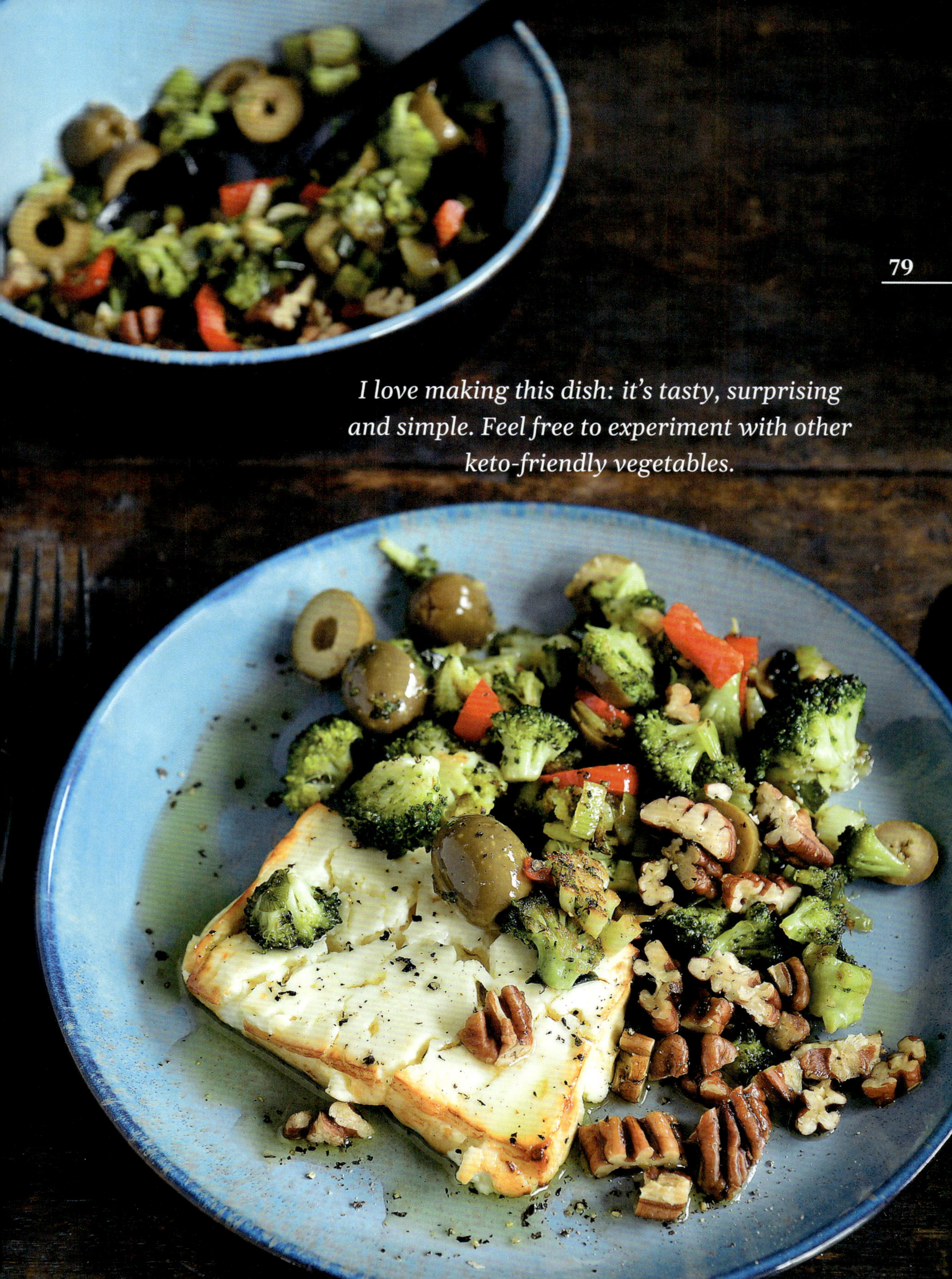

I love making this dish: it's tasty, surprising
and simple. Feel free to experiment with other
keto-friendly vegetables.

Chicken broth

WITH SPINACH

Ready in 2 1/2 hours - serves 4

1 organic chicken (1.3-1.5 kg or approx. 3 pounds) - 2-inch (5 cm) piece of ginger root (1 oz/30 g) - 2-inch (5 cm) piece of turmeric (3/4 oz/20 g) - splash of apple cider vinegar - a little over 1 lb (500 g) spinach

We make extra so we don't have to cook the next day. Put the chicken in a pot and add 2 to 3 quarts of water or enough to submerge the chicken. Add a generous splash of cider vinegar. Put the pot over the heat. Slice the ginger and turmeric—you don't have to peel the turmeric first—and add them to the pot. Season with plenty of sea salt and black pepper. Remove the chicken once the broth has simmered for 1 to 1 1/2 hours. Pull the meat from the chicken and set aside. Put the carcass, the skin and the rest of the chicken pieces back in the broth. Add a little extra water if needed and let the broth simmer gently for at least another hour. Finely chop the spinach. Strain the broth shortly before serving. Return the strained broth to the pan over the heat and add the meat and spinach. Stir briefly until the spinach has wilted. Save the rest for the next day. Serve the other half of the broth.

Tip: which herbs and spices should you use for the broth?
You can add any herbs or spices you like to the broth. I add dried herbs in the beginning and fresh herbs at the end.

Tip: how long do I cook the broth?
Homemade broth is exceptionally nutritious and has made a huge comeback in recent years. The longer you cook the bones, the more nutrients they release into the broth such as calcium and phosphorus. But the connective tissue is also very healthy and rich in glucosamine. The collagen from the bones and the connective tissue is converted into a nutritious form of gelatin during cooking. This is highly beneficial for your gut and body. In a ketogenic diet, drinking broth is recommended because of the many minerals it contains. The extra intake of fluids is also ideal for combating keto flu, and it contains extremely few carbs. A real keto kickstart.

Tip: broth and keto
As you will discover when reading this book, you'll lose a lot of body fluids during a ketogenic diet. This means that you'll also release salt and magnesium. That's why it's highly recommended that you drink lots of fluids. Broth is ideal because it contains plenty of minerals. And don't be too stingy with the salt. You can read more about this in the theory behind the diet.

DAY 1
DINNER   Per serving: 31g P (25%) / 40g F (74%) / 1g NetC (1%)

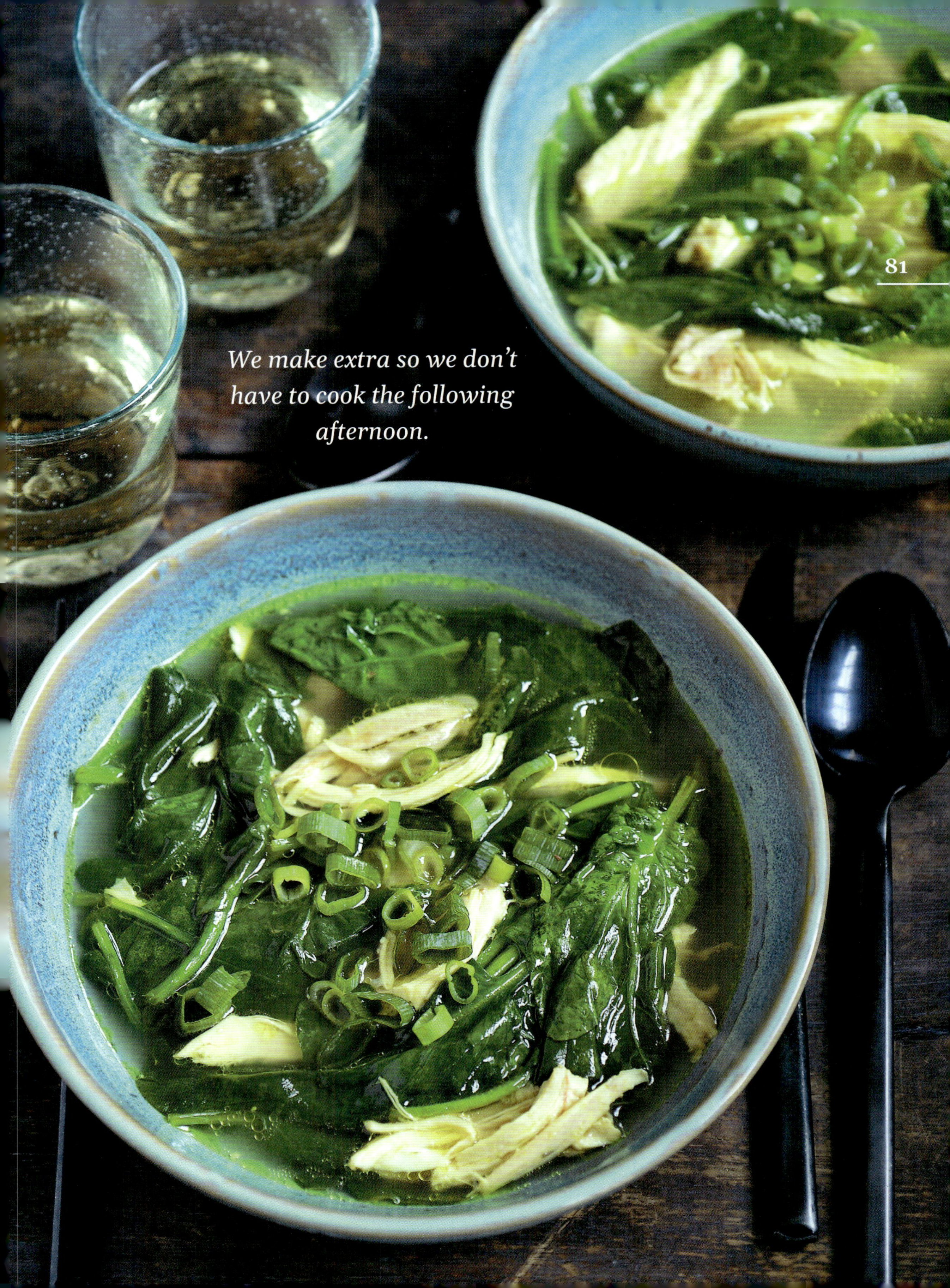
We make extra so we don't
have to cook the following
afternoon.

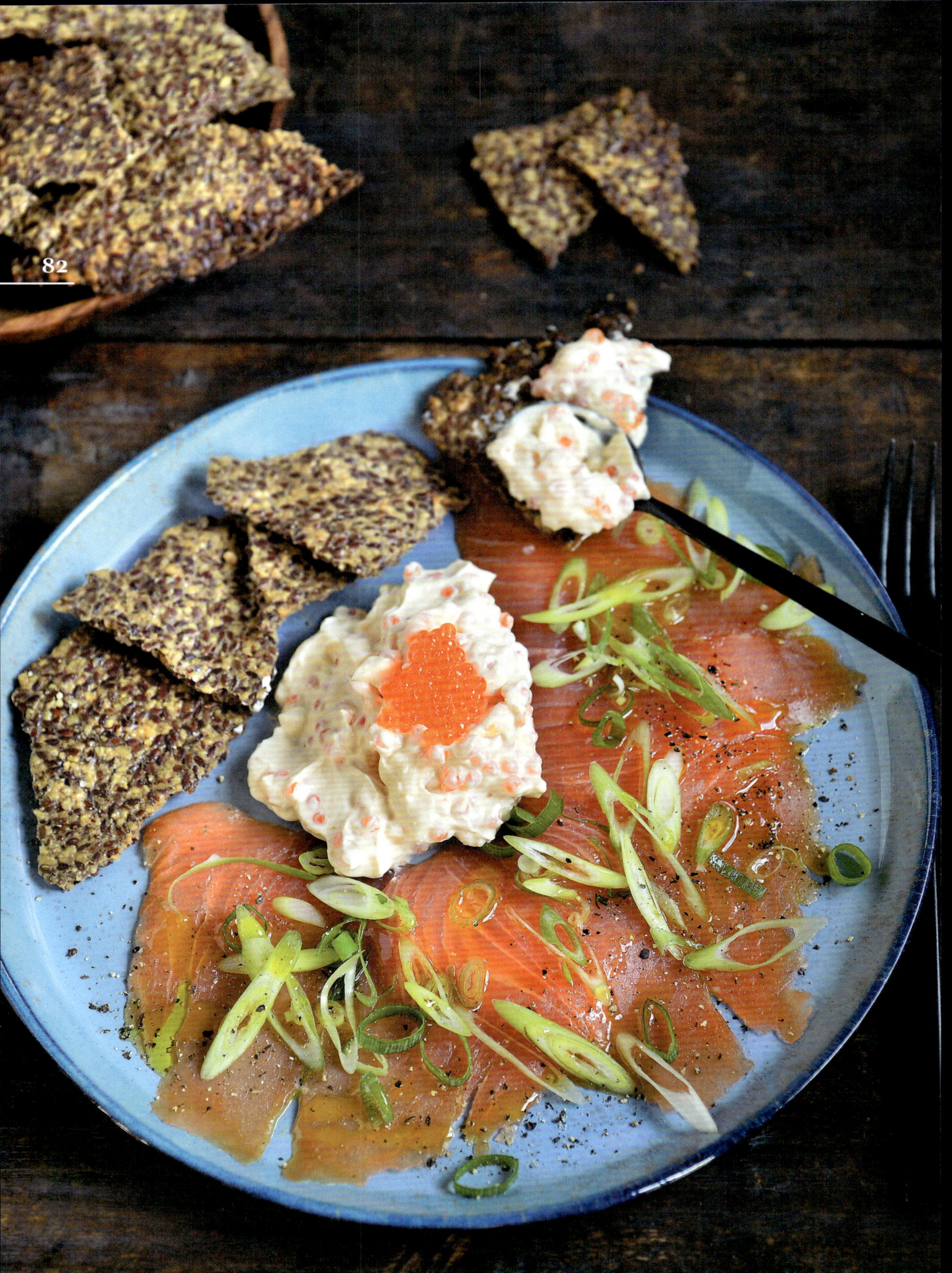

Smoked salmon

WITH MASCARPONE AND FISH EGGS

Ready in less than 10 minutes - serves 2

7 oz (250 g) smoked salmon

3 1/2 oz (100 g) mascarpone

1 3/4 oz (50 g) trout eggs

1 tbsp apple cider vinegar

2 spring onions

+ 1 oz (30 g) keto nut and seed crackers (see page 167)

Combine the mascarpone with three quarters of the trout eggs. Try to crush as many of the eggs as possible to release their color and flavor (see tip). Season with a little salt and the apple cider vinegar. Slice the spring onions diagonally into thin rings. Arrange everything on a plate. Finish with the remaining trout eggs and serve with the crackers.

Tip:
Put the fish eggs in a bowl together with the mascarpone and crush as many eggs as possible with the back of spoon to release their moisture, flavor and color.

Tip: salmon
I hope you like salmon. It is the ideal fish for a keto diet. It is rich in omega-3 fats, allowing you to get plenty of healthy natural fats without having to add extra fat. Another suitable fish is mackerel. I buy wild salmon with the MSC label or farmed salmon.

Per serving with 1 oz (30 g) of the nut and seed crackers: 34.5g P (26%) / 41.2g F (71%) / 3.4g NetC (3%)

DAY 2
BREAKFAST

Chicken broth

FROM PLAIN CHICKEN BROTH
TO ASIAN-STYLE CHICKEN BROTH

Ready in 15 minutes - serves 2

yesterday's chicken broth

2 stalks lemongrass

8 lime leaves (see tip)

juice of 1/2 lemon

3 1/2 fl oz (100 ml) coconut milk

2 garlic cloves

Put the pot of broth over the heat.
Crush the lemon grass stalks by hitting them with the back of a knife sharpener or another heavy object so they release more flavor. Finely chop the fresh garlic.
Add all the ingredients to the broth. Leave to simmer for about 10 minutes.
Serve.

Tip: lime leaves
Lime leaves, also known as kaffir lime leaves, are an ingredient used in Asian cuisine. They are the aromatic leaves of a small type of lime. A few leaves give off a stronger lime flavor than the juice from a normal lime. Sometimes you can find fresh leaves, but dried leaves are more common. You can find them in the supermarket or health food store, and of course in Asian supermarkets.

Per serving: 37g P (26%) / 43g F F (68%) / 8g NetC (6%)

DAY 2
LUNCH

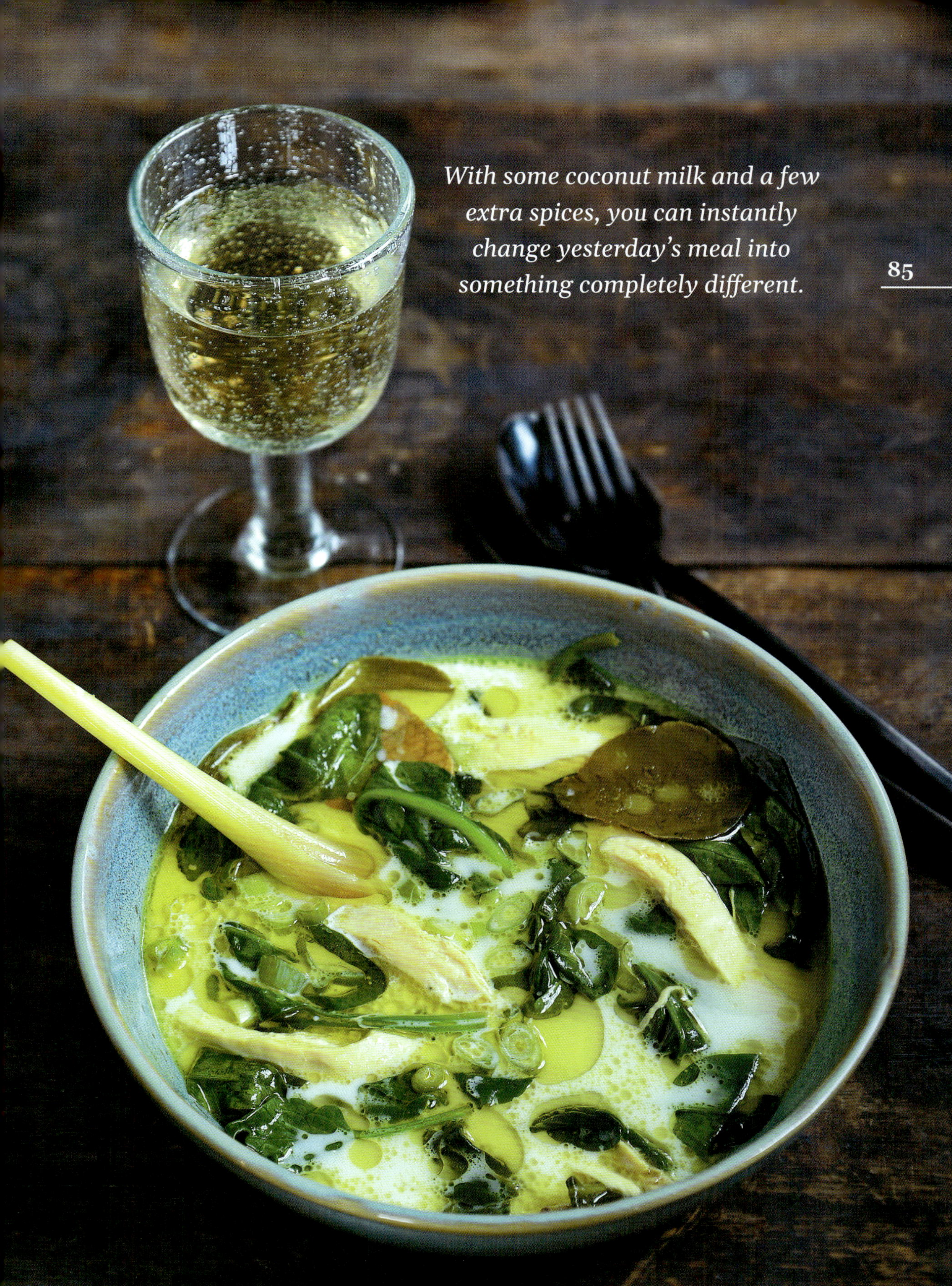

With some coconut milk and a few extra spices, you can instantly change yesterday's meal into something completely different.

Pointed cabbage

WITH SHRIMP

Preparation time: 15 minutes - cooking time: 15 minutes - serves 2

a little over 1 lb (500 g) pointed cabbage
10 1/2 oz (300 g) jumbo shrimp

For the sauce:
1-inch (2 cm) piece of ginger root (3/4 oz/20 g) - 2 cloves of garlic
3/4 oz (20 g) mild soy sauce - 1 lime
1/2 oz (10 g) sesame seeds - 3/4 oz (20 g) cilantro
1 1/2 oz (50 g) coconut oil

Slice the cabbage into 1/2-inch (1 cm) slices. Put them in a pan and pour a generous tablespoonful of coconut oil and a splash of water over the cabbage (to speed up the cooking process). Finely chop the ginger and garlic, add them to the cabbage and season with pepper and a little salt. Sauté the cabbage over gentle heat, stirring occasionally. Once the vegetables are almost done, add a generous splash of soy sauce and some lime juice, followed by the coarsely chopped cilantro and a tablespoon of sesame seeds.
Clean the shrimp but leave the last bit of tail on the end. Sauté the shrimp in the coconut oil until they are no longer translucent. This will take about 6 minutes.
Place the cabbage on the plates and arrange the shrimp on top. Spoon the leftover sauce from the pan over the shrimp. Garnish with some cilantro and sesame seeds.

Per serving: 31.9g P (30%) / 29.4g F (62%) / 8.7g NetC (8%)

DAY 2
DINNER

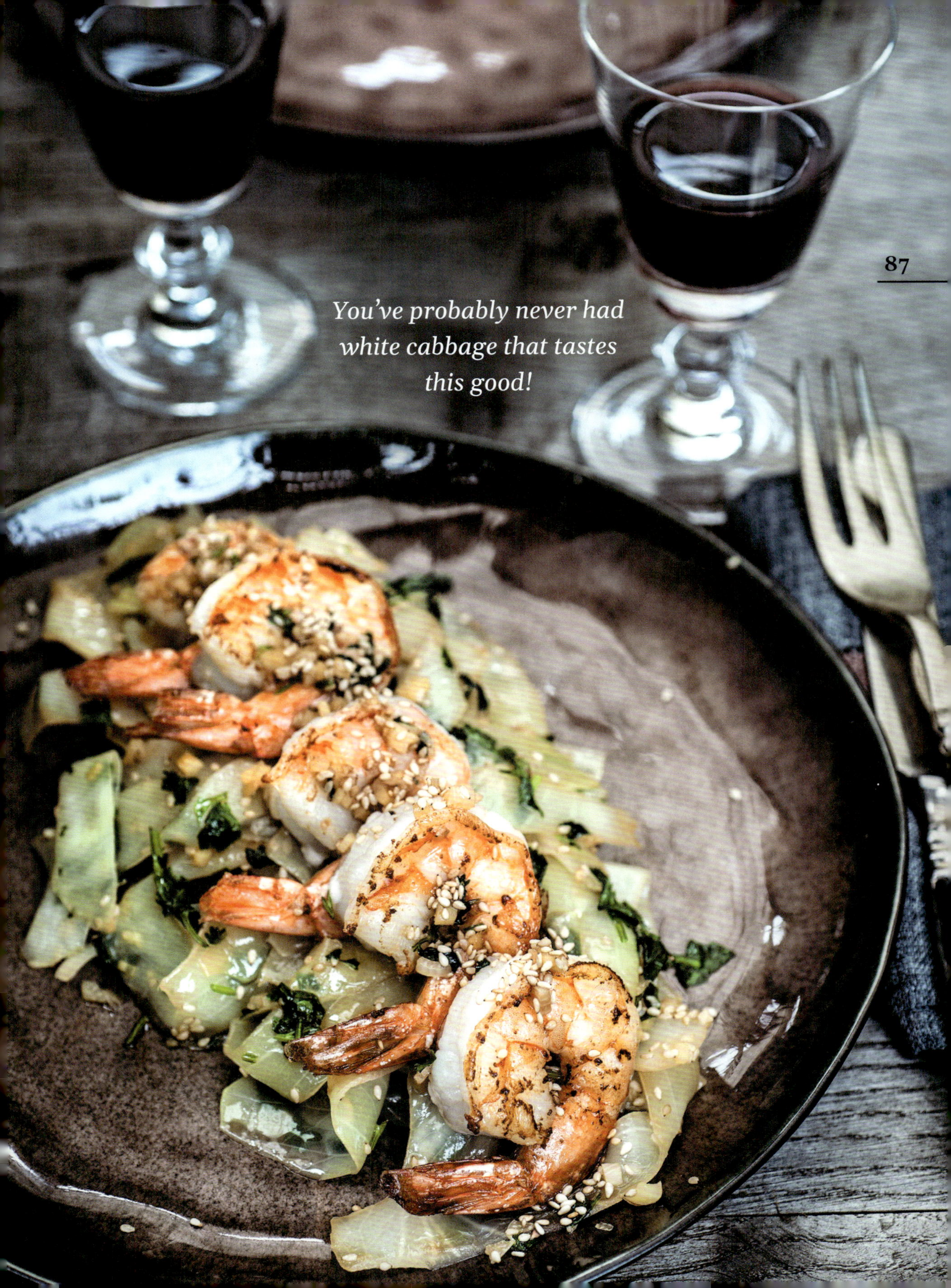
You've probably never had
white cabbage that tastes
this good!

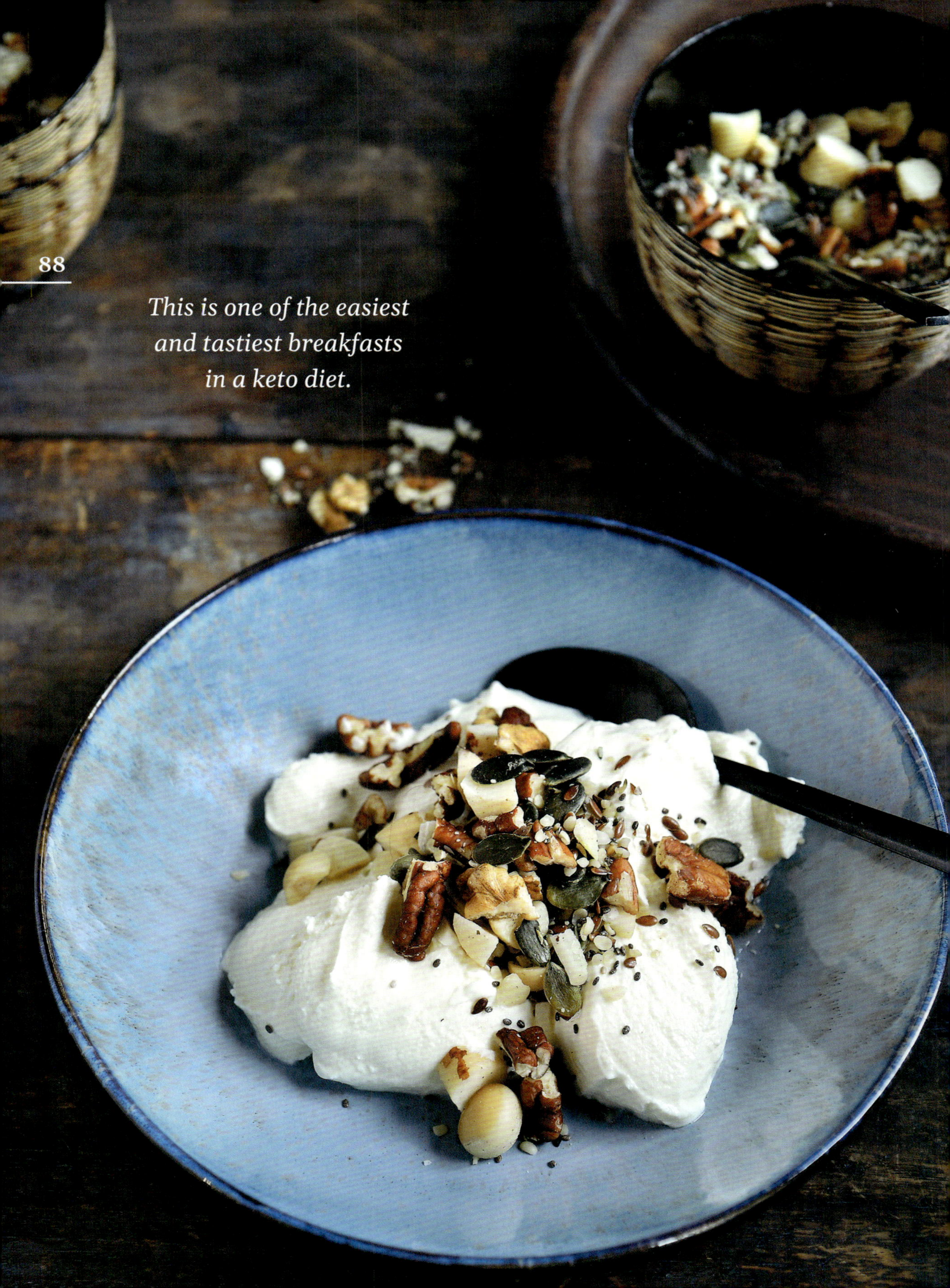

*This is one of the easiest
and tastiest breakfasts
in a keto diet.*

Seeds and nuts

WITH FULL-FAT SOUR CREAM

Ready in 10 minutes - serves 4

1 oz (30 g) flaxseeds

1 oz (30 g) pumpkin seeds

1 oz (30 g) chia seeds

1 oz (30 g) hemp seeds

2 oz (60 g) pecans

1 oz (30 g) Brazil nuts

1 oz (30 g) macadamia nuts

(count about 60 grams of seeds and nuts per person)

1 1/4 lb (600 g) sour cream (5 oz/150 g per person)

This recipe is enough for 2 days, so this includes tomorrow's breakfast.
Part 1 = Day 1 = nuts + sour cream
Part 2 = Day 2 = roasted nuts + sour cream

Coarsely chop the seeds and nuts.
Put 5 oz (150 g) sour cream in a bowl. Sprinkle 2 oz (60 g) of the seed-nut mixture over the top.

Tip: full-fat sour cream and keto
Don't be intimidated by the term sour cream. Sour cream has a fresh, mild, and above all creamy taste. You can also alternate with cheese curds, cottage cheese or full-fat yogurt, but the latter contains slightly more carbs. What is important is that you always choose the full-fat version.

Tip: make more
I always make more of this recipe because it's such a quick and easy breakfast. The seeds and nuts will keep for three or four days in a tightly sealed container. Tomorrow we'll roast 4 ounces (120 grams) of the nuts in the oven with some cinnamon and an egg white for a tasty twist to this breakfast.

Per portion: 13.9g P (7%) / 78.5g F (89%) / 6.9g NetC (4%)

DAY 3
BREAKFAST

Instant cold soup

WITH SPINACH AND AVOCADO

Ready in less than 10 minutes - serves 2

10 1/2 oz (300 g) spinach

2 avocados

7 oz (200 g) cream

1 clove of garlic

14 fl oz (400 ml) water (or vegetable or meat stock)

2 spring onions

Finely chop the fresh garlic.
Put all the ingredients except for the spring onions in a deep bowl and blend to create a thick soup.
Season with salt and black pepper. Divide the soup evenly between two bowls and finish with some finely chopped spring onions, cream and olive oil.

Tip: Fresh herbs
If you have any fresh herbs around the house, like chives, dill or flat-leaf parsley, you can blend them into your soup.

Tip: Feta
If you're feeling hungry, add 1 3/4 oz (50 g) feta to the soup. Crumble the cheese over the soup as a garnish (add 7 g P, 10 g F, 2 g NetC per serving).

Per serving: 8g P (4%) / 78g F (92%) / 7g NetC (4%)

DAY 3
LUNCH

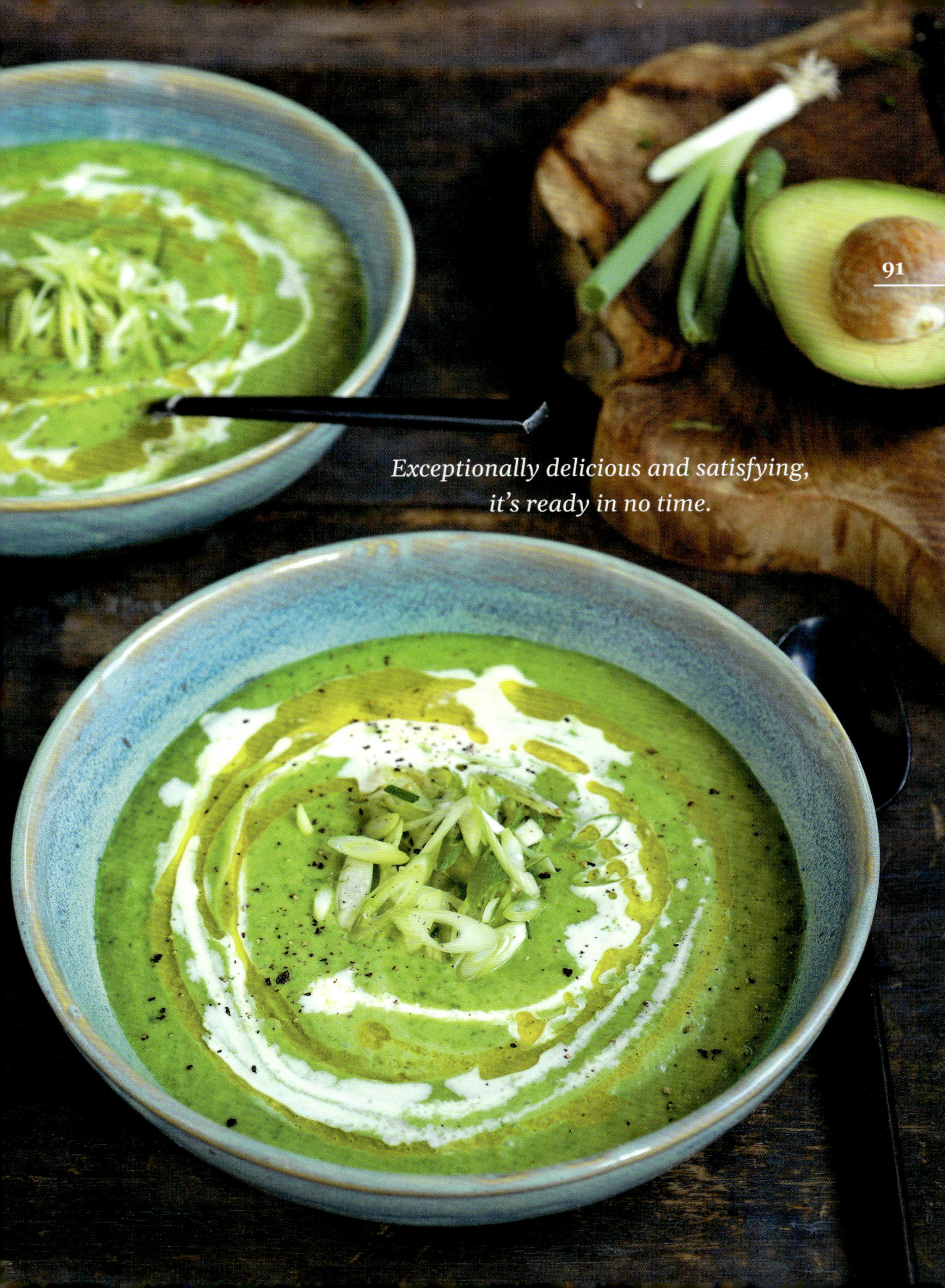
91
Exceptionally delicious and satisfying,
it's ready in no time.

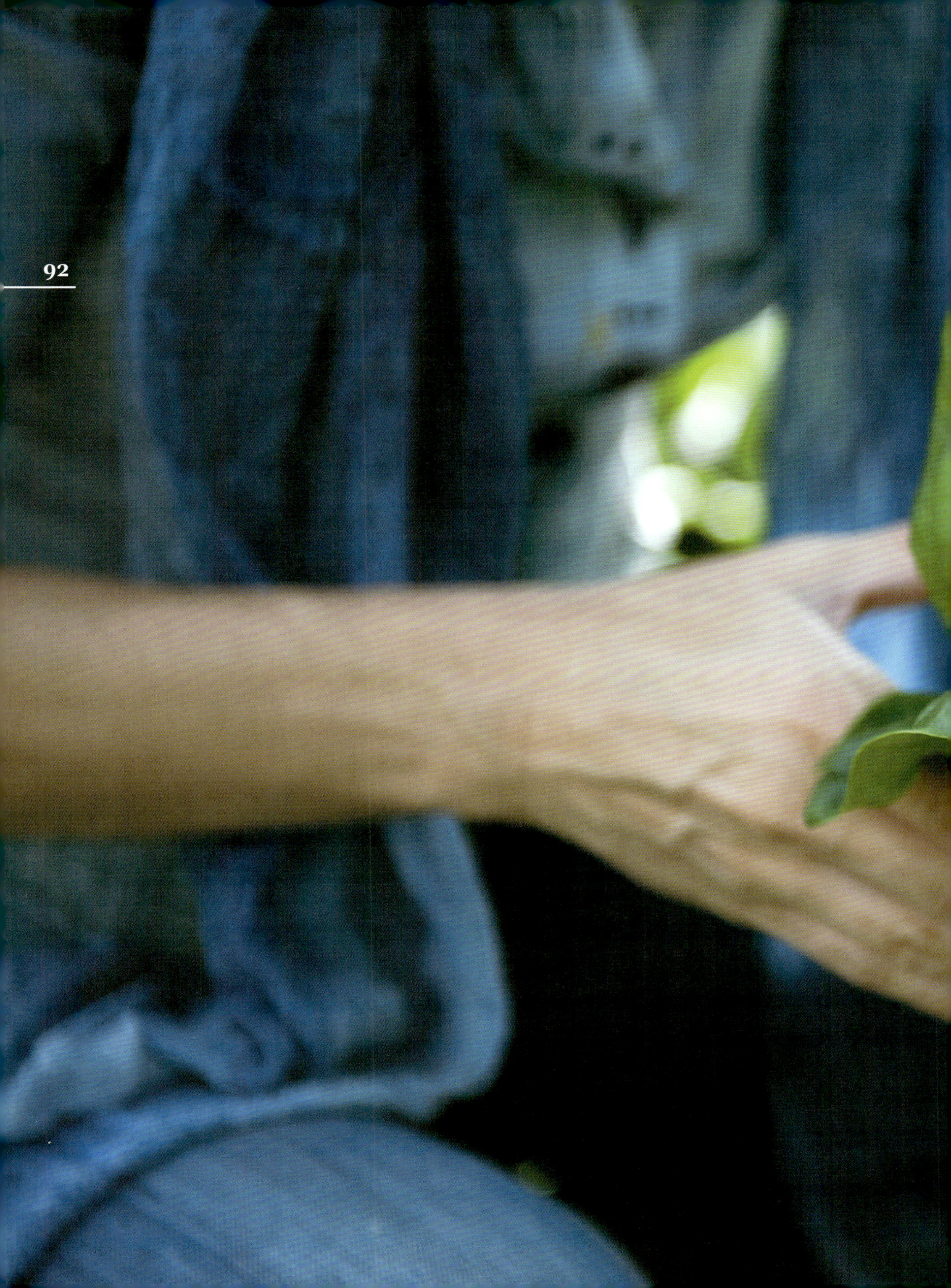

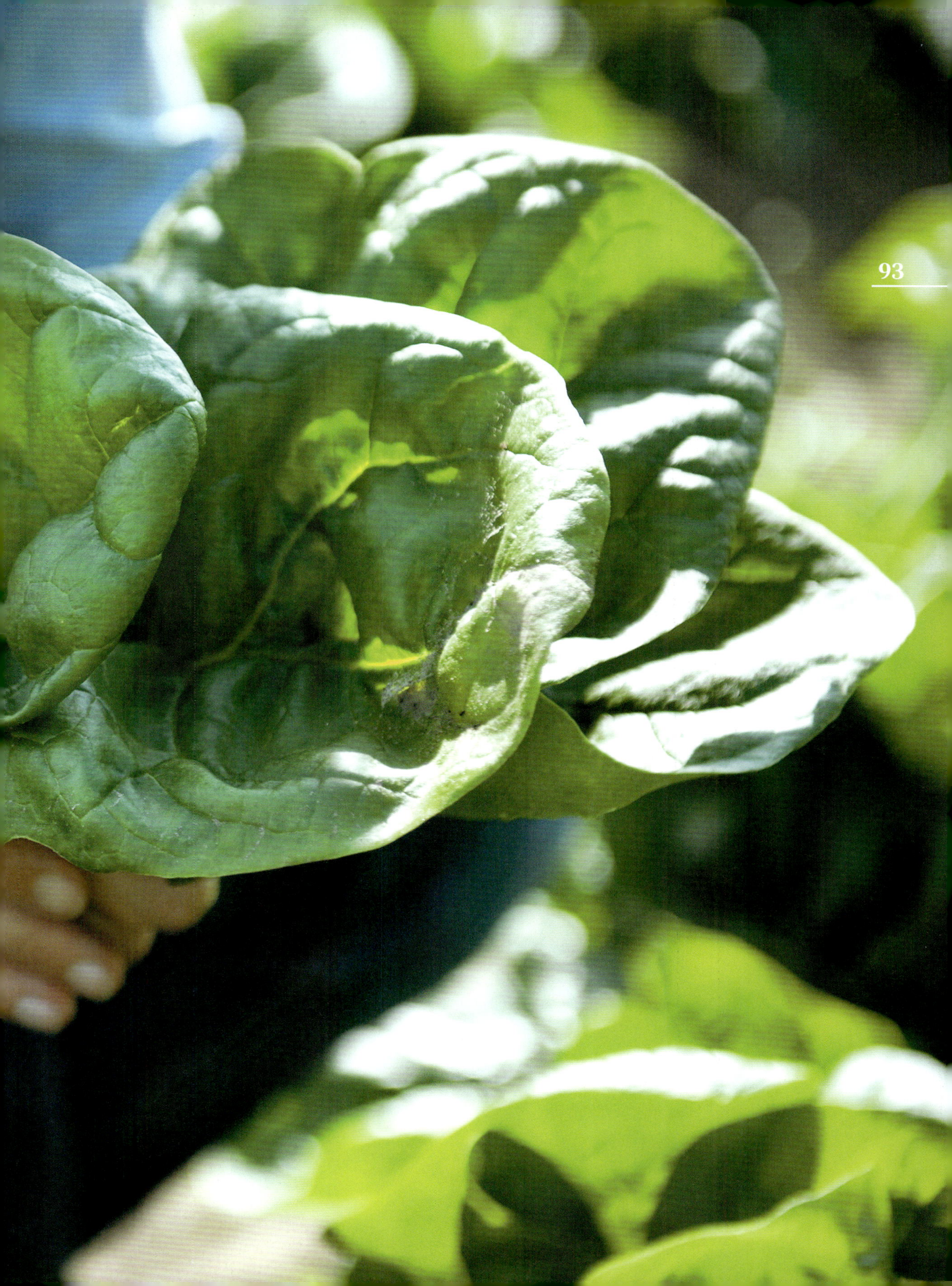

Lamb chops

WITH CREAMED CAULIFLOWER
AND SAUTEED GREEN BEANS

Ready in 20 minutes - serves 2

6 to 8 lamb chops

1/2 head of cauliflower (approx. 1 lb or 500 g)

3 1/2 fl oz (100 ml) cream

3 1/2 oz (100 g) green beans

4 tablespoons red curry paste

Coarsely chop the cauliflower and put the pieces in a cooking pot. Place the green beans next to the cauliflower. Add water until all the vegetables are half submerged and season with a little salt. Add a generous splash of olive oil. Put the pot over the heat and cook, uncovered, for about 7 minutes. Meanwhile, rub the curry paste into the lamb chops, making sure that they are completely coated. Drain the water from the pot containing the vegetables, remove the beans and set them aside. Return the cauliflower over the heat, add the cream and blend to a thick pulp. Season with black pepper and a little salt.
Fry the lamb chops for 1 1/2 minutes on each side in plenty of butter or olive oil. Just before the lamb chops are cooked, add the beans to reheat them and let them soak up some of that delicious sauce.

Per serving: 39g P (27%) / 41g F (65%) / 11g NetC (8%)

DAY 3
DINNER

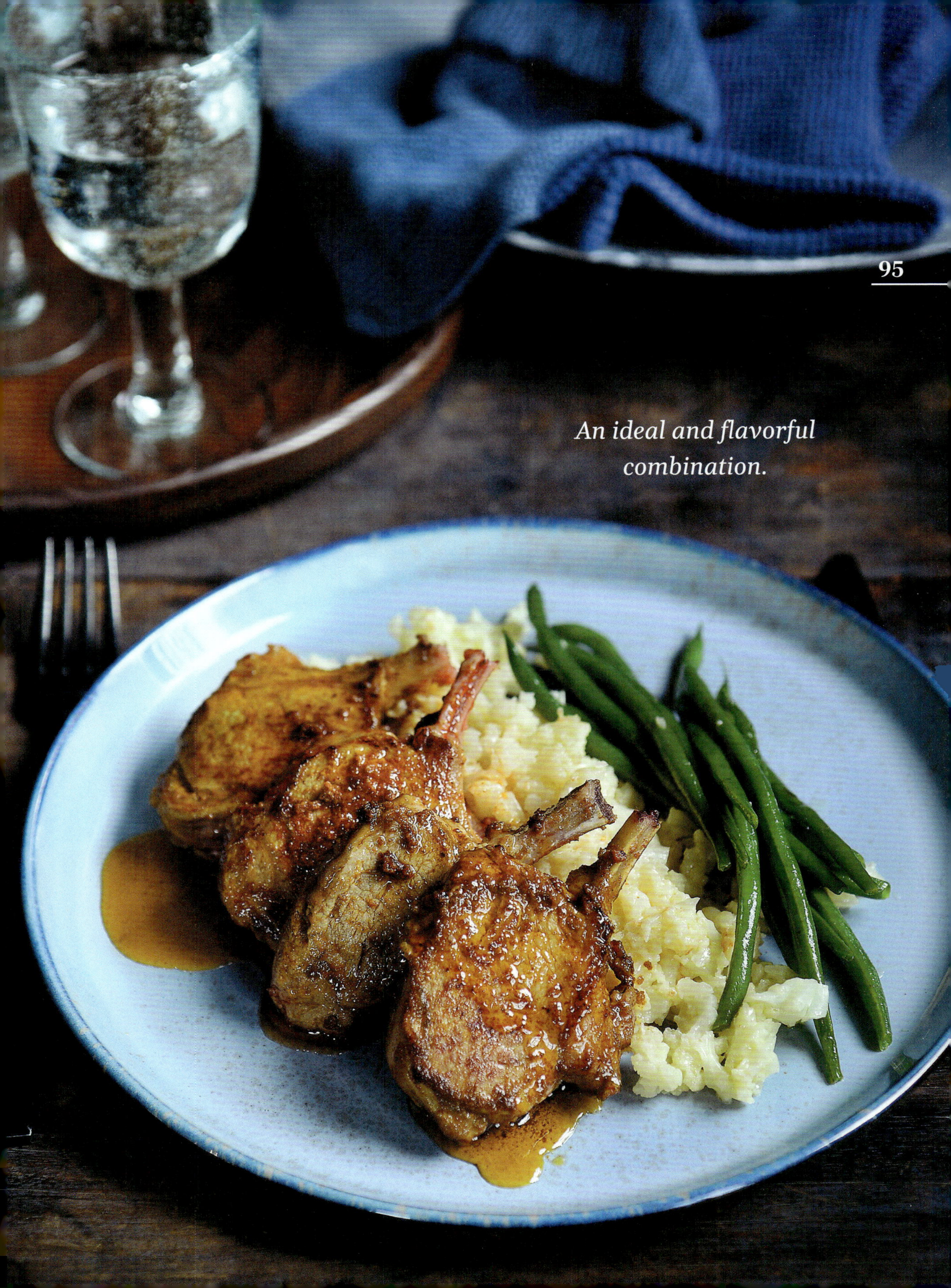

An ideal and flavorful combination.

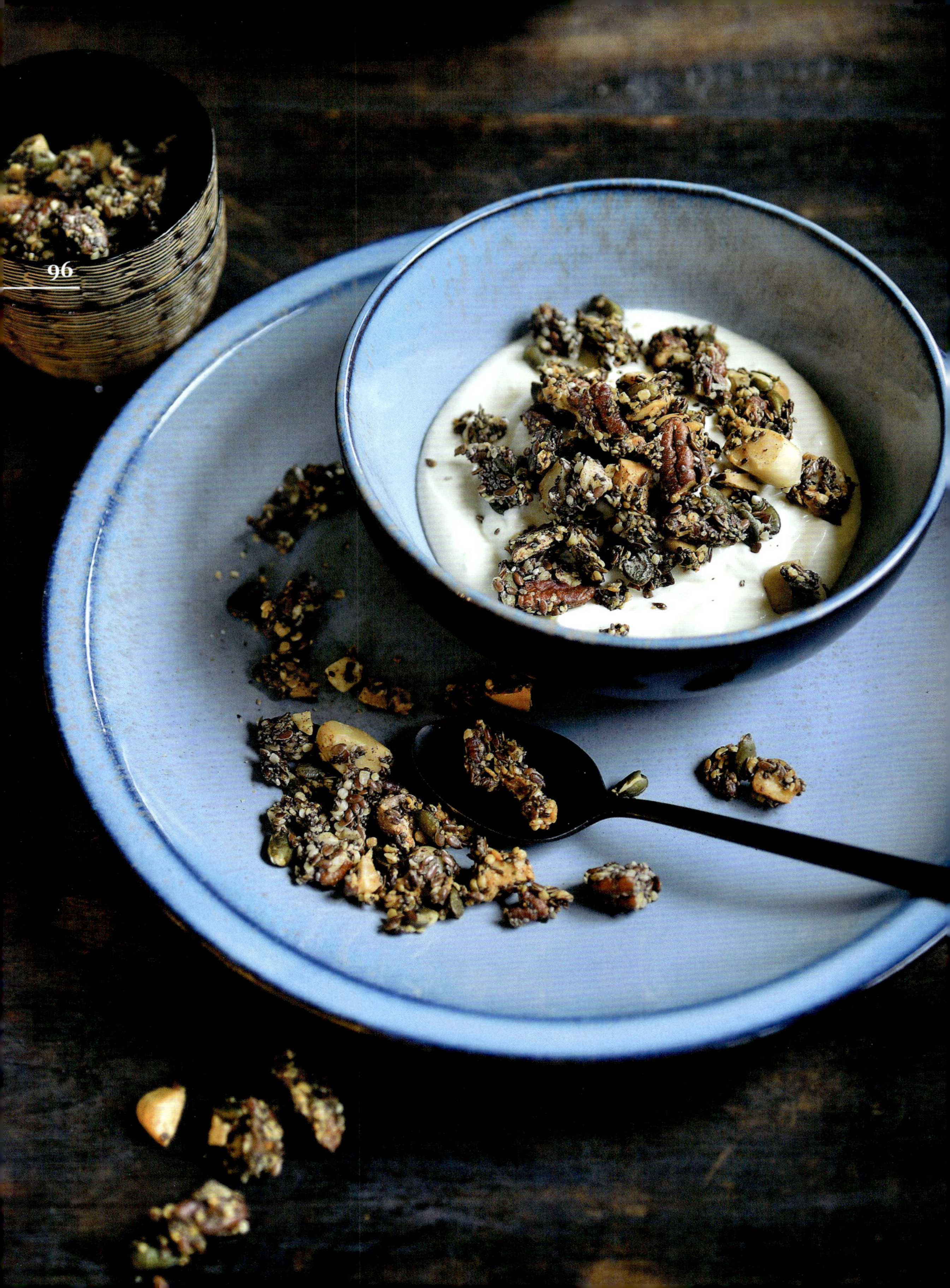
96

Roasted nuts and seeds

WITH FULL-FAT SOUR CREAM

Ready in less than 10 minutes - serves 2

4 oz (120 g) mixed seeds and nuts (from yesterday)

1 egg white

1 teaspoon ground cinnamon

10 1/2 oz (300 g) sour cream (from yesterday)

This is day 2 of a two-part breakfast.
Part 1 = Day 1 = nuts + sour cream
Part 2 = Day 2 = roasted nuts + sour cream

Preheat the oven to 350 °F (180 °C).
Mix the nuts and seeds with the egg white and the cinnamon.
Spread the mixture out on parchment paper on a baking tray.
Bake in the hot oven for about 10 minutes. Keep checking regularly, the nuts must not burn. They are
at their best when they're light brown in color.
Serve the crunchy nuts with the rest of yesterday's sour cream.

Tip: seed and nut cookies
If you make heaps from the nuts and seeds, you can also make cookies, which is always fun to do.
But don't overdo the nuts in a ketogenic diet, especially if you intend to lose weight.

Per 2-oz (60 g) serving of nuts + 5 0z (150 g) sour cream: 15.3g P (8%) / 78.5g F (88%) / 7.8g NetC (4%)

Burrata

WITH TOMATO, CREAM AND PESTO

Ready in less than 10 minutes - serves 2

2 balls of burrata (5 oz/150 g each)

2 tomatoes (14 oz/400 g)

1 3/4 fl oz (50 ml) cream

2 3/4 oz (80 g) green pesto

3/4 oz (20 g) pine nuts

Preheat the oven to 350 °F (180 °C).
Roast the pine nuts in the oven for about 7 minutes.
Break the tomatoes into pieces with your fingers. Arrange the tomato on the plates. Pull the burrata apart into chunks, preferably over the plates so the liquid (cream) inside spills out onto the plate. Divide the cream and the pesto evenly between the plates. Garnish with the pine nuts, drizzle some extra olive oil over the top and season with salt and pepper.

Per serving: 20g P (10%) / 78g F (86%) / 9g NetC (4%)

DAY 4
LUNCH

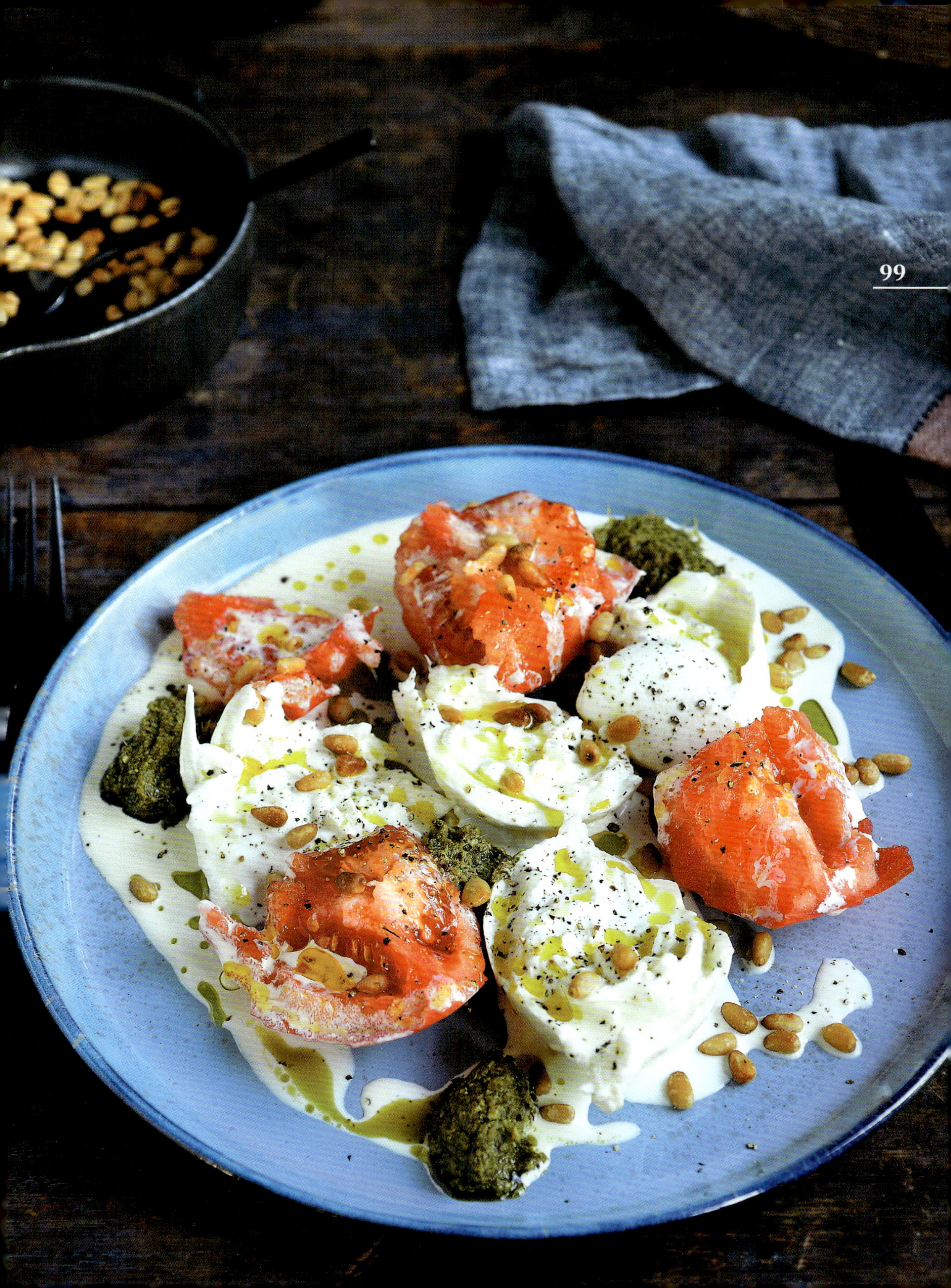

A last-minute recipe for when you have
friends over: it requires absolutely no
effort but tastes unbelievably good.

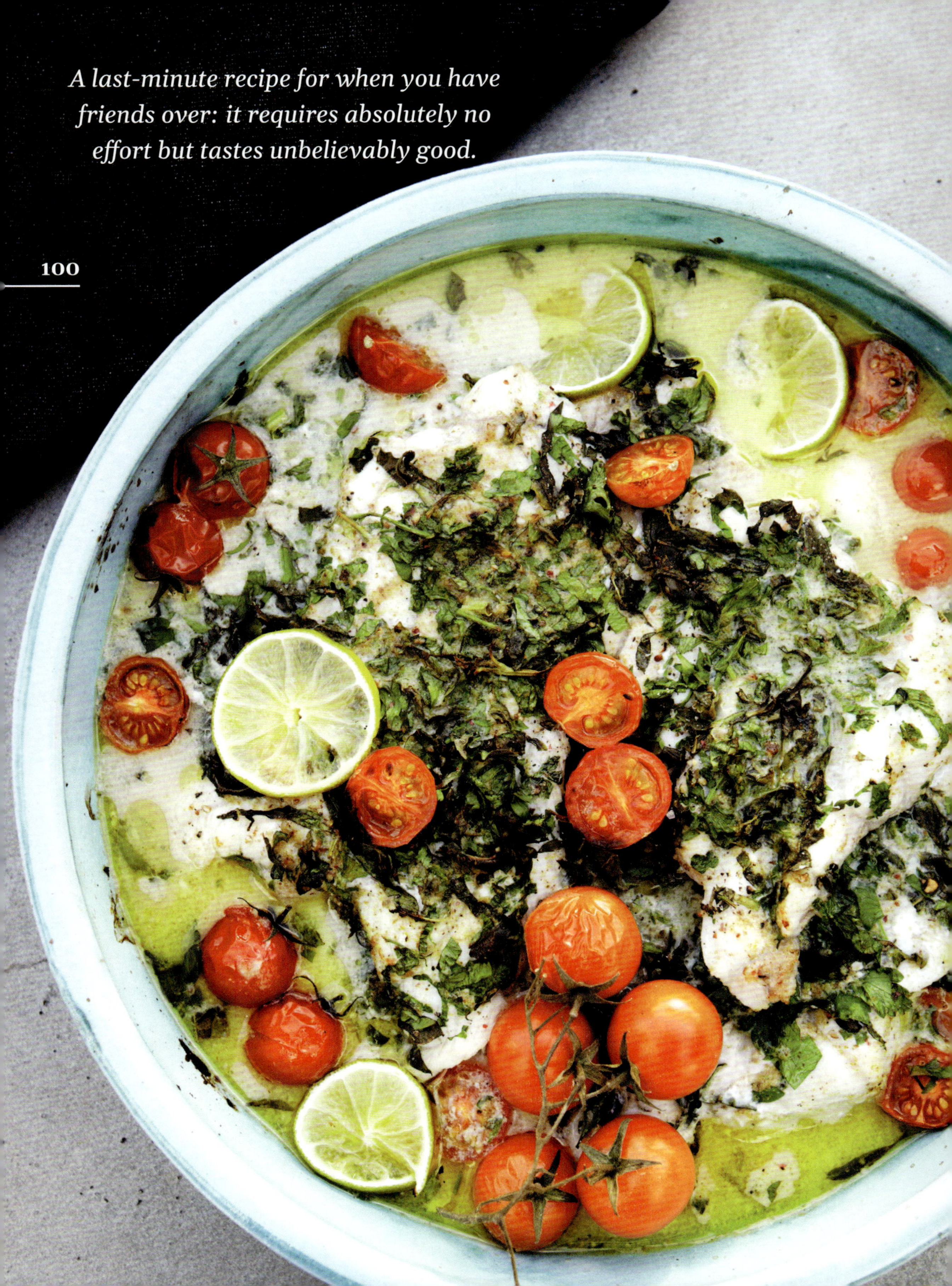

100

Fish

WITH HERBS, COCONUT MILK, LIME AND TOMATOES

Preparation time: 15 minutes - cooking time: 30 minutes - serves 2

14 oz (400 g) firm, flat whitefish fillet

7 oz (200 g) small vine tomatoes

3 1/2 oz (100 g) coconut milk

1 lime

1 large bunch fresh herbs: parsley, dill, cilantro ... 2 oz (60 g)

7 oz (200 g) spinach

1 clove of garlic

2 oz (60 g) olive oil

Combine the coconut milk with the juice of half of the lime and olive oil. Season with salt and pepper and the finely chopped garlic.

Finely chop the herbs and coarsely chop the spinach. Slice the tomatoes in half. Slice the other half of the lime into slices.

Take an ovenproof dish, lay part of the fish fillets in the dish, sprinkle with part of the herb mixture and spinach and some of the sauce. Repeat until you have used up all the fish; finish with the herbs and sauce. Arrange the tomatoes and the slices of lime around the fish. Bake in the oven at 350 °F (180 °C) for about 30 minutes.

Per serving: 37.3g P (28%) / 40.3g F (67%) / 7.2g NetC (5%)

Overnight chocolate mousse

WITH MACADAMIA NUTS

Ready overnight - serves 2

2 oz (60 g) macadamia nuts

4 large teaspoons (1/2 oz/15 g) cocoa powder

7 oz (200 g) coconut milk

20 blueberries

Blend the macadamia nuts with the coconut milk and the cocoa powder until you have a sort of chocolate milk. Divide evenly between two bowls and refrigerate overnight. Serve the next day as breakfast. Garnish with a dusting of cocoa powder and some blueberries on the side.

Tip: breakfast or dessert
You can also serve this as a dessert. It doesn't need any sweetening (for more information about sweeteners, see page 64).

Per serving: 4.4g P (4%) / 40.8g F (91%) / 5.3g NetC (5%)

DAY 5
BREAKFAST

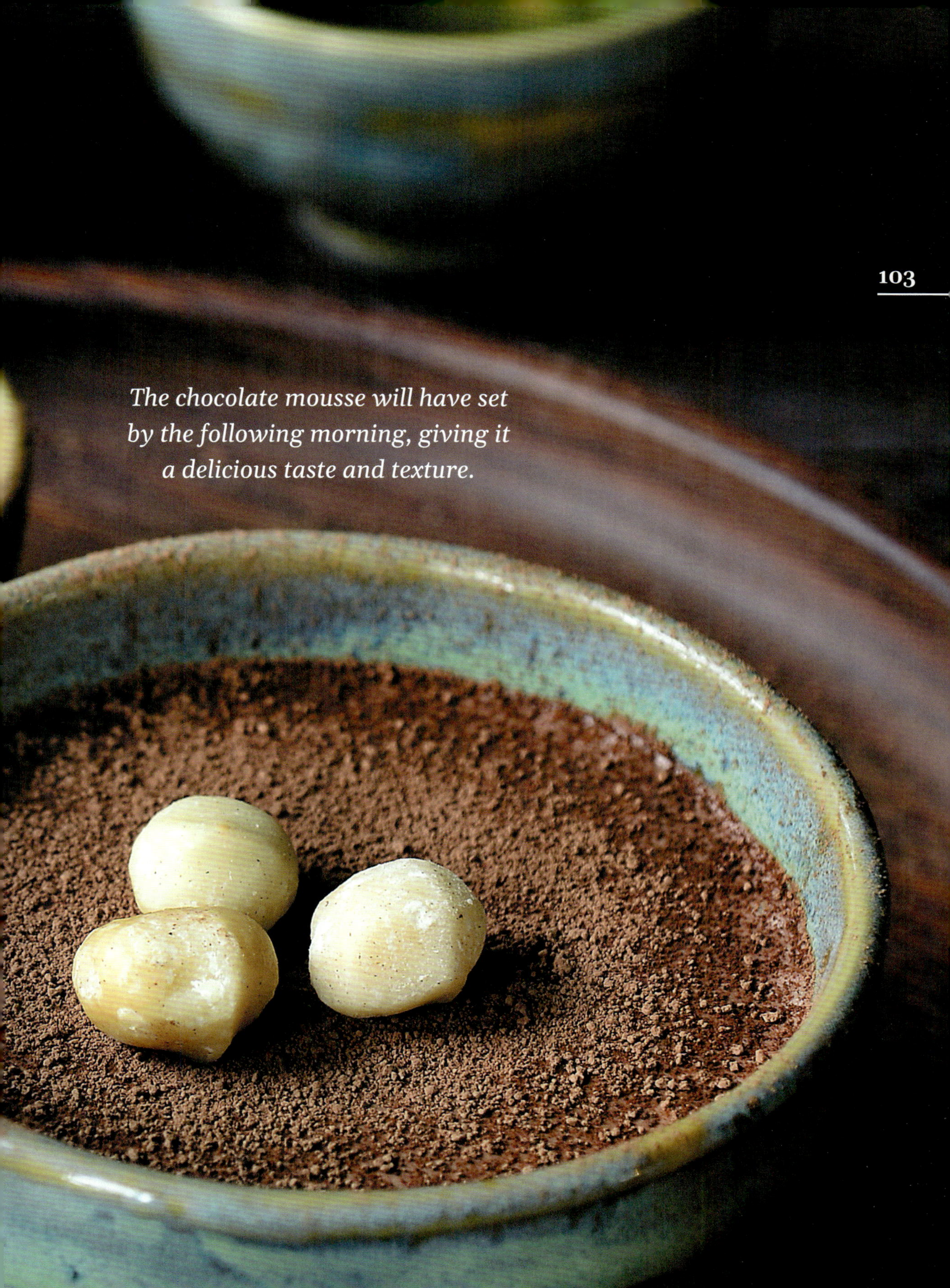

The chocolate mousse will have set
by the following morning, giving it
a delicious taste and texture.

Avocado

WITH BACON AND SNOW PEAS

Preparation time: 7 minutes - cooking time: 10 minutes - serves 2

1 avocado

10 1/2oz (30 g) snow peas

10 1/2 oz (300 g) diced bacon

3 1/2 oz (100 g) lamb's lettuce

Dry-fry the diced bacon in a frying pan until crispy. Briefly cook the snow peas in boiling water with salt and a splash of olive oil. Dice the avocado.
Toss the lamb's lettuce with some olive oil and season with salt and pepper. Divide the lettuce evenly between the plates, arrange the snow peas and diced bacon on top and finish with the avocado. Garnish with a drizzle of olive oil.

Tip: vinaigrette
I think this dish tastes just fine without that hint of sour, but if you prefer, you can make a vinaigrette with some balsamic vinegar or lime and olive oil.

Per serving: 31g P (19%) / 55.9g F (76%) / 7.8g NetC (5%)

DAY 5
LUNCH

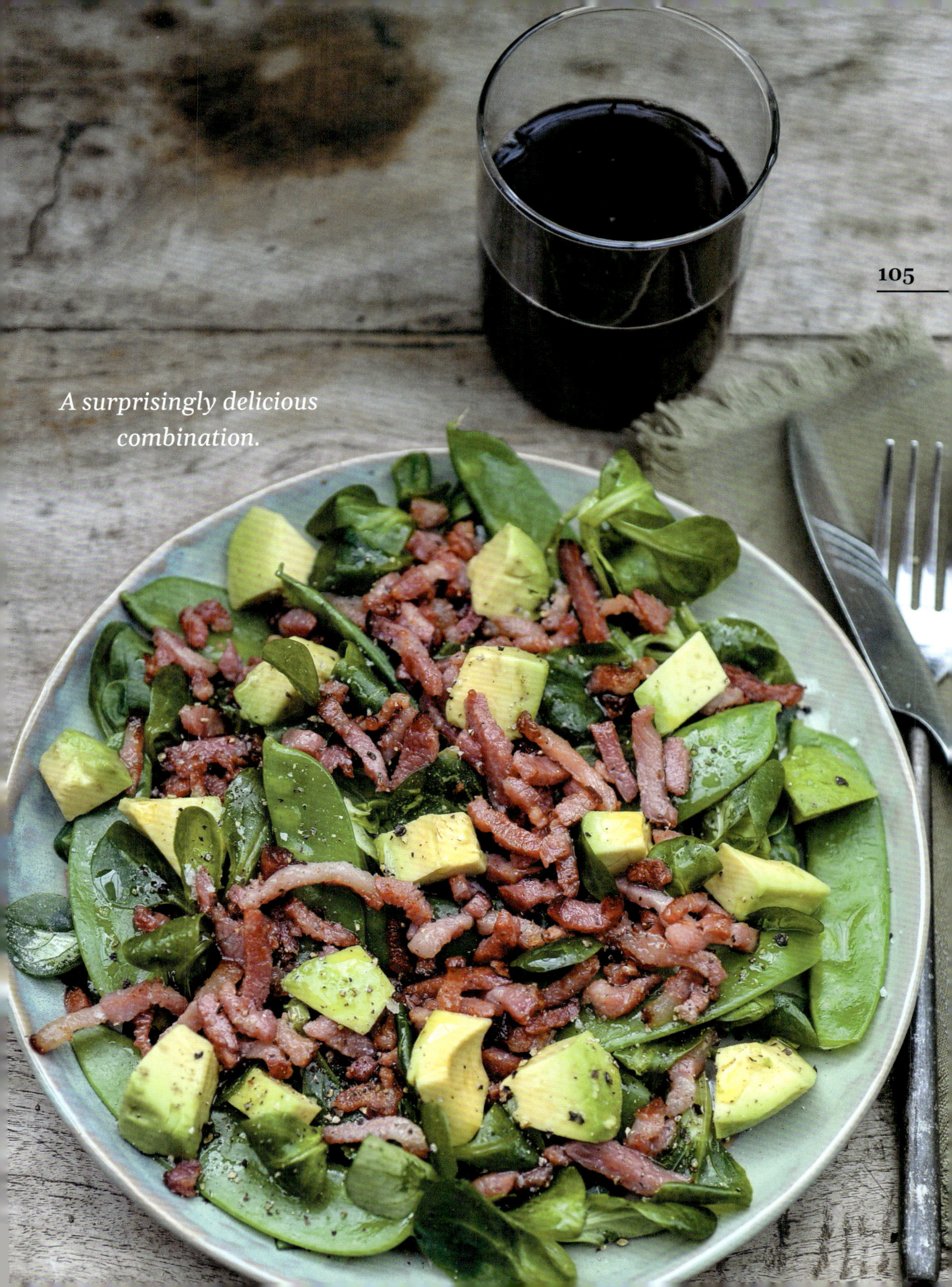
A surprisingly delicious
combination.

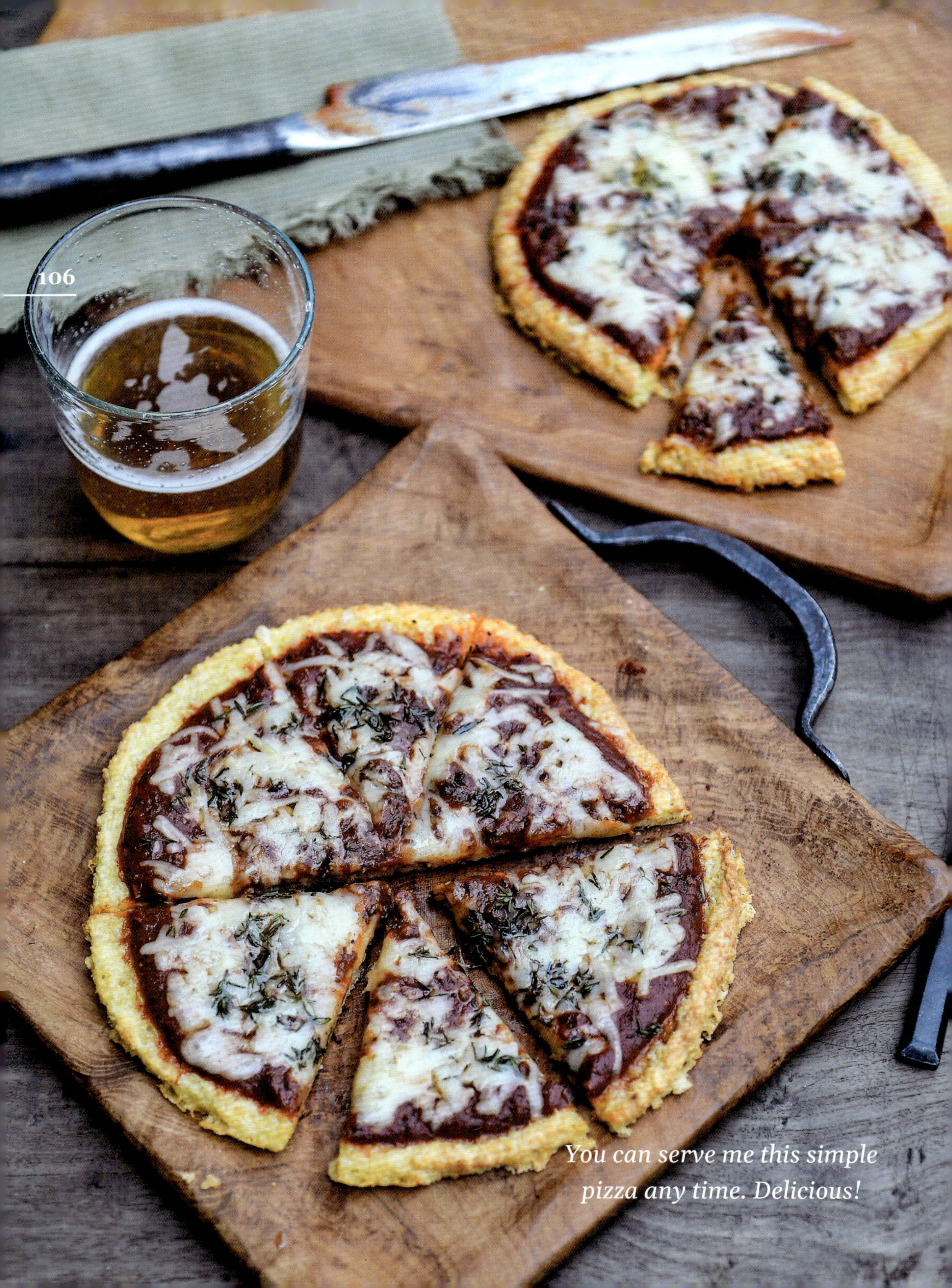

You can serve me this simple
pizza any time. Delicious!

Pizza

Ready in 20 minutes - serves 2

3 1/2 oz (100 g) ground almonds

2 eggs

3 1/2 oz (100 g) grated gruyere cheese

7 oz (200 g) strained tomatoes

or thick tomato sauce

Dried herbes de Provence:

(oregano, thyme, rosemary ...)

1 oz (30 g) olive oil

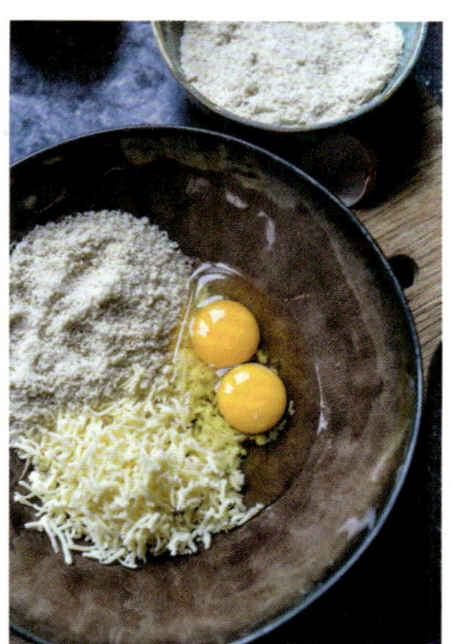

Preheat the oven to 350 °F (180 °C).

Mix half the gruyere cheese with the ground almonds and the eggs. Knead into a dough and split into two balls. Place them on a sheet of parchment paper. Place a second sheet of parchment paper on top and flatten using a tea towel to make a "crust" about 1/4 inch (1/2 cm) thick. Remove the top sheet of parchment paper. If the edges of the pizza crust have cracked a little, press them in slightly towards the middle. Bake the bases in the oven for 7 minutes until the dough is light brown in color and cooked through.

Add a generous splash of olive oil to the strained tomatoes and season with black pepper, a little salt and plenty of herbes de Provence.

Spread the sauce out over the pizza bases and divide the remaining cheese over the top of each pizza. Sprinkle with some extra herbes de Provence and bake the pizzas another 3 minutes in the oven until the cheese has melted.

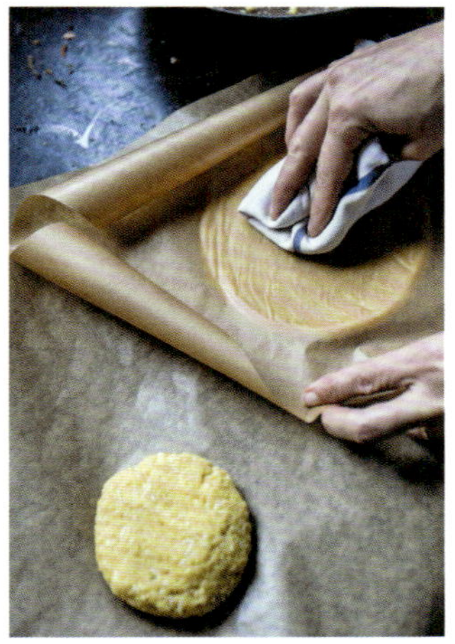

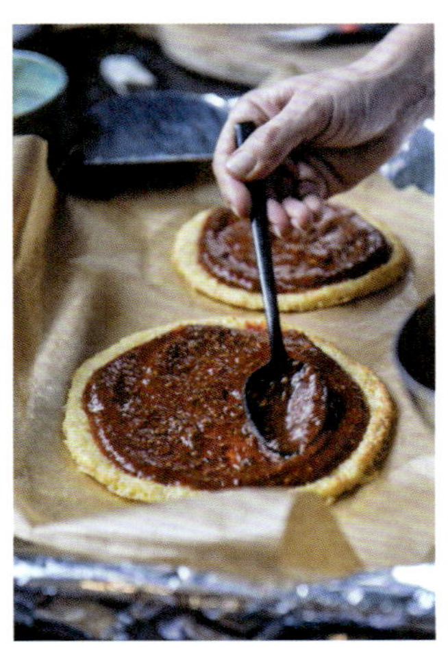

Per serving: 32.4g P (18%) / 63.2g F (78%) / 6.7g NetC (4%)

DAY 5
DINNER

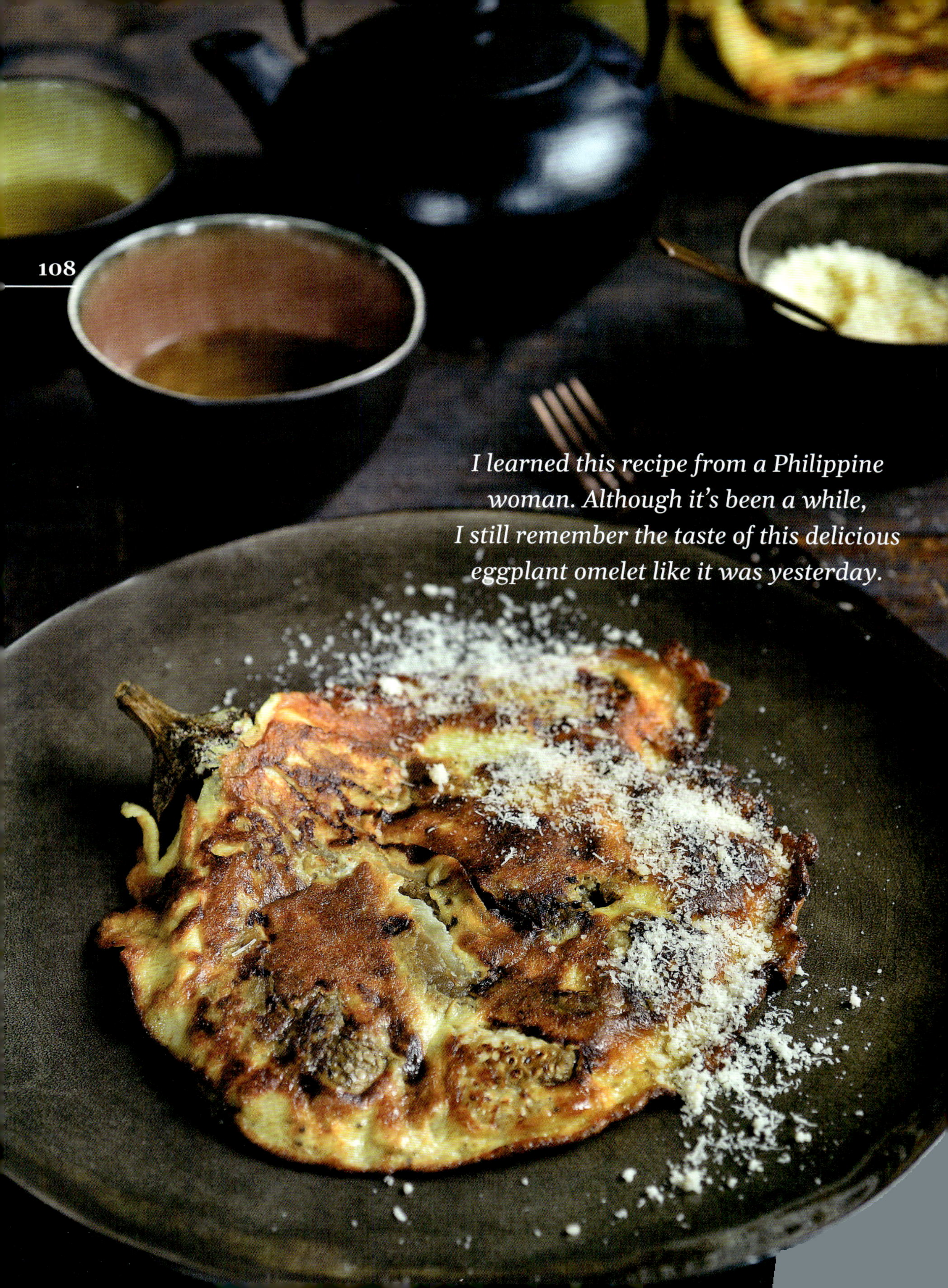

I learned this recipe from a Philippine woman. Although it's been a while, I still remember the taste of this delicious eggplant omelet like it was yesterday.

Eggplant

PHILIPPINE-STYLE

Ready in 45 minutes (30 minutes of which in the oven) - serves 2

2 small eggplants (approx. 1 lb /500 g)

2 eggs

3 1/2 fl oz (100 ml) cream

2 oz (60 g) Parmesan cheese

1 1/2 oz (40 g) coconut oil

Preheat the oven to 400 °F (200 °C).

Poke two holes into each eggplant and bake them in the hot oven for 30 minutes.

Whisk the eggs together with the cream and 1 1/2 oz (40 g) of the Parmesan cheese. Season with salt and black pepper. Remove the eggplants from the oven and remove the skin. Place each eggplant in a deep dish and flatten the flesh, fanning the eggplant out to create a fan shape. Divide the egg mixture over the eggplants. Flatten the eggplant out a bit more. Leave for about 5 minutes so the eggplant can soak up the egg mixture. Put some coconut oil (or butter) in a small pan just big enough to hold the fanned-out eggplant, heat the oil and quickly and carefully place the eggplant in the pan. Cover the pan and cook. Carefully turn the eggplant omelet over and cook the other side.

Place the omelet on a plate (or put in an oven preheated to 120 °F (50 °C) to keep warm).

Fry the other omelet. Serve the eggplant omelets with the remaining Parmesan cheese.

Tip: Philippine dish "tortan talong"

I learned this recipe from a Philippine woman with whom I lived in Hong Kong when I was still working as a model. That was a long time ago, but I remember the taste of this delicious omelet like it was yesterday. This dish is called "tortan talong".

Tip: keto

Eggplants contain quite a lot of carbs, but half of those come from fiber. This makes eggplant a suitable vegetable for keto dishes.

Per serving: 22.1g P (15%) / 54.2g F (80%) / 8g NetC (5%)

DAY 6
BREAKFAST

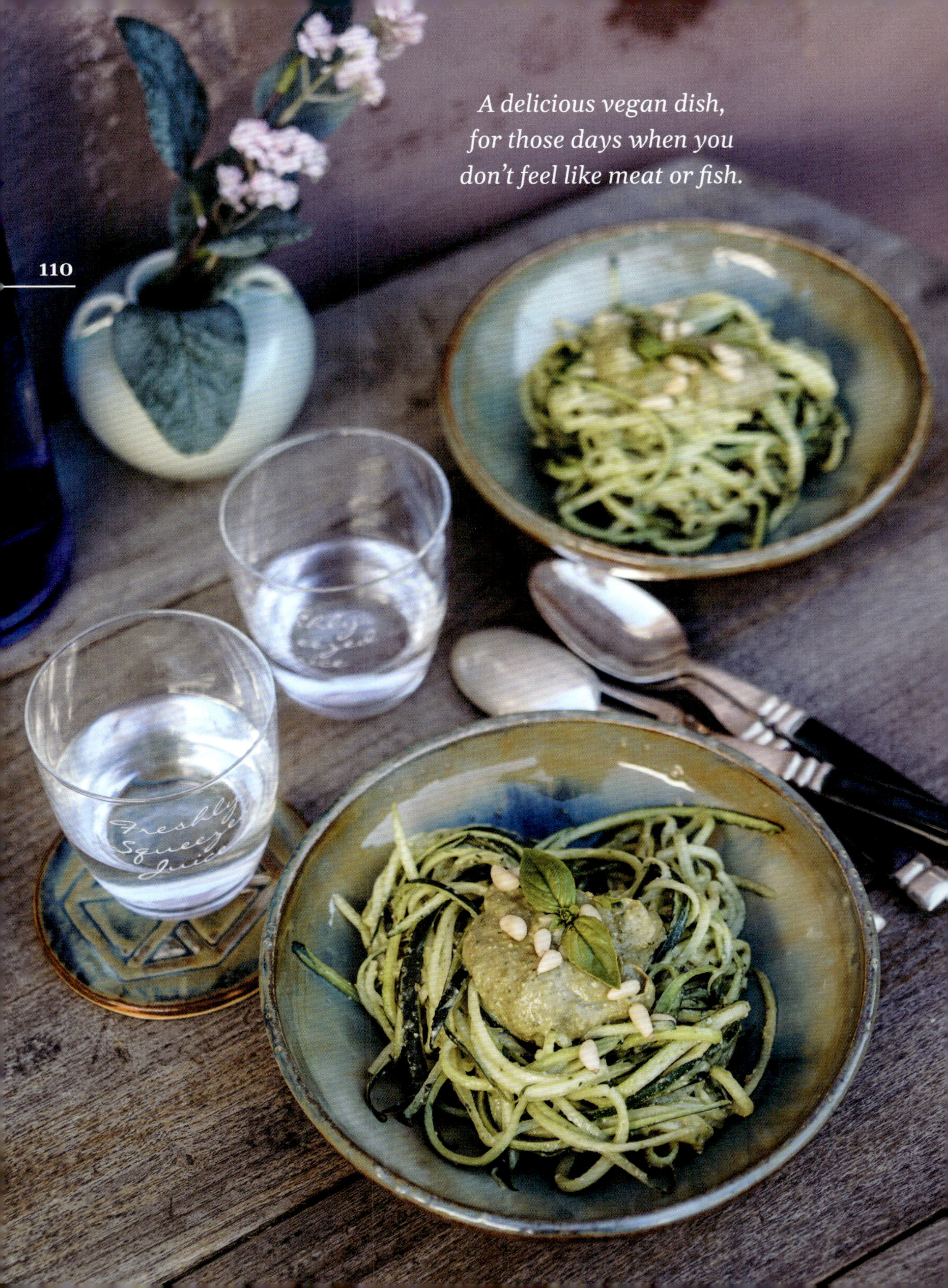
A delicious vegan dish,
for those days when you
don't feel like meat or fish.

Zucchini noodles

WITH PINE NUTS AND BASIL PESTO

Ready in 15 minutes - serves 2

10 1/2 oz (300 g) zucchini noodles (tip)

1 avocado

1 3/4 oz (50 g) pine nuts

1 clove of garlic

1 1/2 oz (40 g) fresh basil

1 oz (30 g) olive oil

Blend all the ingredients except the zucchini noodles together to a thick paste. Add a splash of water to make a creamy sauce. Season with salt and pepper.
Stir the sauce gently into the zucchini noodles. Garnish with some extra pine nuts and a few basil leaves.

Tip: Zucchini noodles
Take two medium-sized zucchini and slice them into spaghetti strands with a julienne peeler or a spiralizer. We call these zucchini noodles, or zoodles. Once you get to the seeds, you will no longer be able to peel them. You can use the leftover zucchini in soups, for instance. Two medium-sized zucchini will give you about 10 1/2 oz (300 g) zucchini noodles.

For 1 serving: 7g P (6%) / 50g F (90%) / 5g NetC (4%)

Cod

WITH GREEN CURRY AND CHERRY TOMATOES

Preparation time: 5 minutes - cooking time: 25 minutes - serves 2

2 cod fillets (10 1/2 oz/300 g)

1 oz (30 g) green curry paste

3 oz (90 g) cherry tomatoes

7 fl oz (200 ml) white wine

10 1/2 oz (300 g) spinach

2 oz (60 g) olive oil

Take a heatproof dish. Pour in 2 tablespoons of olive oil and place the cod fillets in the dish.
Combine the curry paste with 3 tablespoons of olive oil and coat the fish with this mixture.
Cut the cherry tomatoes in half and arrange them around the fish fillets. Drizzle 2 tablespoons
olive oil over the fish and season with salt and pepper. Pour the white wine over the mixture until
everything is submerged by about 1/4 inch (less than 1 cm). Bake the fish in the oven at 350 °F
(180 °C) for 25 minutes.
Wilt the spinach in a pan with 3 tablespoons of olive oil and season with salt and pepper.
Arrange the fish and vegetables on the plates.

Tip: olive oil
Don't be stingy with the olive oil. The oil is the most important source of fat in this dish. Use at least
2 oz (60 g), which amounts to about 7 large tablespoons. That isn't even that much. When you're
cooking, you will use that amount quite easily.

Per serving: 28.3g P (26%) / 34.3g F (70%) / 4.5g NetC (4 %)

DAY 6
DINNER

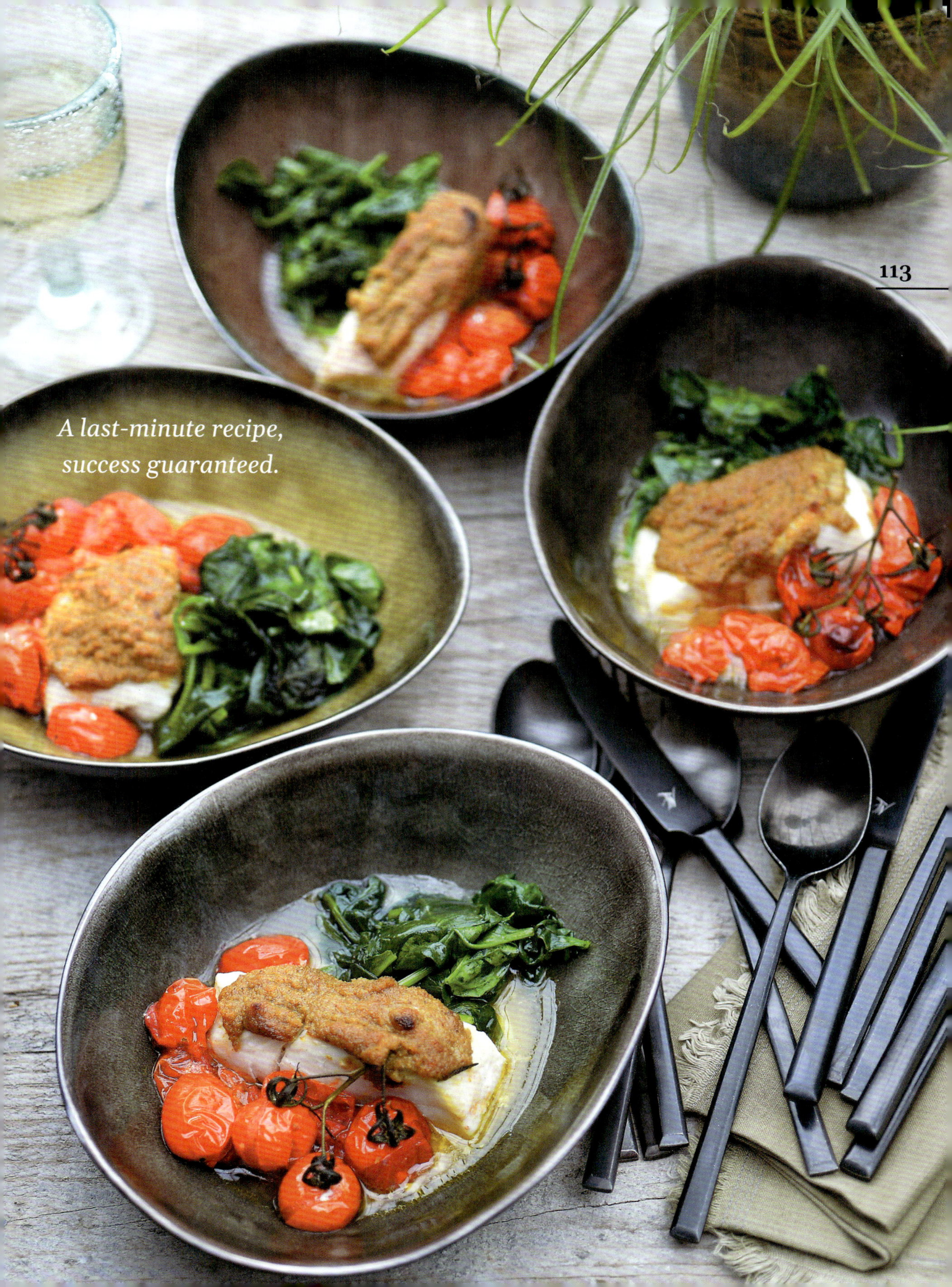
A last-minute recipe,
success guaranteed.

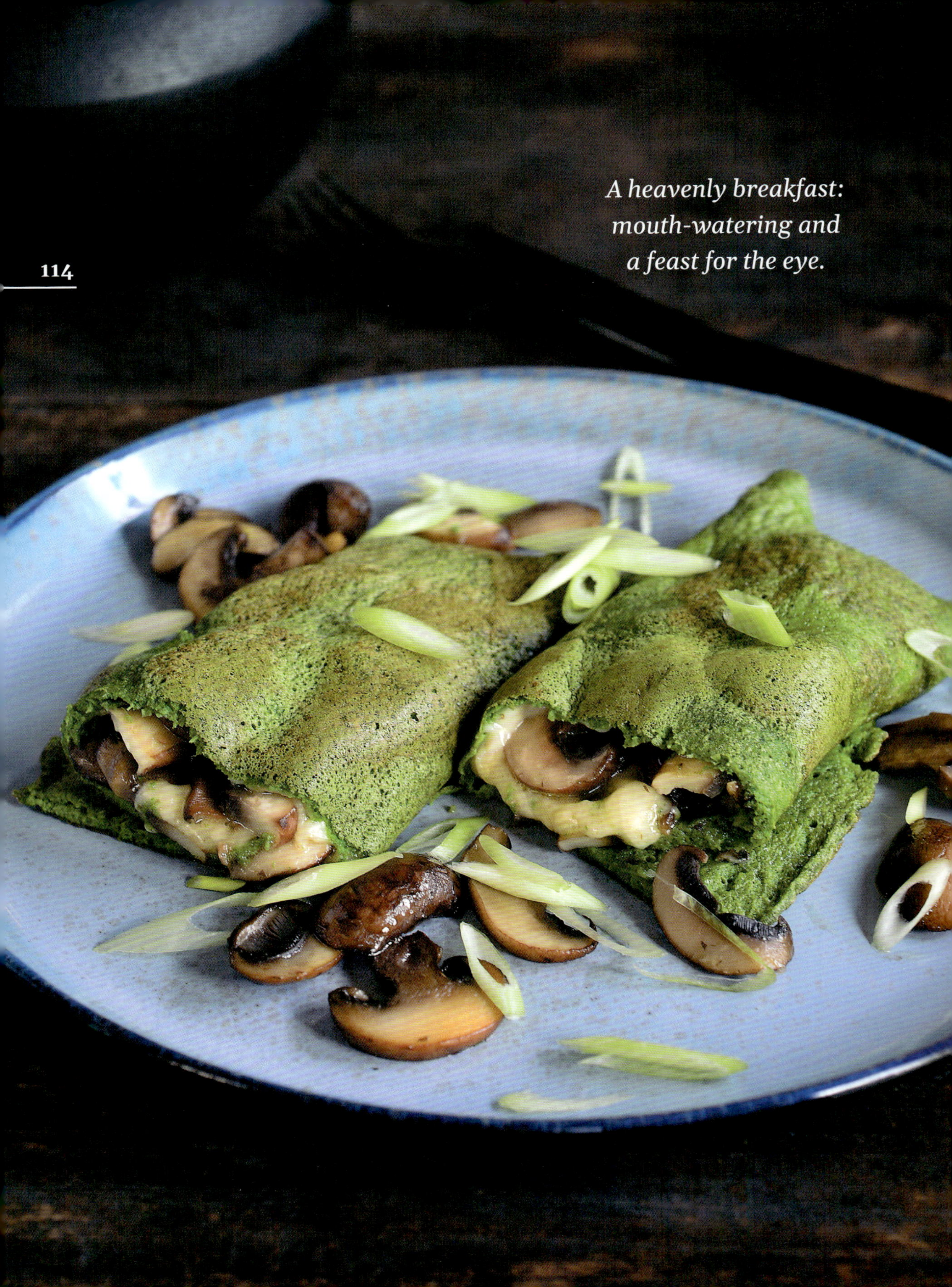

114

Spinach omelet roll-up

WITH MUSHROOMS AND CHEESE

Ready in 25 minutes - serves 2

4 eggs

3 1/2 oz (100 g) spinach

7 oz (200 g) mushrooms

5 1/2 oz (160 g) grated Emmentaler cheese (or other melty cheese)

2 spring onions

Slice the mushrooms and sauté them in plenty of olive oil; don't be stingy with the oil.
Put the eggs and spinach in a blender and blend until the spinach has practically dissolved and you're
left with a thick, green, eggy mixture. Season with salt and black pepper.
Drizzle a bit of olive oil in a pan and pour half the egg mixture into the pan. You do not have to turn
the omelet over. Wait until the top is just dry and then place half the mushrooms and half the cheese
on top. Roll the omelet up and transfer to a plate. Do the same with the second omelet. Serve the
omelets with some finely chopped spring onion.

Per serving: 38g P (26%) / 47g F (73%) / 2g NetC (1%)

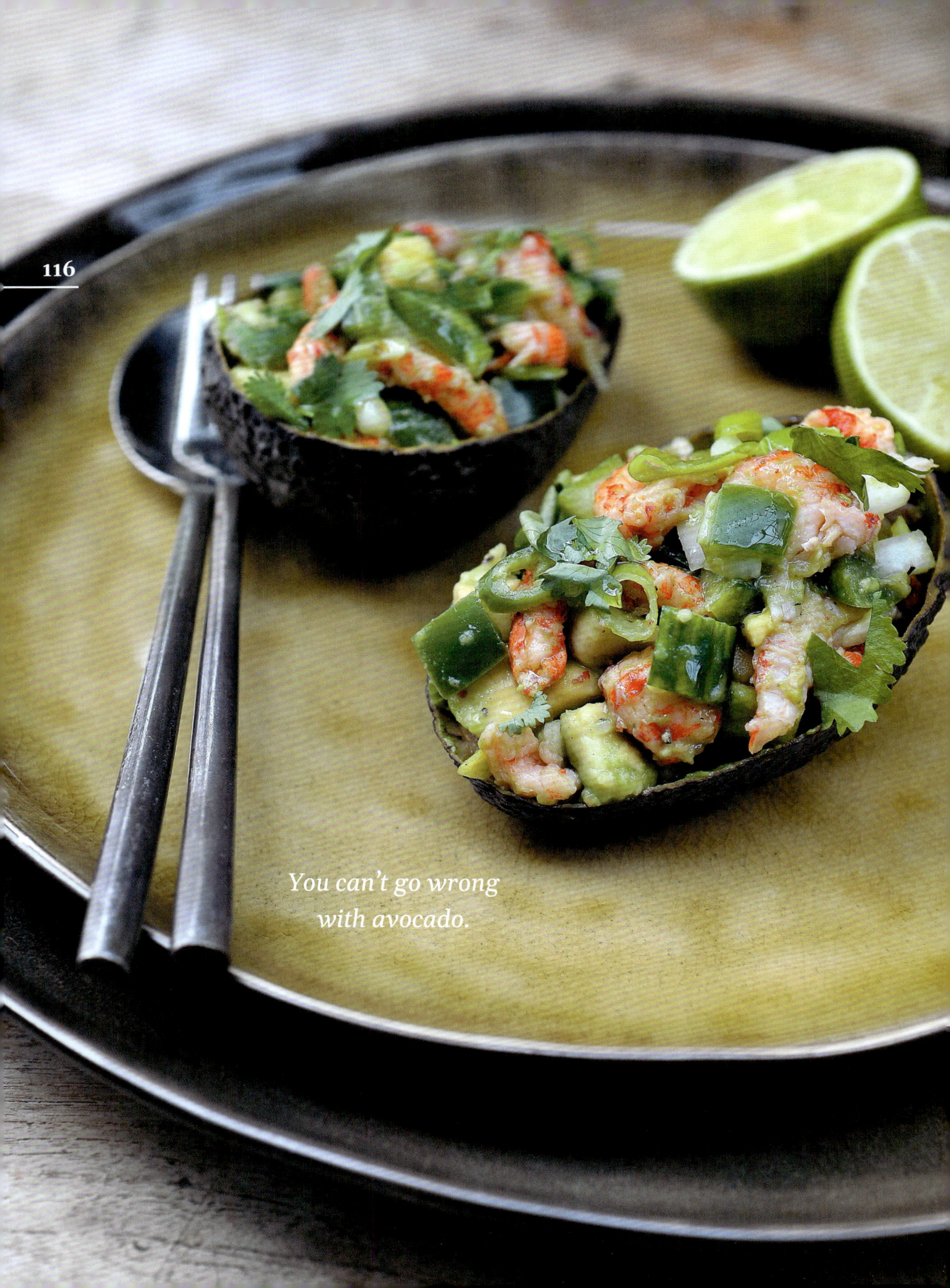
116
You can't go wrong
with avocado.

Stuffed avocado

WITH CRAWFISH

Preparation time: 15 minutes - cooking time: none - serves 2

9 oz (250 g) peeled, precooked crawfish

2 nice, ripe avocados

4 1/4 oz (120 g) green bell pepper

2 3/4 oz (80 g) white onion

1/2 green chili pepper

1 lime

2 sprigs cilantro

2 sprigs fresh mint

Cut the avocado in half, remove the pit and spoon out the flesh. Keep the skins. Finely dice the avocado, bell pepper and onion and combine in a bowl. Add the finely chopped chili pepper, mint and coriander. Drizzle the mixture with the juice of half a lime and some olive oil. Season with sea salt and pepper and combine well.
Finally, spoon the crawfish into the salad and fill the avocado skins with the mixture.
Drizzle the juice from the other lime half over the top and serve.

Per serving: 26.6g P (20%) / 42.2g F (73%) / 8.5g NetC (7%)

Chicken

WITH OLIVES AND MUSHROOMS

Preparation time: 15 minutes - cooking time: 25 minutes - serves 2

14 oz (400 g) chicken breasts, with skin

5 1/4 oz (150 g) mixed olives, pitted

14 oz (400 g) baby bella or cremini mushrooms

1 oz (30 g) butter

1 sprig of rosemary

Coarsely chop the olives and slice the mushrooms.
Cook the chicken breasts until browned on both sides over medium heat in some coconut oil or other type of fat.
Continue to cook the chicken breasts on a wire rack in the oven at 350 °F (180 °C).
Pour the fat out from the pan (see tip). Add some fresh fat to the pan (olive oil or butter). First sauté the mushrooms for a few minutes and then add the olives. Season with salt and pepper and the finely chopped rosemary. Let the vegetables cook for a few more minutes, then add half a glass of water. Let the mixture simmer briefly so that all the flavors are well combined. Remove the pan from the heat, add the diced butter and fold the butter into the sauce. Slice the chicken and serve with those deliciously tasty vegetables and olives.

Tip: which olives should you use during cooking?
You can use any type of olive: marinated olives, dried olives, olives from a can... There's only one rule: taste the olives, and if you like them, you'll be sure to love them in these dishes. Bear in mind that pitted olives are easier to work with.

Tip: why should you pour the fat out from the pan?
I don't like fat that's been heated too much, even fats with a high melting point such as coconut oil or butter. When you heat them to a moderate temperature, these fats taste better, and they're healthier too. That's why I always pour off the brown fat after cooking and return the pan to the heat with fresh fat for cooking the vegetables. The chicken drippings are then scraped into the fresh fat to give the vegetables some extra flavor.

Per serving: 51.1g P (31%) / 49.6g F (68%) / 1.6g NetC (1%)

DAY 7
DINNER

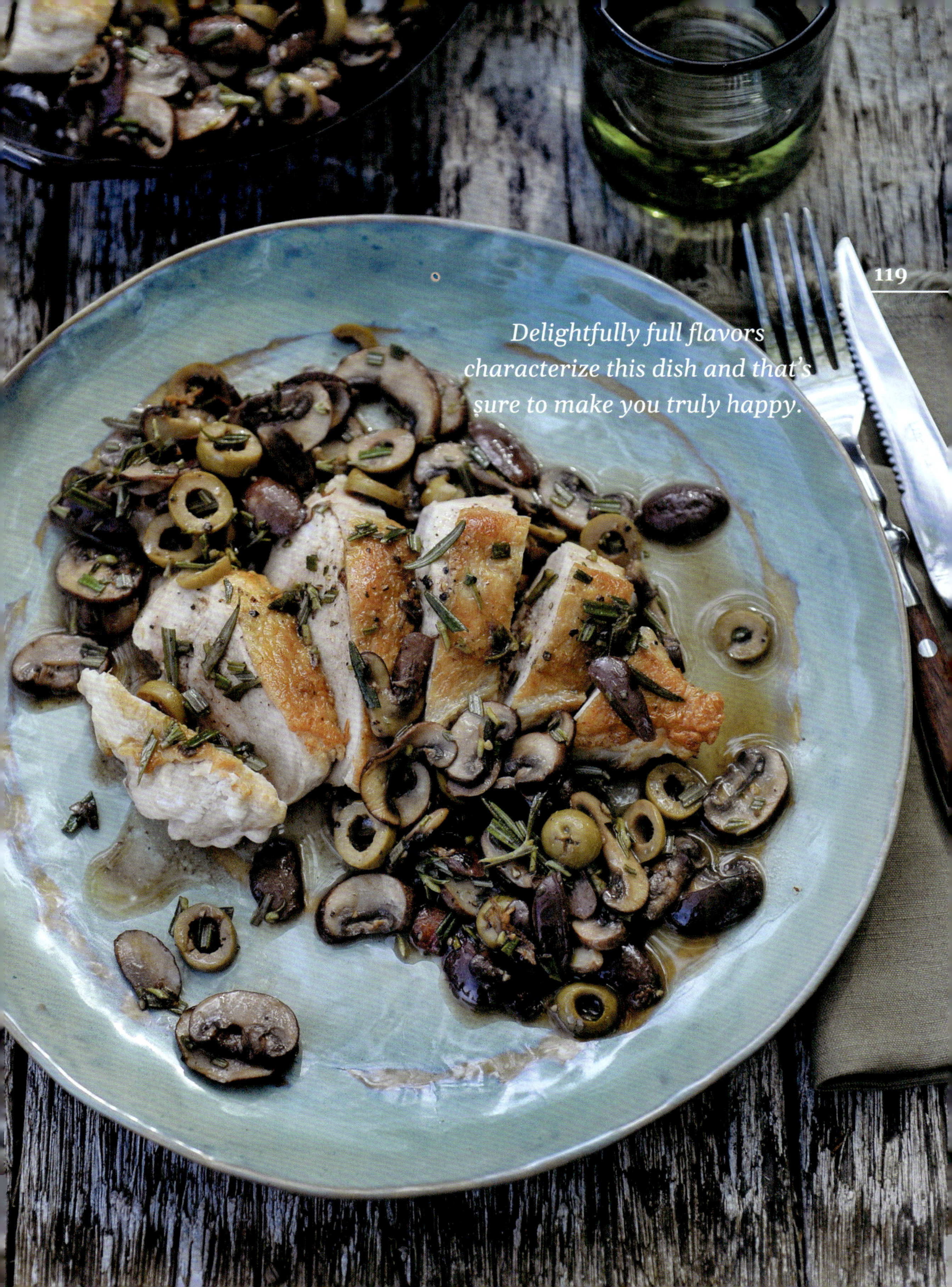
Delightfully full flavors
characterize this dish and that's
sure to make you truly happy.

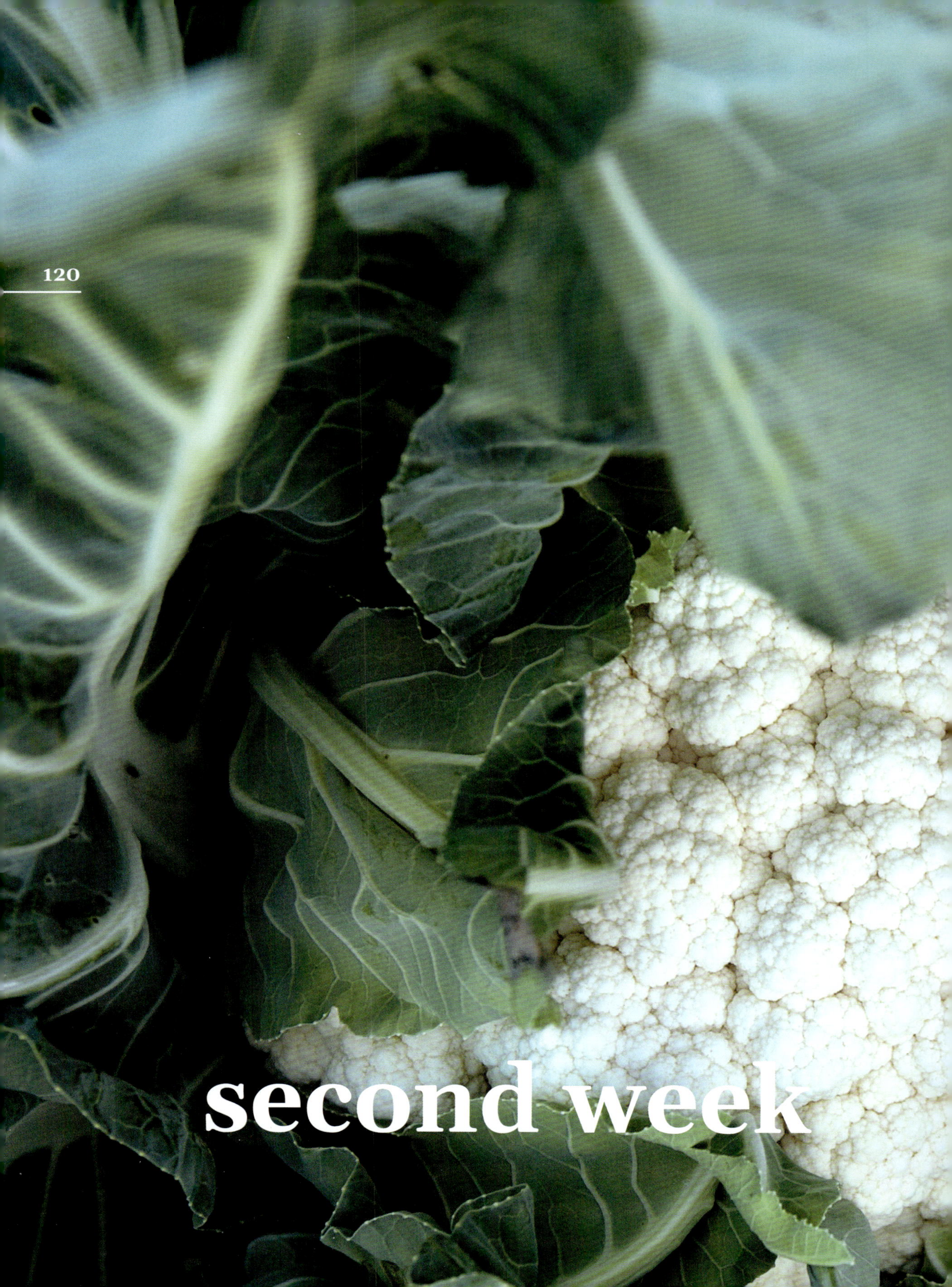
second week

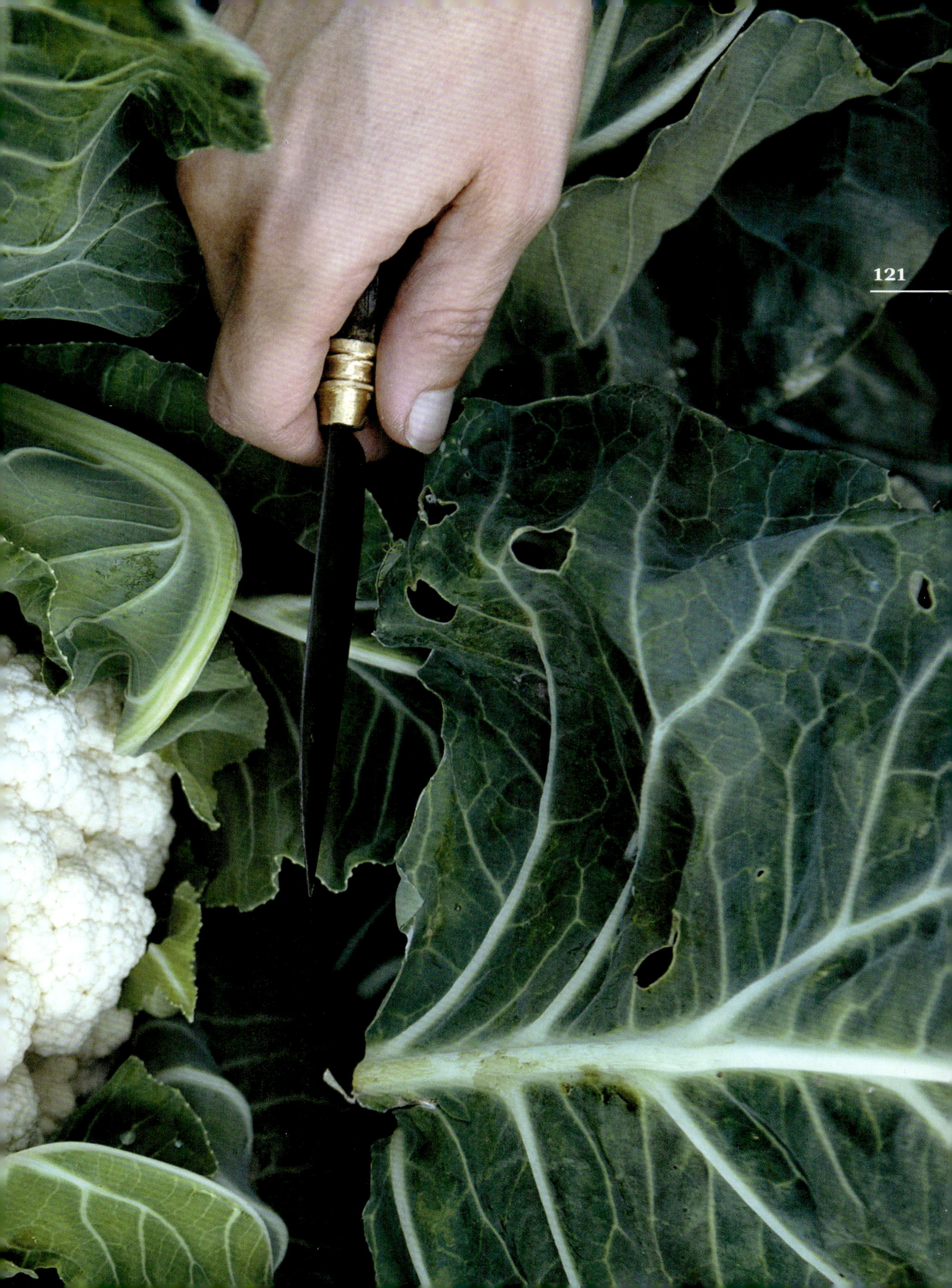

Mini-quiche

WITH HAM

Preparation time: 10 minutes - cooking time: 15 minutes - makes 8 quiches
We make four quiches for today; the other four we save for tomorrow.

24 slices of ham (for example, dry-cured ham) (14 oz/400 g)

8 eggs

8 tablespoons mascarpone (7 oz/200 g)

1 1/2 oz (40 g) chives

Extra: molds

Preheat the oven to 212 °F (100 °C).
We'll make an extra-large batch so we'll have some for tomorrow as well:
day 1: 4 mini-quiches
day 2: 4 mini-quiches

Place three slices of ham in each mold, making sure to cover the sides and bottom of the mold.
Finely chop the chives. Briefly place the mascarpone in the oven to soften it up. Raise the oven
temperature to 350 °F (180 °C).
Beat each egg separately with 1 tablespoon mascarpone, some chives, salt and pepper. The mixture
doesn't have to be completely smooth. If it contains some mascarpone lumps, that's fine. Pour the
egg mixture into the molds and bake for 15 minutes in the oven. Serve slightly warm.

Tip: quantities
I usually make enough for two quiches per person for breakfast, but if you think that may be too
much, just have one quiche. The idea is simple: adjust the quantities to match your needs. If you are
full, stop eating; if you're still hungry, eat more.

Per piece: 22g P (30%) / 21.9g F (68%) / 1.5 g NetC (2%)
Per 2 pieces: 44g P (30%) / 43.8g F (68%) / 3g NetC (2%)

DAY 8
BREAKFAST

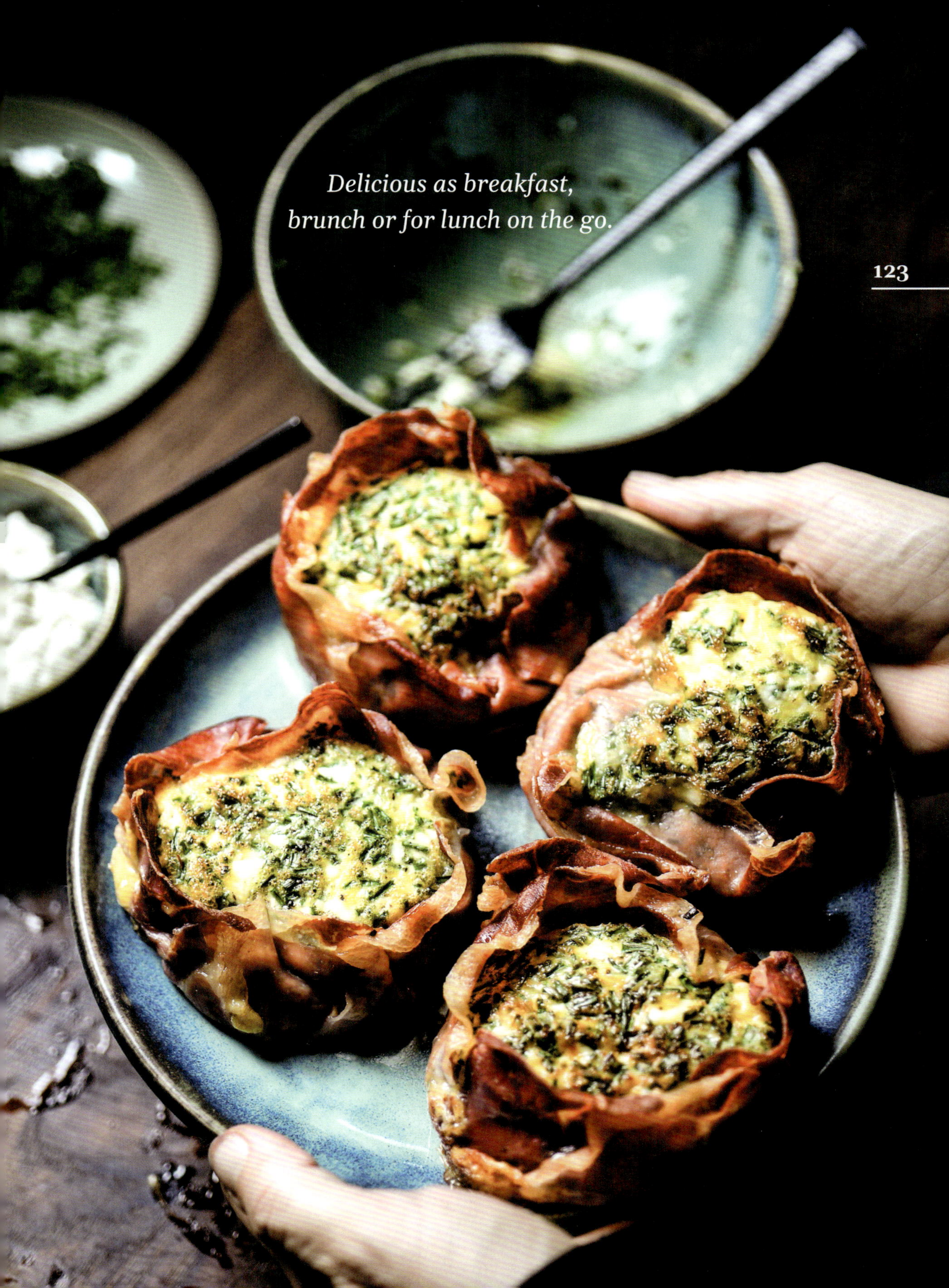

Delicious as breakfast,
brunch or for lunch on the go.

Brown shrimp

WITH GUACAMOLE

Preparation time: 20 minutes - cooking time: none - serves 2

10 1/2 oz (300 g) small, precooked brown shrimp

2 ripe avocados

bunch of fresh cilantro (3/4 oz/20 g)

bunch of chives (3/4 oz/20 g)

a few sprigs of fresh dill (3/4 oz/20 g)

1 clove of garlic

juice of 1 lemon

salt and pepper

1 oz (30 g) olive oil

Finely chop the garlic and fresh herbs.
Slice the avocados in half, remove the pit and spoon the flesh out of the skin. Put the avocado flesh in a bowl and mash together with some lemon juice, garlic, olive oil and chopped herbs (set some herbs aside to garnish). Season with salt and pepper.
Arrange the guacamole on a plate and sprinkle the brown shrimp over the top. Garnish with remaining fresh herbs.

Per serving: 38.4g P (23%) / 53.8g F (73%) / 6.6g NetC (4%)

DAY 8
LUNCH

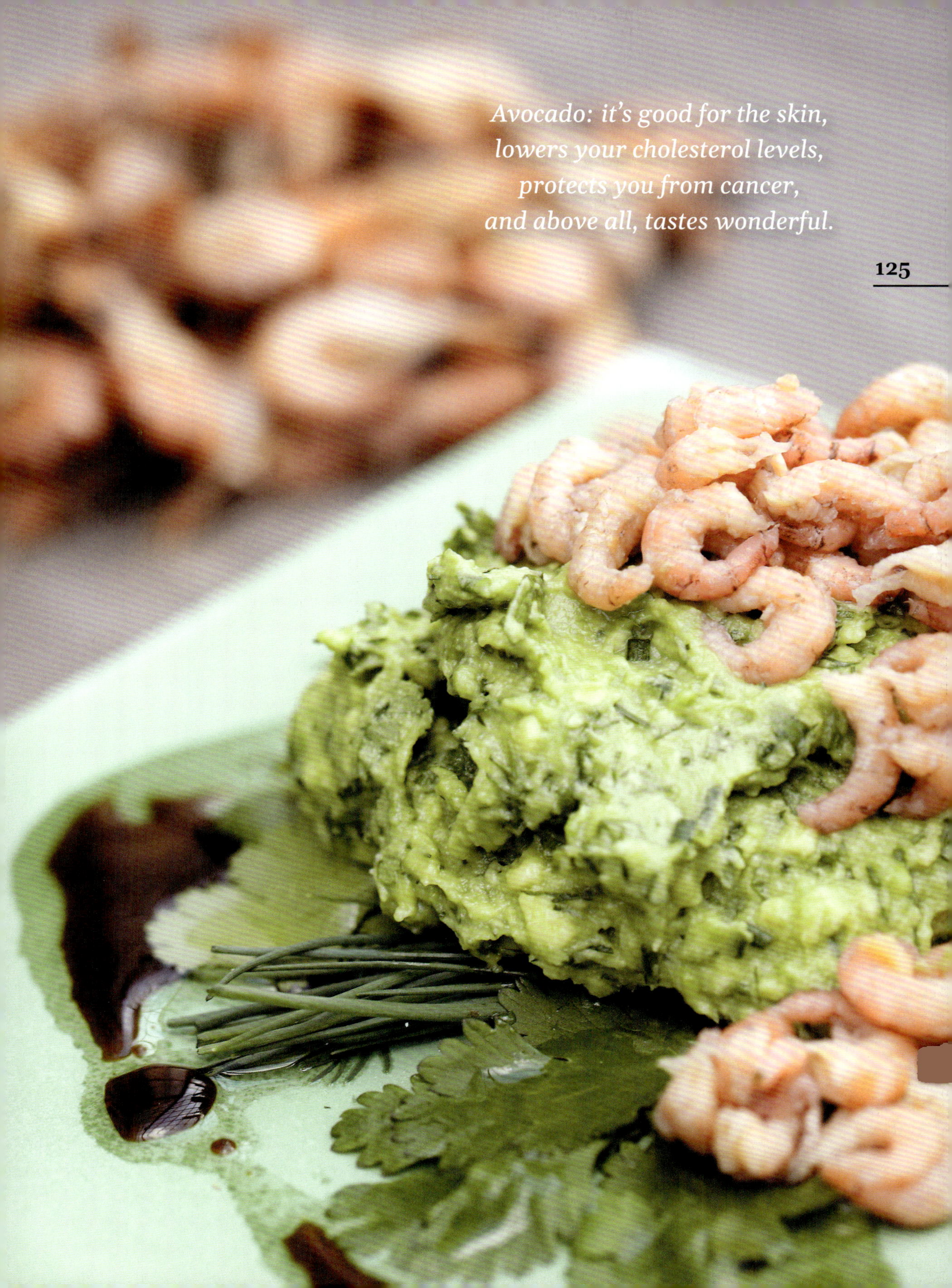
Avocado: it's good for the skin,
lowers your cholesterol levels,
protects you from cancer,
and above all, tastes wonderful.

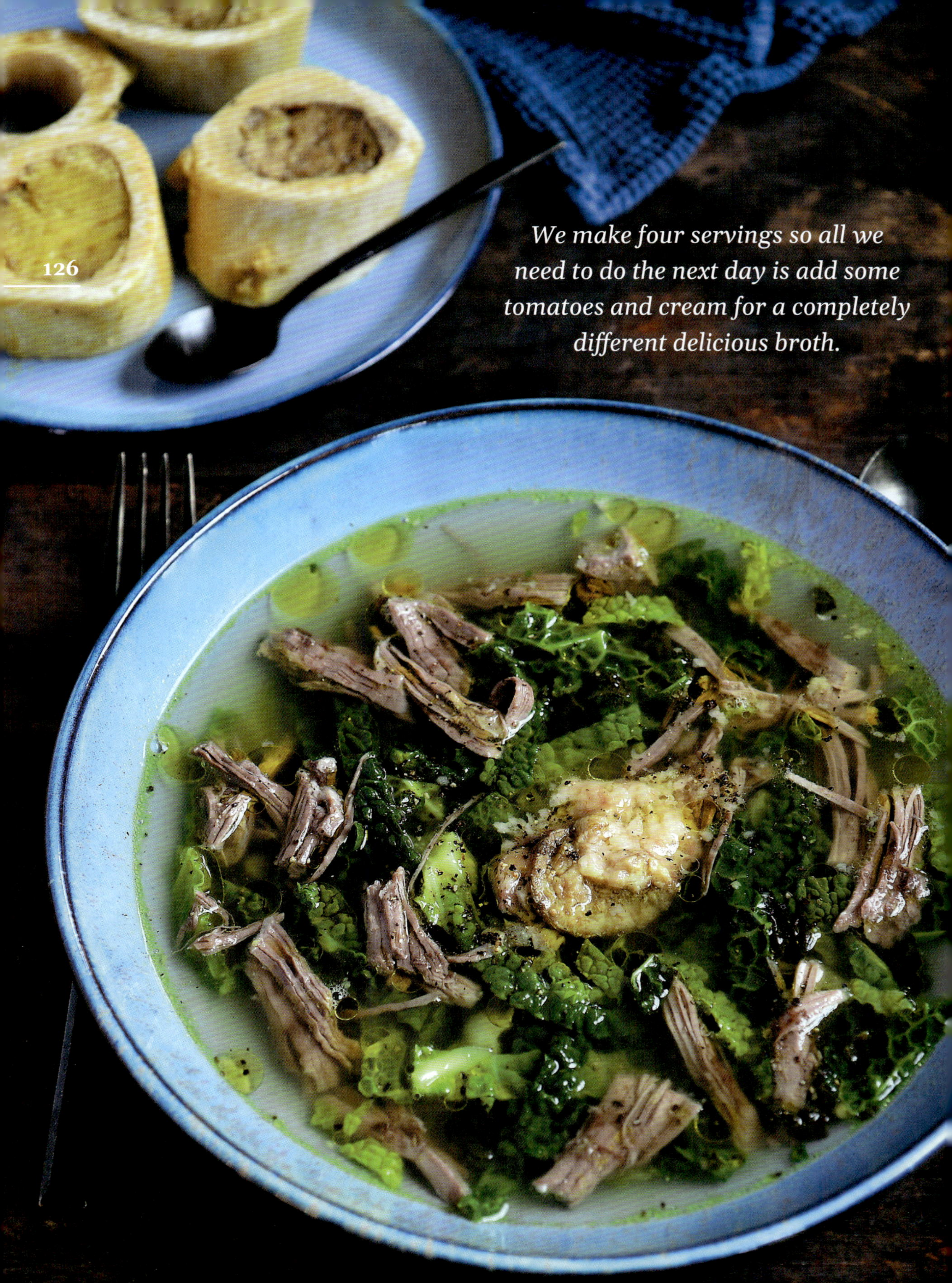

We make four servings so all we
need to do the next day is add some
tomatoes and cream for a completely
different delicious broth.

Beef broth

WITH SAVOY CABBAGE AND MARROW BONES

Ready in 3 1/2 hours - serves 4

4 marrow bones - about 2 lbs (800 g - 1 kg) beef scraps with bones
2-inch (5 cm) piece of ginger root (1 oz/30 g) - 2-inch (5 cm) piece
of turmeric root (3/4 oz/20 g)
14 oz (400 g) savoy cabbage - splash of apple cider vinegar

On day 1, we eat half of the broth + all four marrow bones.
On day 2, we eat the other half of the broth + tomatoes + cream (see p. 131)

Put the meat and the marrow bones into a large pot and add 2 to 3 quarts of water and a splash of apple cider vinegar. Slice the ginger and turmeric (you don't have to peel them) and add them to the pot. Season with plenty of sea salt and black pepper. Allow to simmer for 3 hours. Slice the savoy cabbage into thin strips (see tip). Remove the meat and the marrow bones from the broth and add the savoy cabbage. You can now pull the beef scraps apart into pieces. Throw the bones and any fatty or tough pieces away. Return the meat to the broth. Check the seasoning. Once the savoy cabbage is cooked, fill two deep dishes with the broth. Spoon the marrow out of the bones and divide evenly between the two plates. Serve immediately.
Save the rest for the next day.

Tip: savoy cabbage strips
The strips are sometimes difficult to eat. If you prefer, you can shred the savoy cabbage even more thinly, making it easier to eat. Personally, I like letting my teeth do the work.

Tip: broth
Homemade broth is exceptionally nutritious and has made a huge comeback in recent years. The longer you cook the bones, the more nutrients they release into the broth, including calcium and phosphorus. But the connective tissue is also healthy and rich in substances such as glucosamine. The collagen from the bones and the connective tissue is converted into a nutritious form of gelatin during cooking. This is highly beneficial to your gut and body. In a ketogenic diet, drinking broth is recommended because of the many minerals it contains, and the extra intake of fluids is an ideal remedy for the keto flu.

Per serving: 46.8g P (31%) / 43.2g F (66%) / 4.1g NetC (3%)

DAY 8
DINNER

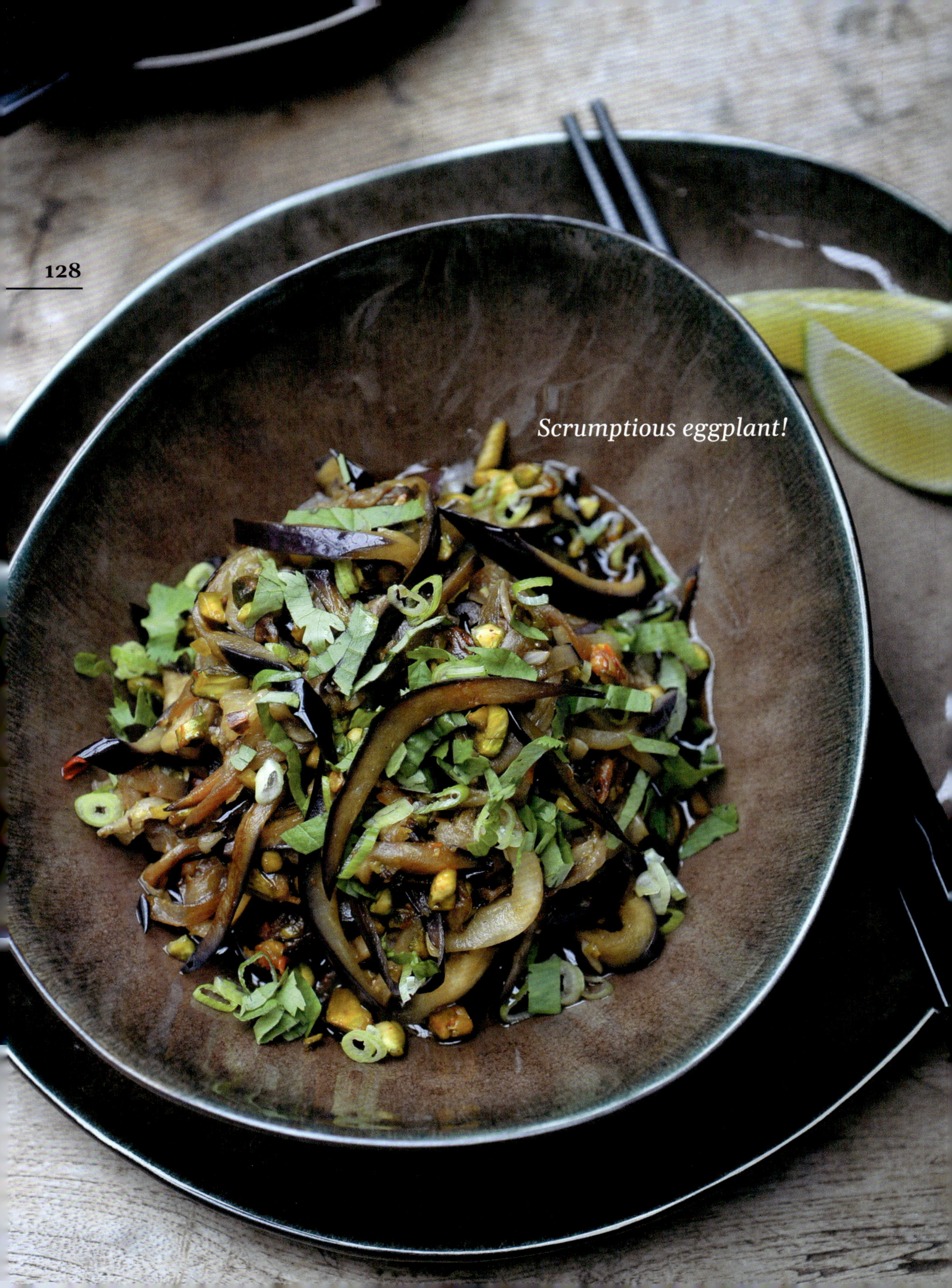

Scrumptious eggplant!

EGGPLANT
NOODLES

Preparation time: 10 minutes - cooking time: 5 minutes - serves 2

1 1/4 lb (600 g) eggplant

2 garlic cloves

1 tablespoon sambal oelek

3 1/2 oz (100 g) peanuts

2 sprigs basil

4 sprigs cilantro

5 spring onions (2 3/4 oz/80 g)

2 to 3 tablespoons olive oil (3/4 oz/20 g)

3 to 4 tablespoons roasted sesame seed oil (1 oz/30 g)

Remove the stems from the eggplants, slice vertically into thin slices and then into thin noodles.
Finely chop the garlic and combine with the sambal oelek. Heat the olive oil and sesame seed oil
in a wok.
Add the eggplant noodles to the wok and stir-fry 3-4 minutes until the noodles are tender and have
colored slightly.
Add extra oil if required. Now add the garlic-chili paste and combine.
Divide the eggplant noodles evenly between the plates and sprinkle the chopped peanuts and finely
chopped basil, coriander and spring onion over the top. Drizzle some sesame oil over the noodles
and serve immediately.

Per serving: 17.2g P (12%) / 48.9g F (78%) / 13.9g NetC (10%)

DAY 9
LUNCH

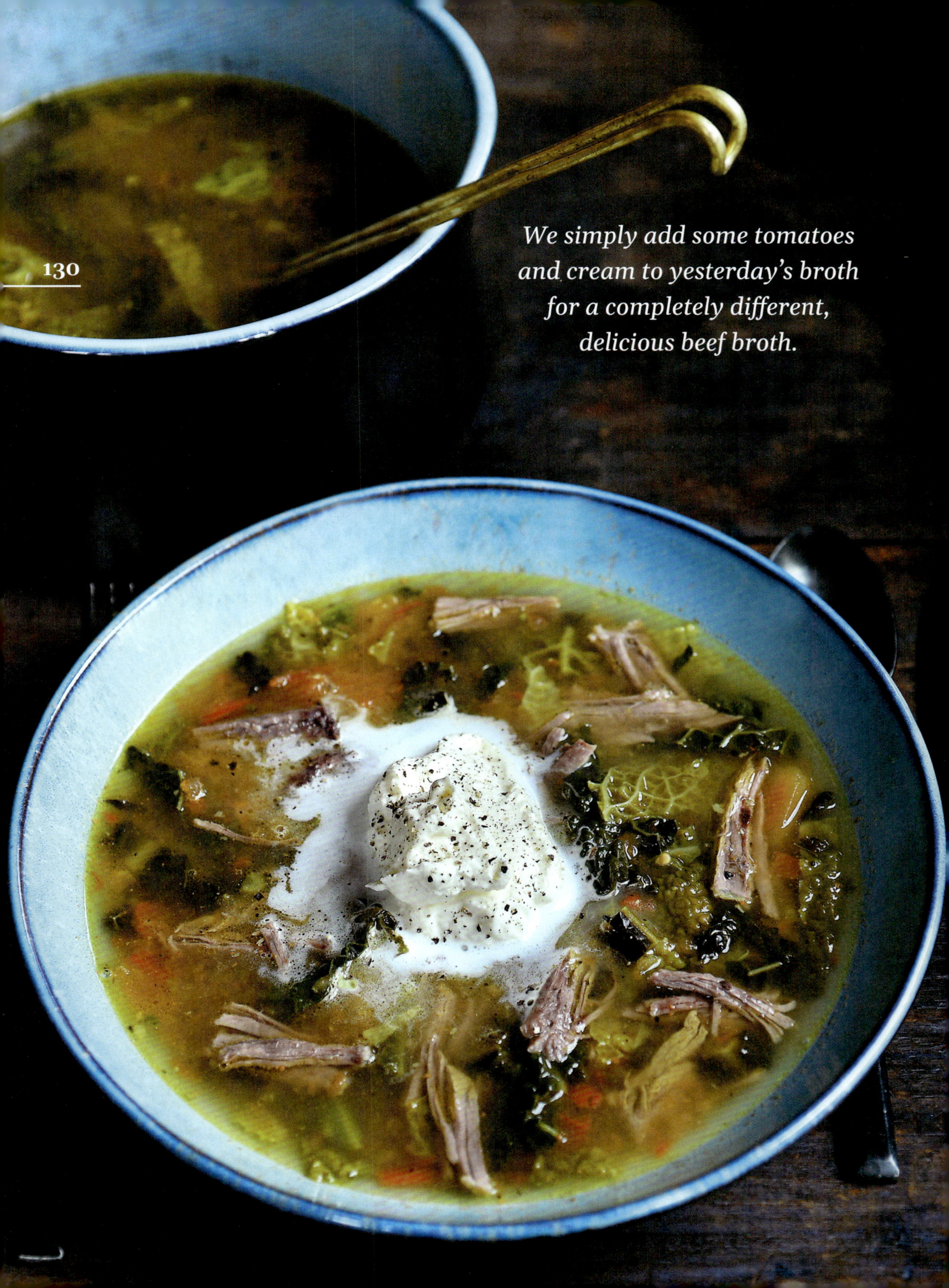

We simply add some tomatoes and cream to yesterday's broth for a completely different, delicious beef broth.

Beef broth

WITH TOMATO AND CREAM

Ready in 10 minutes - serves 2

yesterday's beef broth
10 1/2 oz tomatoes (300 g)
5 1/2 fl oz (150 ml) cream

Put the pan with the broth over the heat. Blend the tomatoes to a puree and add to the broth.
Whisk the cream until peaks form.
Once the broth is warm, divide it evenly between two bowls and spoon a dollop of whipped cream
in the middle. Season with black pepper.

Per serving: 50g P (29%) / 50g F (65%) / 10g NetC (6%)

DAY 9
DINNER

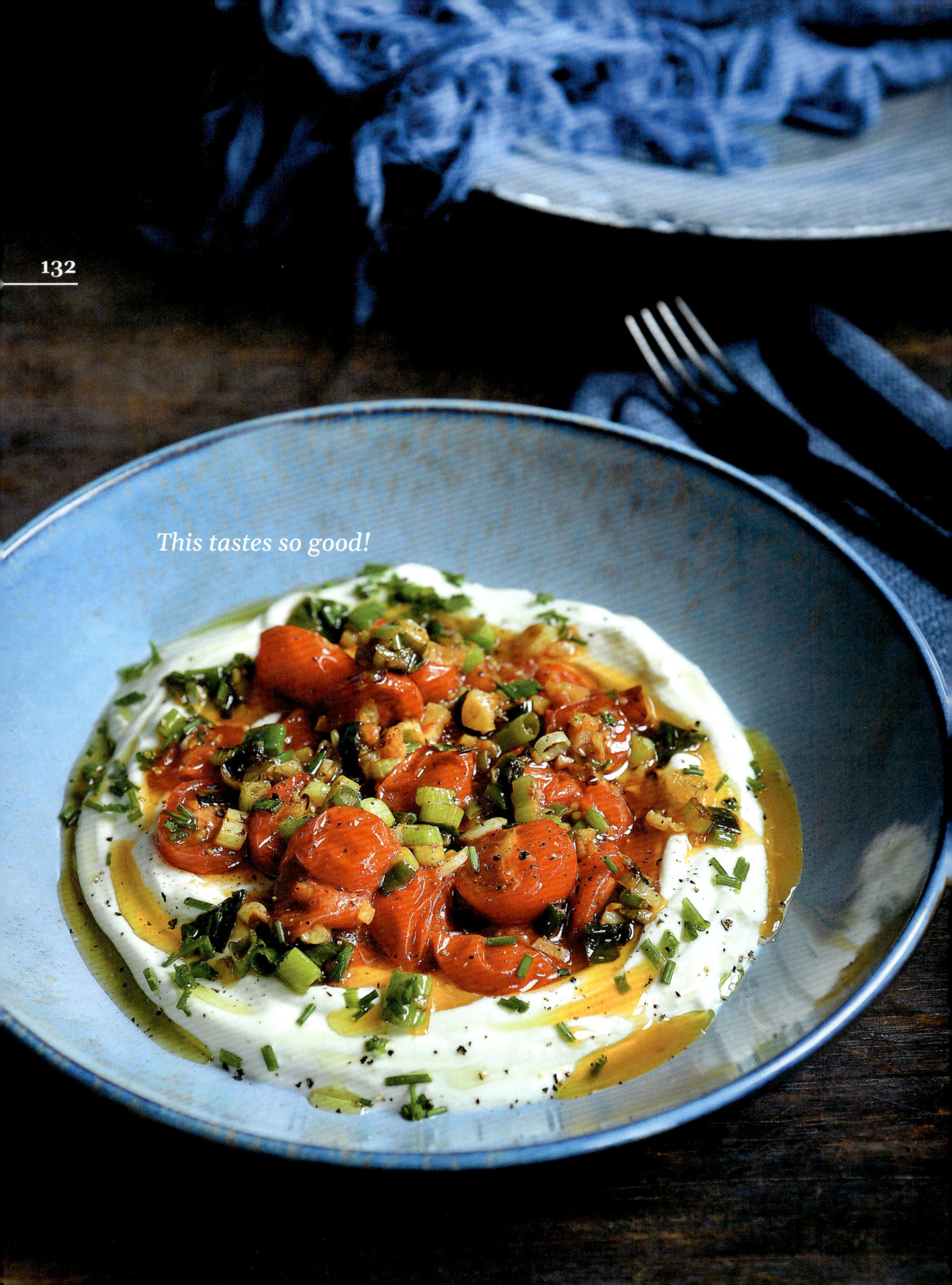
This tastes so good!

Creamy cheese

WITH ROAST TOMATOES AND FRESH HERBS

Ready in 15 minutes - serves 2

14 oz (400 g) full-fat, fresh cheese (quark cheese)

20 cherry tomatoes

2 spring onions

2 garlic cloves

chives

2 oz (60 g) olive oil

Slice the tomatoes in half. Slice the spring onions into rings and finely chop the garlic. Sauté them in 1 1/2 oz (40 g) of the olive oil. Let the vegetables cook for about 5 minutes, stirring occasionally. Season with salt and black pepper. Divide the fresh cheese evenly between the plates and make a well in the middle with a spoon. Divide the vegetables evenly and spoon them over the cheese. Garnish with the finely chopped chives, olive oil and black pepper

Tip: keto
Choose full-fat, fresh cheese with as few carbs as possible and don't overdo the cherry tomatoes. If you have trouble reaching ketosis, I recommend not exceeding these quantities. If you are already fully fat-adapted, you might be able to eat a larger serving.

Per serving: 17.5g P (13%) / 48.5g F (79%) / 10.6g NetC (8%)

DAY 10
BREAKFAST

Avocado

WITH MUSHROOMS AND DRY-CURED HAM

Preparation time: 15 minutes - cooking time: 20 minutes - serves 2

10 1/2 oz (300 g) dry-cured ham - 2 ripe avocados

7 oz (200 g) mushrooms - lemon juice

2 sprigs rosemary - 1 1/2 oz (40 g) olive oil

Extra: 2 cooking rings

Preheat the oven to 350 °F (180 °C).

Place the slices of dry-cured ham on a broiler pan and put the pan in the oven for about 7 minutes.

Remove the rosemary leaves from the stems. Chop the mushrooms into tiny pieces and sauté them together with the rosemary in a hot pan with olive oil. Season with salt and pepper.

Slice the avocados in half and remove the pit. Spoon the soft flesh out of the skin and transfer to a plate. Sprinkle a little lemon juice over the avocado (to prevent discoloration) and mash with a fork to a homogenous whole. Season with salt and pepper.

Keep a couple of mushroom pieces aside to garnish and combine the rest with the mashed avocado pulp. Season with salt and pepper.

Remove the ham from the oven and put the slices between two layers of paper towels.

Put a cooking ring on each plate and spoon the avocado mixture into the ring.

Remove the cooking ring. Tear the ham up into large pieces and place them on top of the avocado mixture.

Per serving: 45.9g P (21%) / 75.2g F (77%) / 4.1g NetC (2%)

DAY 10
LUNCH

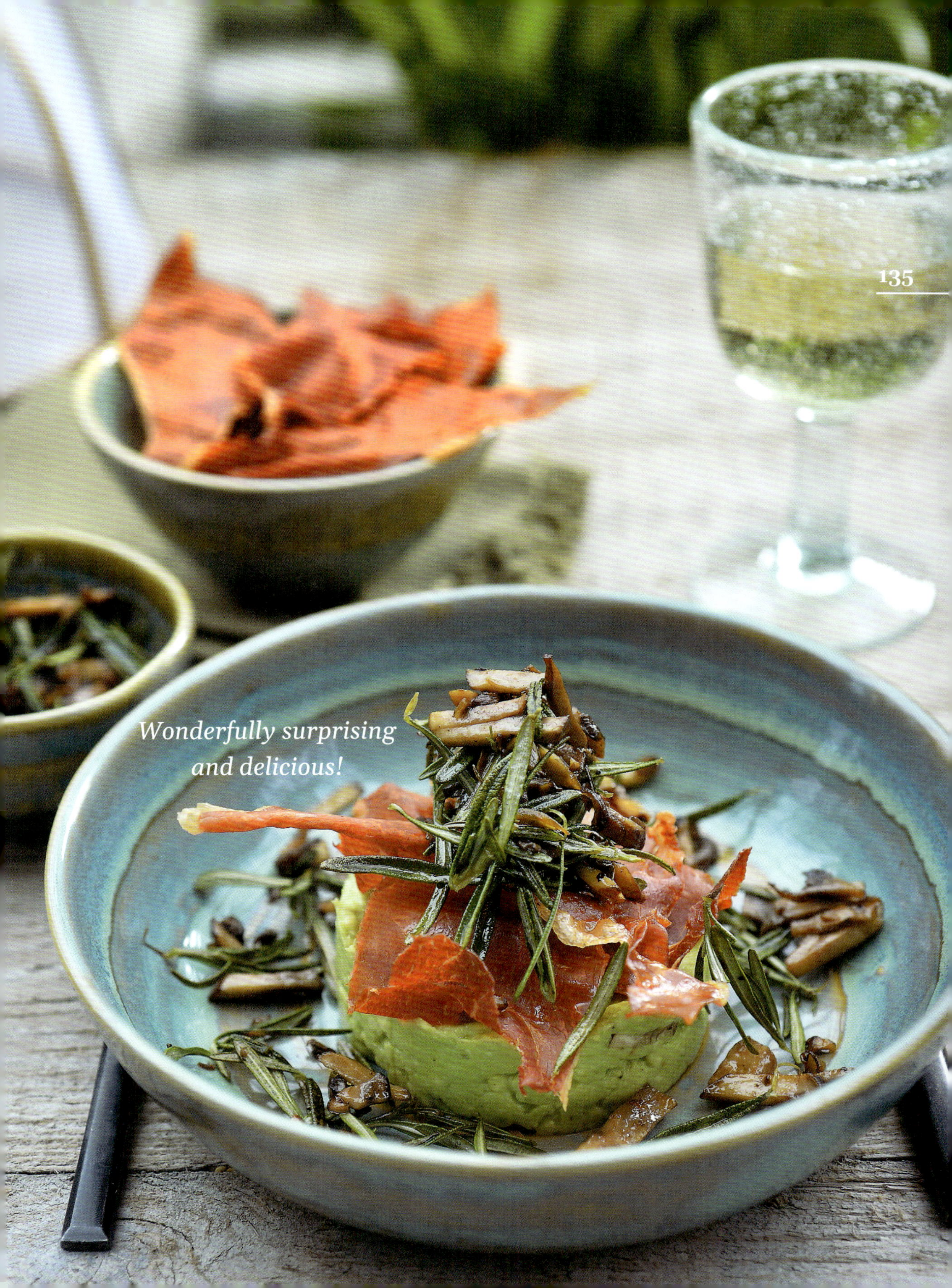
Wonderfully surprising
and delicious!

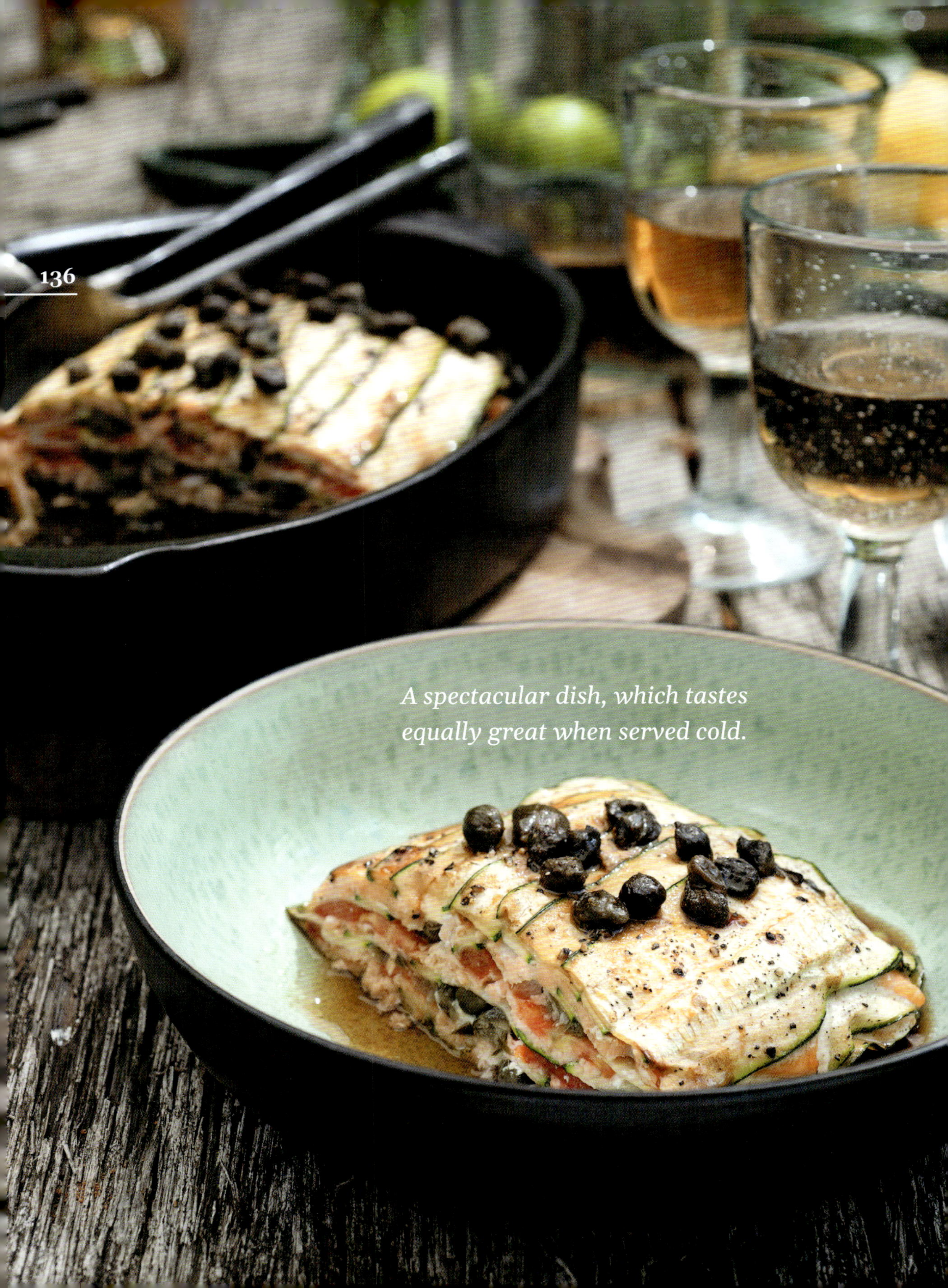
A spectacular dish, which tastes
equally great when served cold.

Zucchini

WITH SMOKED SALMON, SOY SAUCE AND CAPERS

Preparation time: 10 minutes - cooking time: 20 minutes - serves 4

4 zucchini (2 lbs/1kg)

1 1/4 lb (600 g) smoked salmon slices

2 tomatoes (10 1/2 oz/300 g)

3 1/2 oz (100 g) capers

light soy sauce

3 1/2 oz (100 g) olive oil

We make twice the quantity needed. Half the recipe is for tonight, while the other half will be eaten cold the next day. This dish might even taste better cold :-).

Slice the tomato into wafer-thin slices. Thinly slice the zucchini with a vegetable peeler. Coat the zucchini slices with olive oil.
Arrange a few zucchini slices in a baking dish, place a few slices of smoked salmon on top and spoon some capers over the salmon. Cover with another layer of the zucchini, a layer of salmon, a layer of tomatoes (there is only one layer with tomatoes, otherwise your dish will be too soggy) and some capers and finish with a layer of zucchini and some capers. Pour a generous splash of olive oil and soy sauce over the top and season with pepper only (the soy sauce and smoked salmon are salty enough).
Bake the dish in the oven at 350 °F (180 °C) for 20 minutes.
After 10 minutes, spoon the sauce that has built up on the sides over the rest of the dish. Just before serving, drizzle a bit of the sauce over the top.

Per serving: 34.1g P (26%) / 39.2g F (69%) / 6.7g NetC (5%)

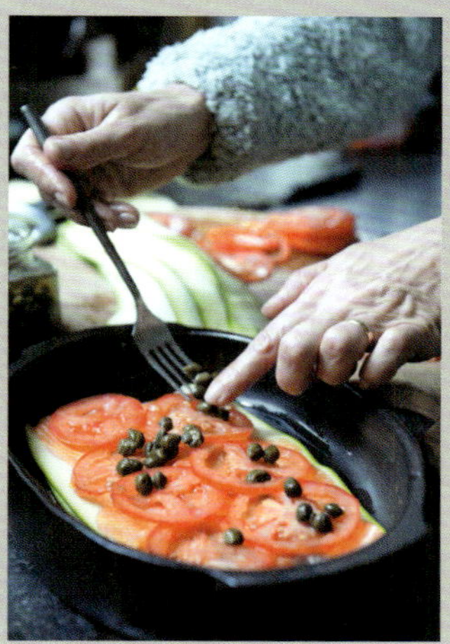

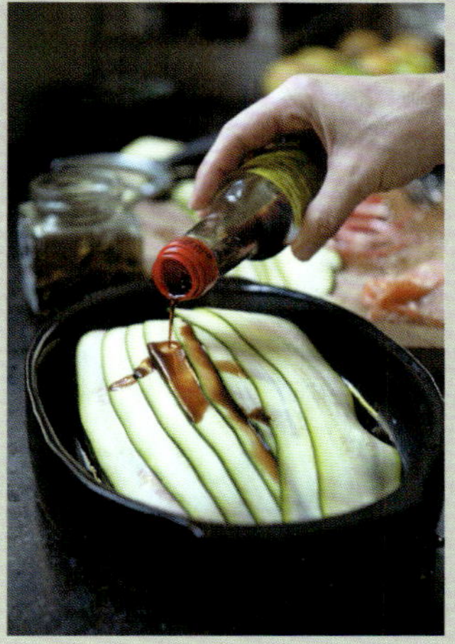

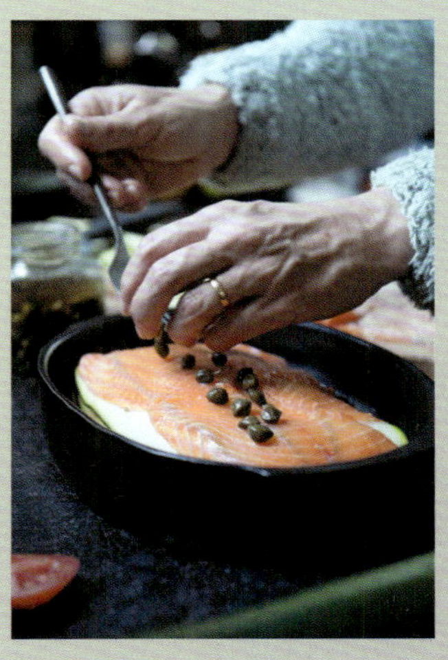

DAY 10
DINNER

DAY 11 BREAKFAST
The same as day 3. Seeds and nuts with full-fat sour cream, see p. 89

Zucchini

WITH SMOKED SALMON, SOY SAUCE AND CAPERS

We eat the other half of yesterday's dish as a cold lunch.
I personally think this dish tastes even better when
served cold.
Also ideal for when you're on the go.

Tip: freezing
You can also freeze this dish, so you will always have a
keto dish on hand for those unexpected moments.

Per serving: 33g P (29%) / 34g F (67%) / 5g NetC (4%)

DAY 11
LUNCH

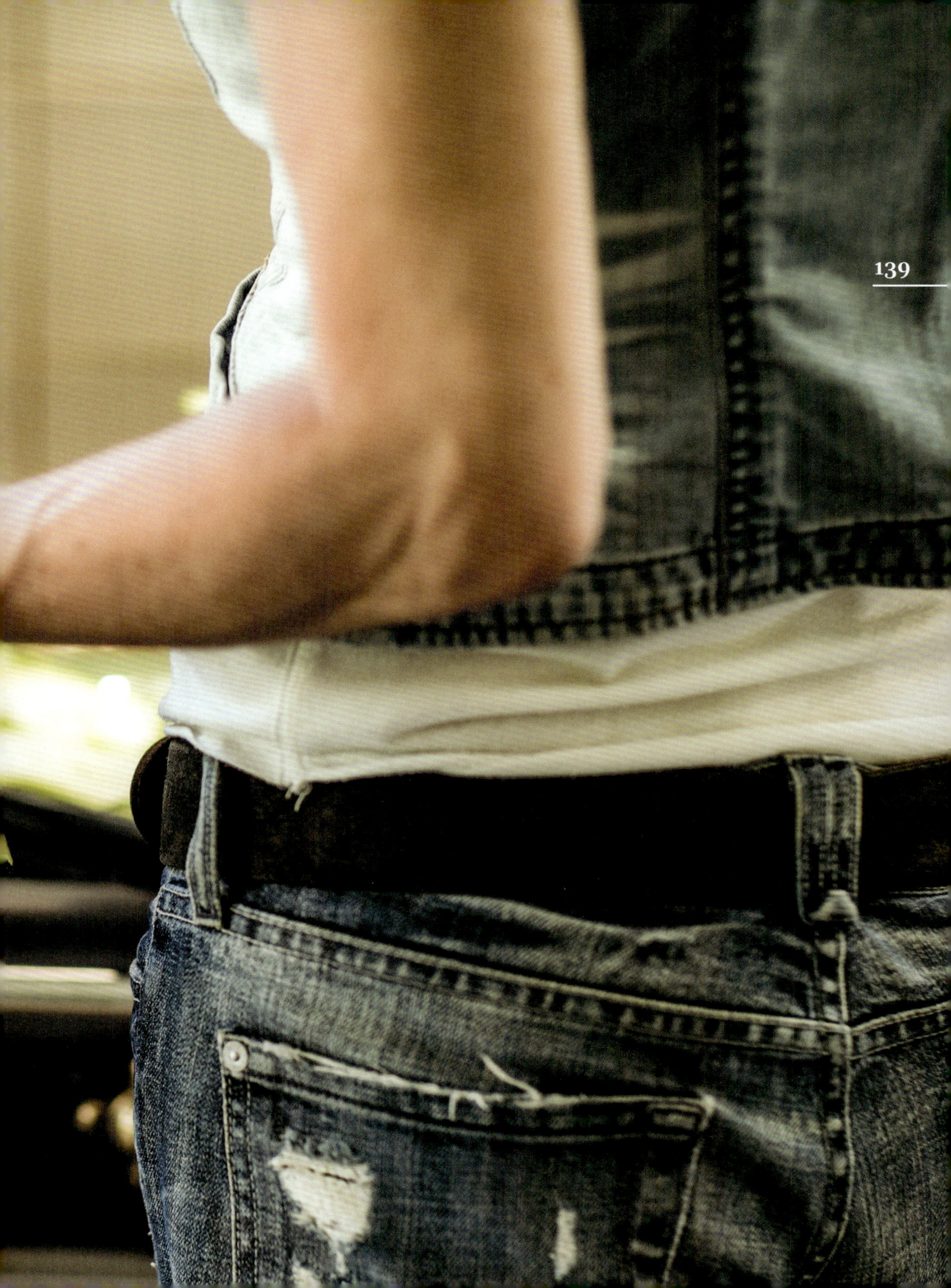

Cod

WITH SPINACH, TOMATO, EGGPLANT AND PISTACHIO PESTO

Preparation time: 15 minutes - cooking time: 25 minutes - serves 2

1 cod fillet (10 1/2 oz/300 g)

10 1/2 oz (300 g) fresh spinach

7 oz (200 g) tomatoes

7 oz (200 g) eggplant

1 1/2 oz (40 g) basil

1 1/2 oz (40 g) pistachios

1 clove of garlic

1 3/4 oz (50 g) olive oil

This is one of those dishes that always makes my husband happy. He loves spinach and cod and the herbed crust adds something special to the fish. The eggplant and tomato give the spinach its creamy texture.

Quarter the tomatoes, remove the liquid and seeds from the inside, and dice the flesh.
Dice the eggplant into small cubes. Finely chop the garlic. Drizzle the olive oil in a pan and add the diced eggplant. Stir-fry the eggplant for two minutes before adding the diced tomato. Stir-fry for another 2 minutes, then add the garlic and spinach. Let the vegetables simmer for about 20 minutes, stirring regularly. Add some extra oil if the mixture becomes too dry. Season with salt and pepper.
Put the nuts, basil, salt and pepper and 5 tablespoons of oil in a blender and blend to form a thick tapenade. Add some extra oil if needed.
Slice the cod lengthwise in two and place the two halves in a baking dish.
Spoon the tapenade over the two halves, rub it into the fish and place the dish in a hot oven at 350 °F (180 °C) for about 15 minutes. Arrange the fish on top of the vegetables.

Per serving: 34.2g P (28%) / 35.6g F (65%) / 8.1g NetC (7%)

DAY 11
DINNER

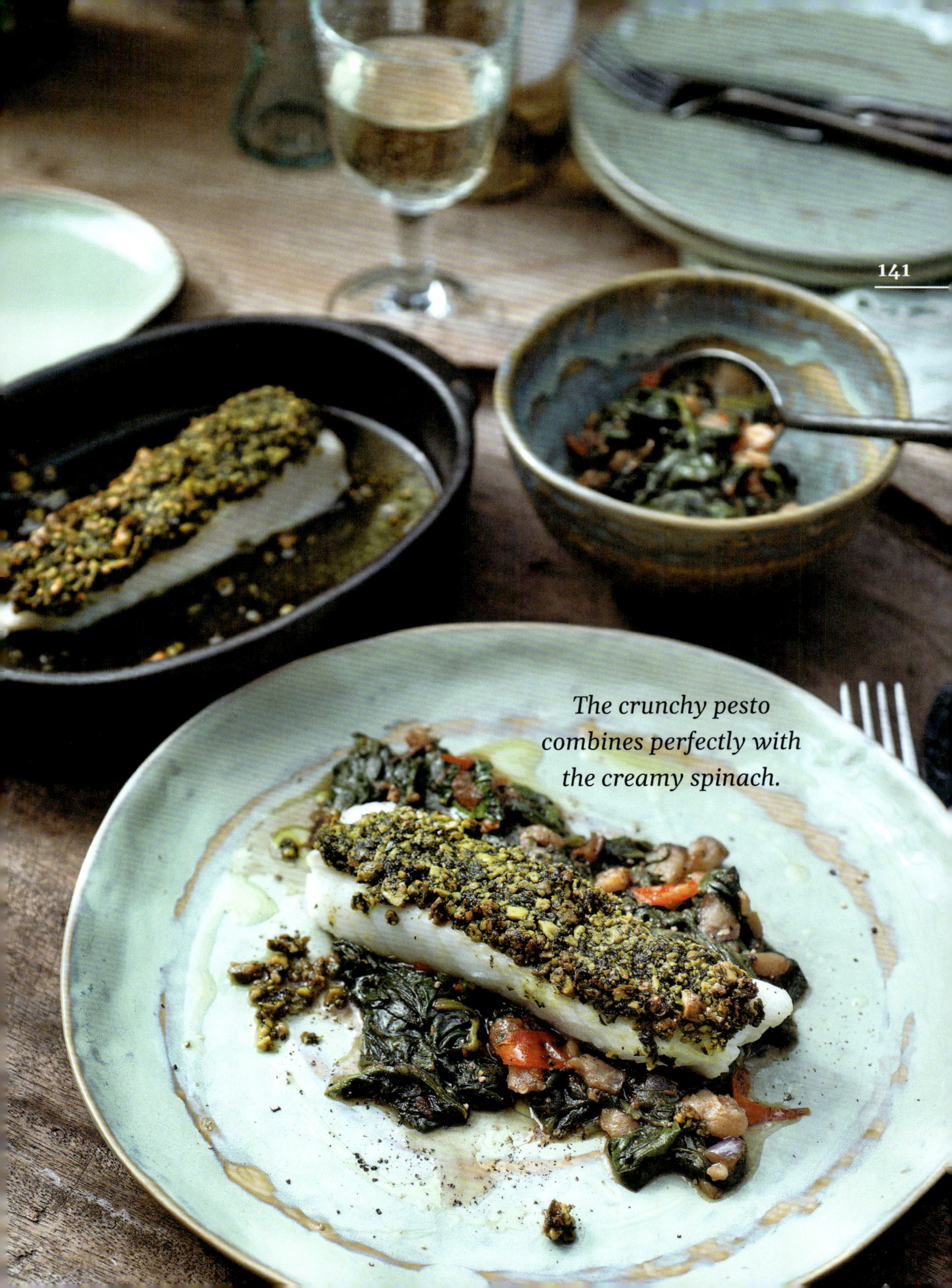

The crunchy pesto
combines perfectly with
the creamy spinach.

DAY 12 BREAKFAST
The same breakfast as day 4.
Roasted nuts and seeds with
full-fat sour cream, see p. 97

142

Spinach soup

WITH SLICED ALMONDS
AND A BOILED EGG

Preparation time: 20 minutes - cooking time: 15 minutes - serves 2

a little over 1 lb (500 g) spinach

1 small onion (1 1/2 oz/40 g)

3 1/2 fl oz (100 ml) cream

2 eggs

a handful of sliced almonds (1 oz/30 g)

1 oz (30 g) olive oil (4 tablespoons)

A simple soup can taste heavenly, and this creamy
spinach soup is no exception. It's an ideal dish for when
you're not feeling particularly hungry and still need a
boost of vitamins, minerals and healthy fats.

Finely chop the onion and sauté in olive oil. Add the
spinach and let it wilt. Remove some of the spinach for
the garnish and set aside.
Add the cream, season with salt and pepper and cook
for a little bit longer. Blend the soup.
Boil the eggs for 5 minutes.
Roast the sliced almonds for about 6 minutes in an oven
preheated to 350 °F (180 °C).
Divide the soup evenly between two bowls, place the
spinach and peeled eggs in the soup and garnish with
the sliced almonds.

Per serving: 15.3g P (12%) / 51.2g F (86%) / 2.8g NetC (2%)

DAY 12
LUNCH

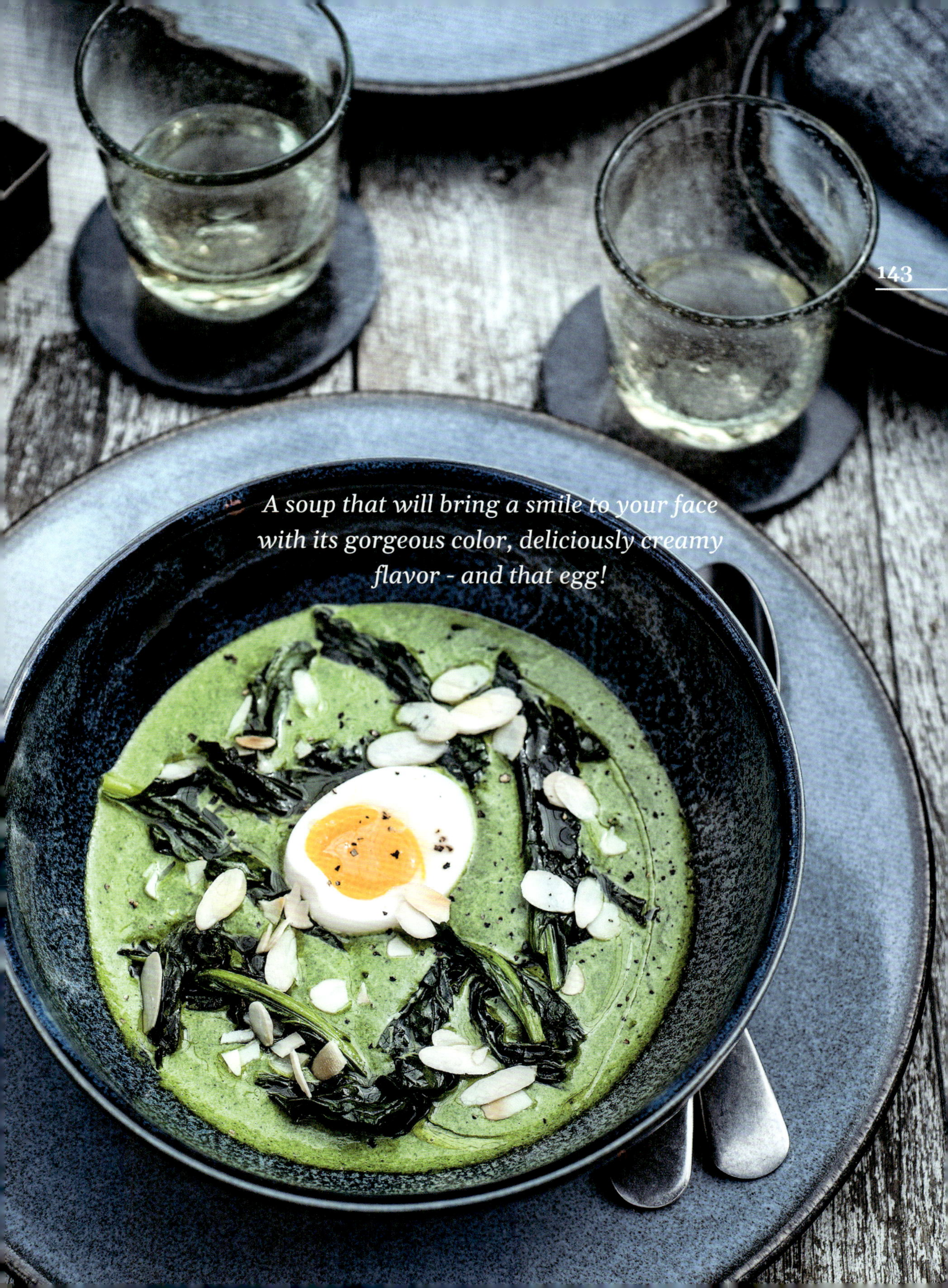
A soup that will bring a smile to your face
with its gorgeous color, deliciously creamy
flavor - and that egg!

Vegetables

WITH HAZELNUTS

Ready in 30 minutes - serves 2

4 celery stalks (7 oz/200 g)

1/3 green bell pepper (3 1/2 oz/100 g)

1/4 red bell pepper (2 oz/60 g)

1 large tomato (5 oz/150 g)

2 garlic cloves

1/3 onion (1 3/4 oz/50 g)

2 oz (60 g) hazelnuts

1 tablespoon turmeric (1/2 oz/15 g)

chili seasoning to taste (optional)

1 3/4 fl oz (50 ml) olive oil

tender leafy greens (arugula, flat-leaf parsley) to serve

Coarsely chop the vegetables and finely chop the garlic. Put the garlic in a pan, sauté first the celery for a few minutes and then add the bell peppers, tomato, onion, and garlic. Let the vegetables cook for about 6 minutes.

Add 7 fl oz (200 ml) water and the hazelnuts, cover, and let the mixture stew over low heat for 15 minutes.

Add the turmeric, plenty of black pepper, salt, and some chili seasoning if you like your dishes spicy. Let the mixture cook a little longer.

Serve with some tender leafy greens.

Per serving: 8.8g P (7%) / 45.3g F (87%) / 7.1g NetC (6%)

DAY 12
DINNER

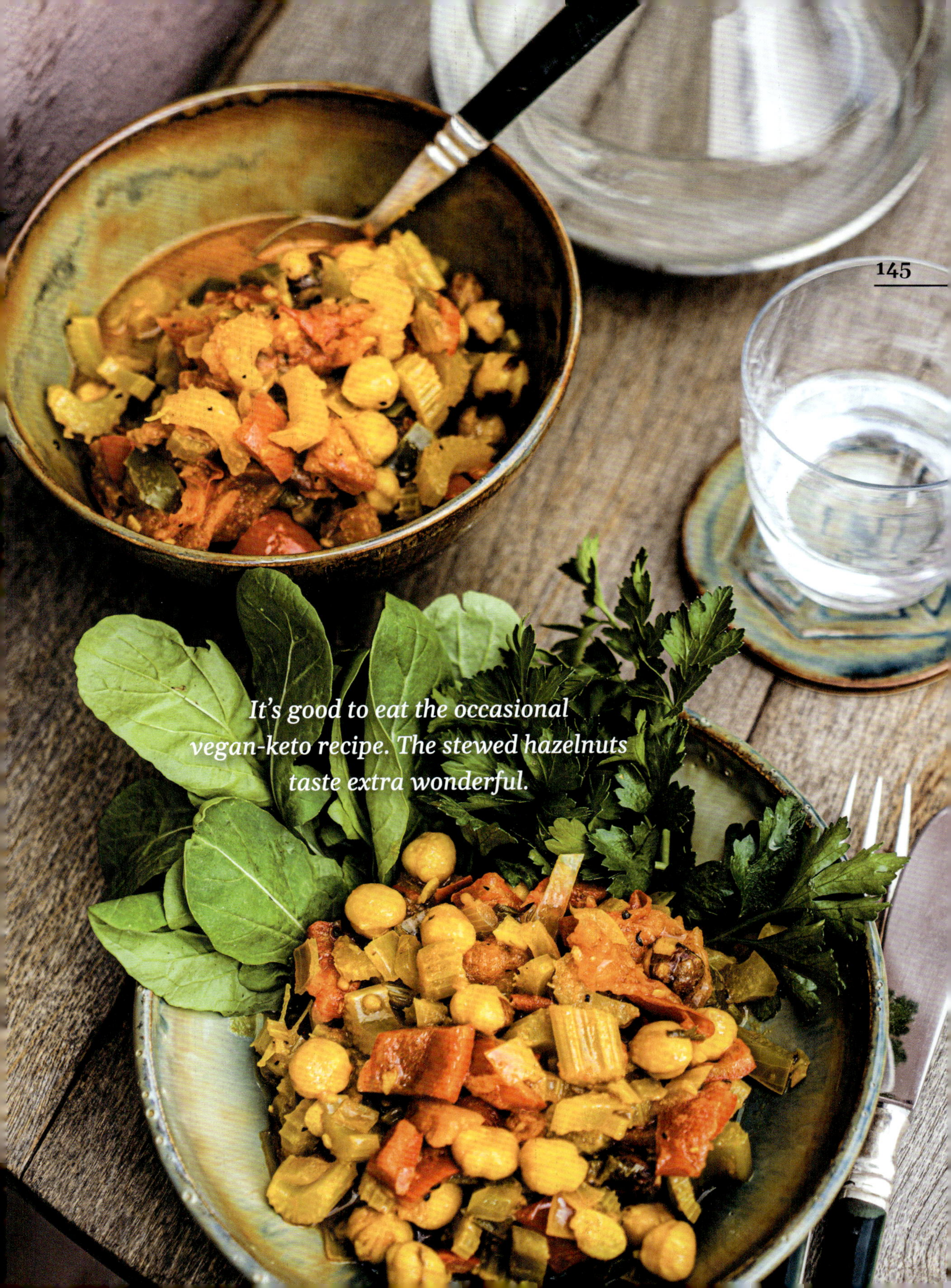
It's good to eat the occasional
vegan-keto recipe. The stewed hazelnuts
taste extra wonderful.

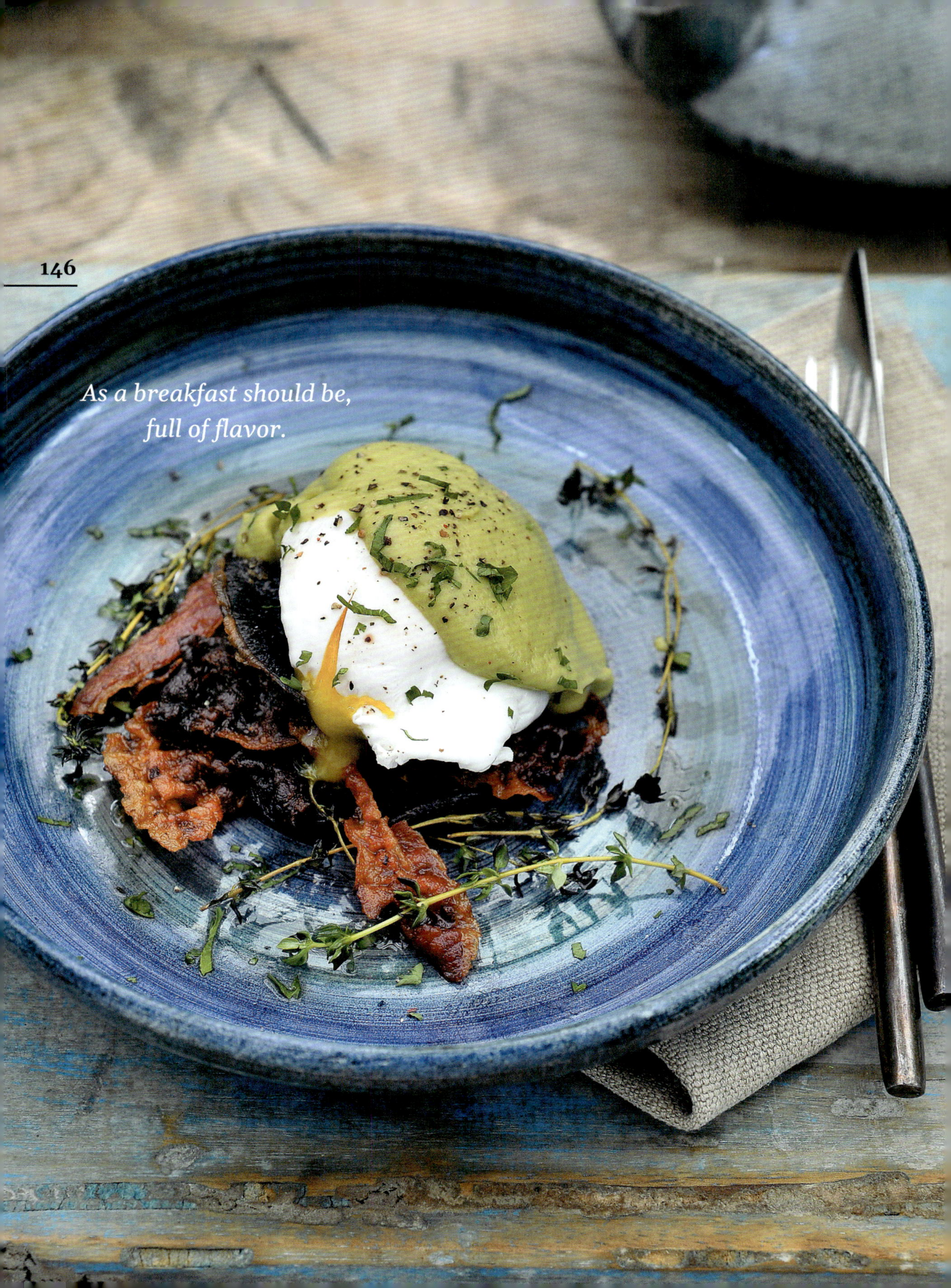
As a breakfast should be,
full of flavor.

Brown mushrooms

WITH POACHED EGG AND AVOCADO SAUCE

Preparation time: 30 minutes - cooking time: 20 minutes - serves 2

10 1/2 oz (300 g) large brown mushrooms (cremini, portobella)

1 avocado

juice of 1/2 lemon

pinch cayenne pepper

2 market-fresh, free-range eggs

7 oz (200 g) bacon

white vinegar

chives

1 1/2 oz (40 g) olive oil

Preheat the oven to 350 °F (180 °C).

Remove the stalks from the mushrooms and drizzle them with olive oil. Season with freshly ground pepper and sea salt and put them together with the bacon in a baking dish. Bake in the oven for about 15 minutes.

Bring 5 1/2 fl oz (150 ml) salted water to a boil together with the lemon juice, a generous splash of olive oil and the cayenne pepper. Spoon the flesh from the avocado into a food processor or blender. Add the boiling water and blend to a smooth sauce.

Bring a pan with water and a generous splash of vinegar to the boil. Break each egg into a cup. Stir the water in a circular motion, creating a whirlpool, and carefully slide the eggs into the water, one by one. Keep the water at a gentle boil and poach the eggs for 3 minutes.

Remove the mushrooms from the oven, arrange the poached eggs on top and finish with the bacon and the avocado sauce. Sprinkle some finely chopped chives over the top.

Per serving: 28.5g P (17%) / 60.4g F (81%) / 3.8g NetC (2%)

DAY 13
BREAKFAST

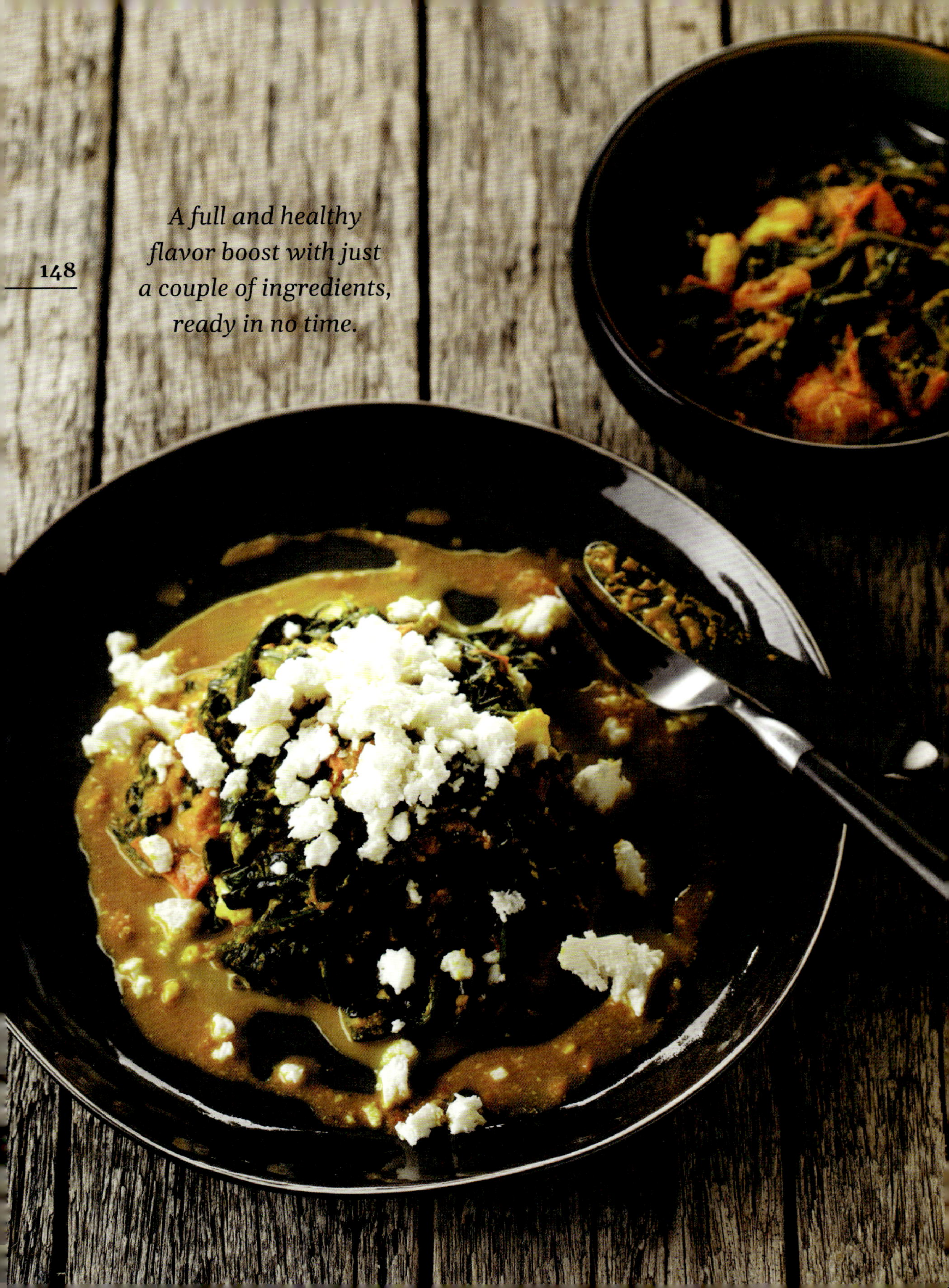

A full and healthy
flavor boost with just
a couple of ingredients,
ready in no time.

Spinach

WITH TOMATO, TURMERIC AND FETA

Preparation time: 3 minutes - cooking time: 15 minutes - serves 2

10 1/2 oz (300 g) spinach

10 1/2 oz (300 g) feta

14 oz (400 g) tomatoes

1 teaspoon turmeric

1 1/2 oz (40 g) olive oil

Chop the tomatoes into large chunks. Remove only the white, hard core. Add a generous splash of olive oil to a pan and cook the tomatoes in the oil. After 5 minutes, add the fresh spinach and another splash of olive oil. Once the spinach has wilted, stir in the turmeric and plenty of black pepper. Crumble half the feta over the vegetables. Stir well so the feta partially melts.
Serve on plates and crumble the rest of the feta over the top. Finish with black pepper.

Tip: salt
Use salt sparingly; feta already contains plenty of salt.

Per serving: 27.7g P (17%) / 56.6g F (78%) / 7.7 g NetC (5%)

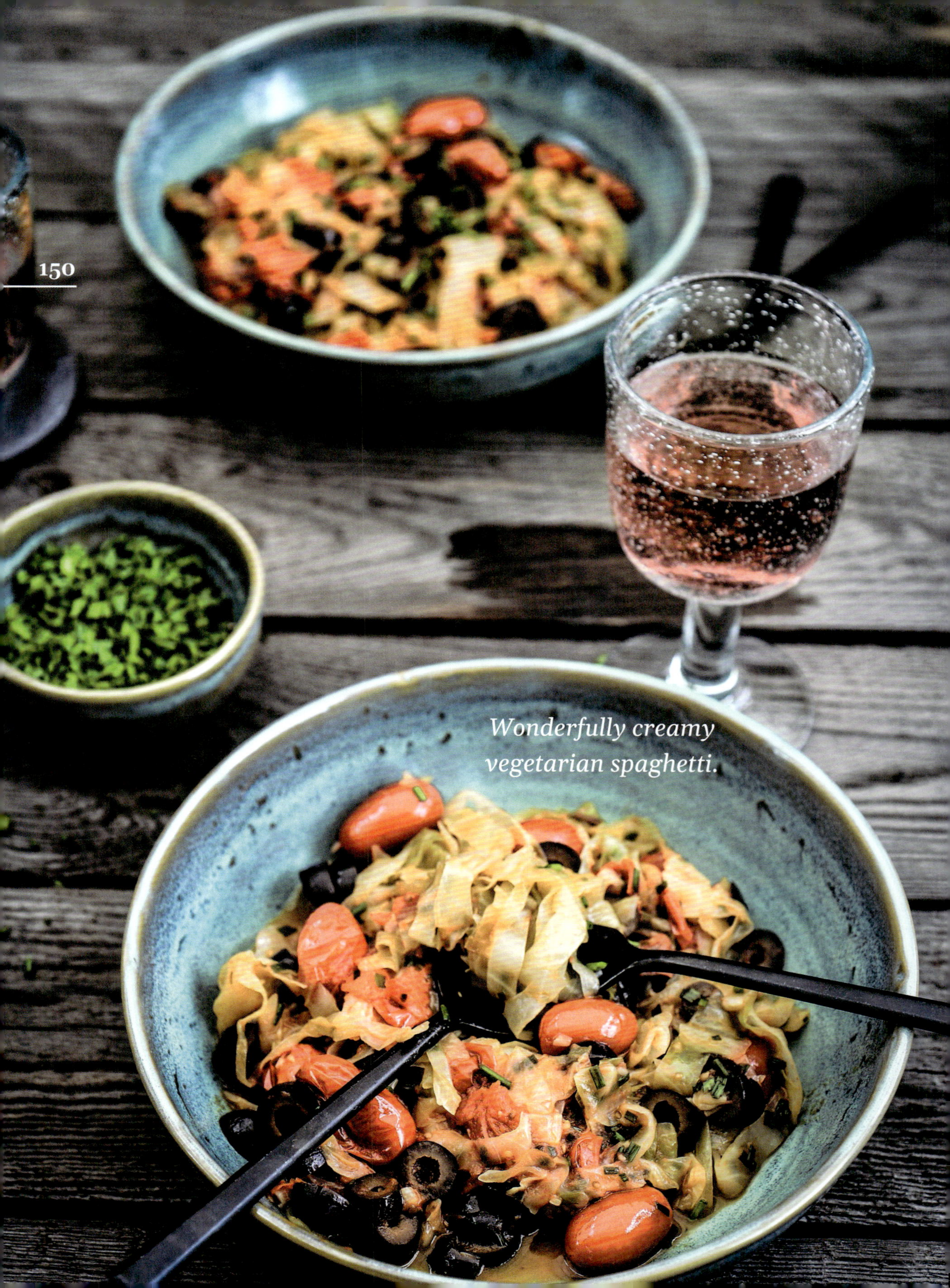
Wonderfully creamy
vegetarian spaghetti.

Pointed cabbage spaghetti

WITH TOMATOES AND OLIVES

Ready in 15 minutes - serves 2

14 oz (400 g) pointed cabbage

7 oz (200 g) tomatoes

7 oz (200 g) pitted olives (your favorite olives)

1 bunch of chives (3/4 oz/20 g)

2 garlic cloves

1 3/4 oz (50 g) coconut oil

Slice the pointed cabbage into long strips. Start at the top of the cabbage to get nice, long, strips.
Halve three-quarters of the tomatoes and finely chop the garlic.
Melt the coconut oil in a pan and add the pointed cabbage, tomatoes and garlic.
Add half a glass of water, cover the pan, and cook the cabbage for about 5 minutes. Make sure that
the cabbage doesn't burn. Add a little coconut oil if necessary.
Meanwhile, slice the olives into rings and finely chop the chives. Add the olives, the remaining
tomatoes and the chives to the cabbage, but keep some of the chives aside to garnish. Stir everything
well, season with salt and pepper and cook for another two minutes. Serve in a deep plate or pasta
bowl and garnish with some chives.

Per serving: 8.4g P (8%) / 40.7g F (85%) / 7.3g NetC (7%)

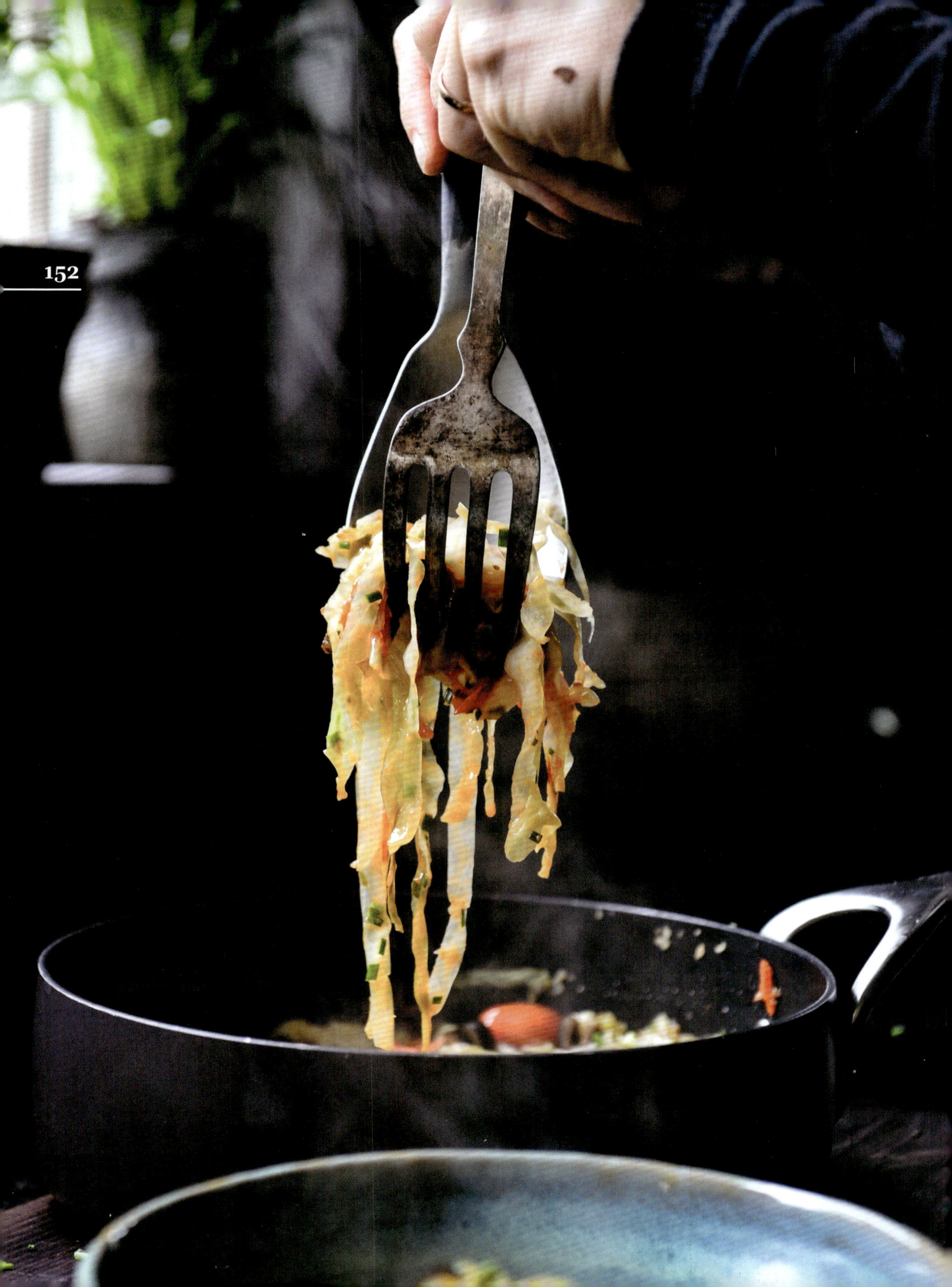

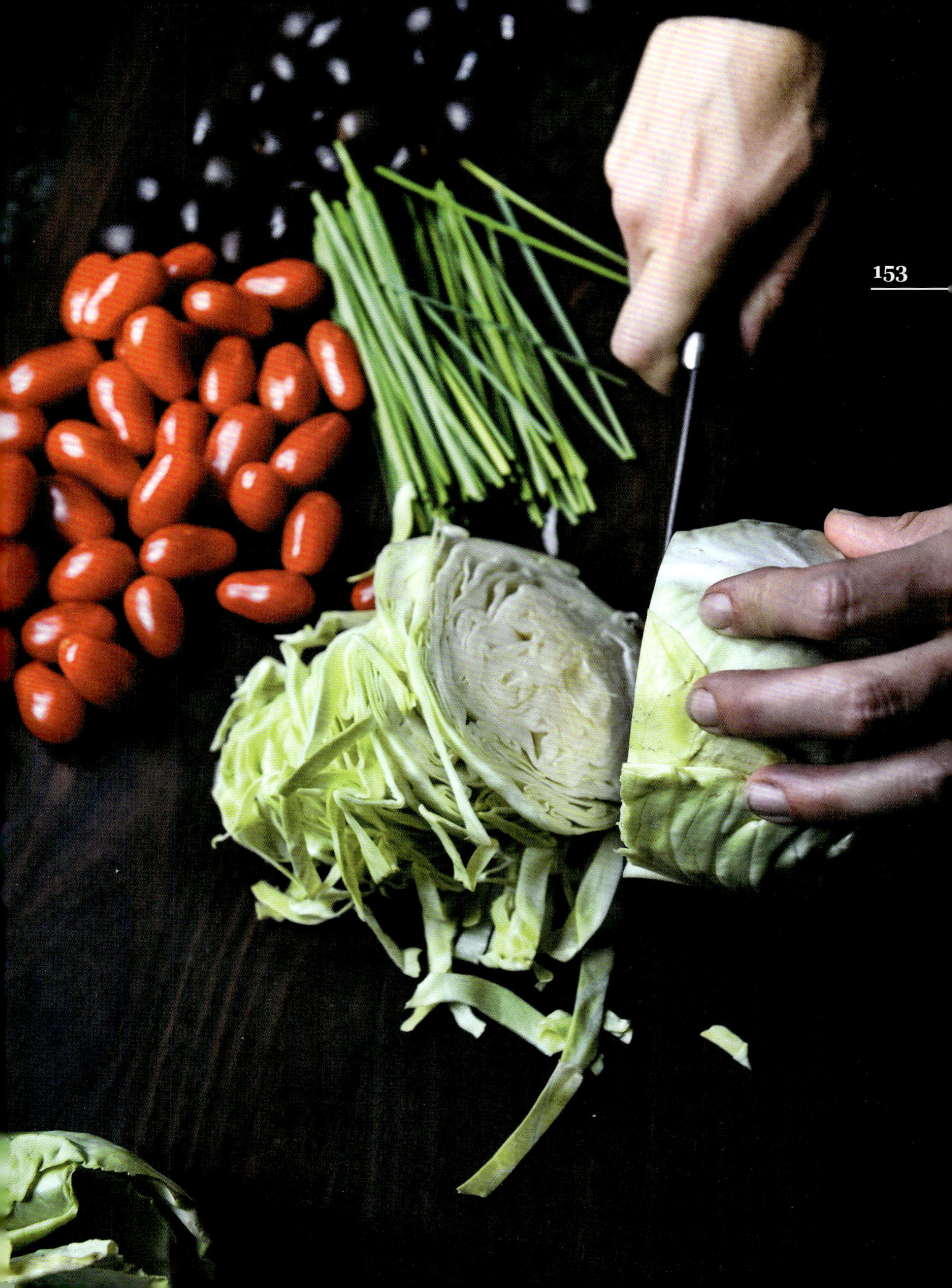

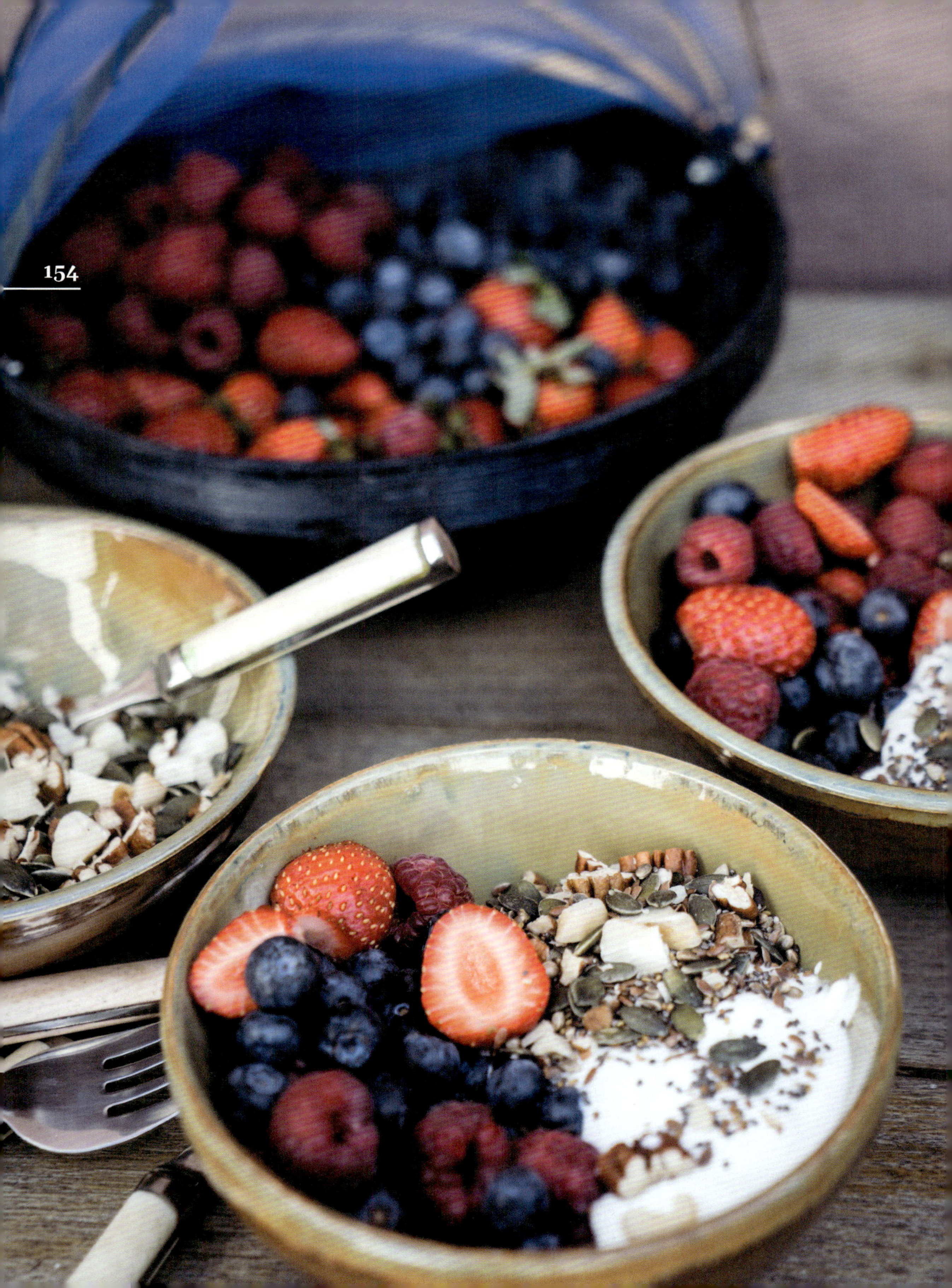

Greek yogurt

WITH BERRIES AND SEEDS

Ready in 10 minutes - serves 2

10 1/2 oz (300 g) Greek yogurt

7 oz (200 g) strawberries - 7 oz (200 g) raspberries

3 1/2 oz (100 g) blueberries

Mixed seeds and nuts: 4 1/2 oz (120 g) (= 2 servings)

1/2 oz (15 g) flaxseed - 1/2 oz (15 g) pumpkin seeds

1/2 oz (15 g) chia seeds - 1/2 oz (15 g) hemp seeds

1 oz (30 g) pecans - 1/2 oz (15 g) Brazil nuts

1/2 oz (15 g) macadamia nuts

This breakfast contains more carbs, but after two weeks of a ketogenic diet, your body should be able to process it. Read the tip.

Put the Greek yogurt in a bowl and serve with fruit, seeds and nuts.

Tip: keto
This breakfast contains more carbs than other breakfasts, but after two weeks of eating keto, most of you should be fully fat-adapted. This is the moment to test whether you can have more carbs. This breakfast doesn't kick me out of ketosis, but it's different for everyone. Try it, enjoy it, and measure your ketone levels to see what happens. Consider it a treat after two weeks of keto. Congratulations!

Per serving: 22.5g P (14%) / 48.5g F (70%) / 25.2g NetC (16%)

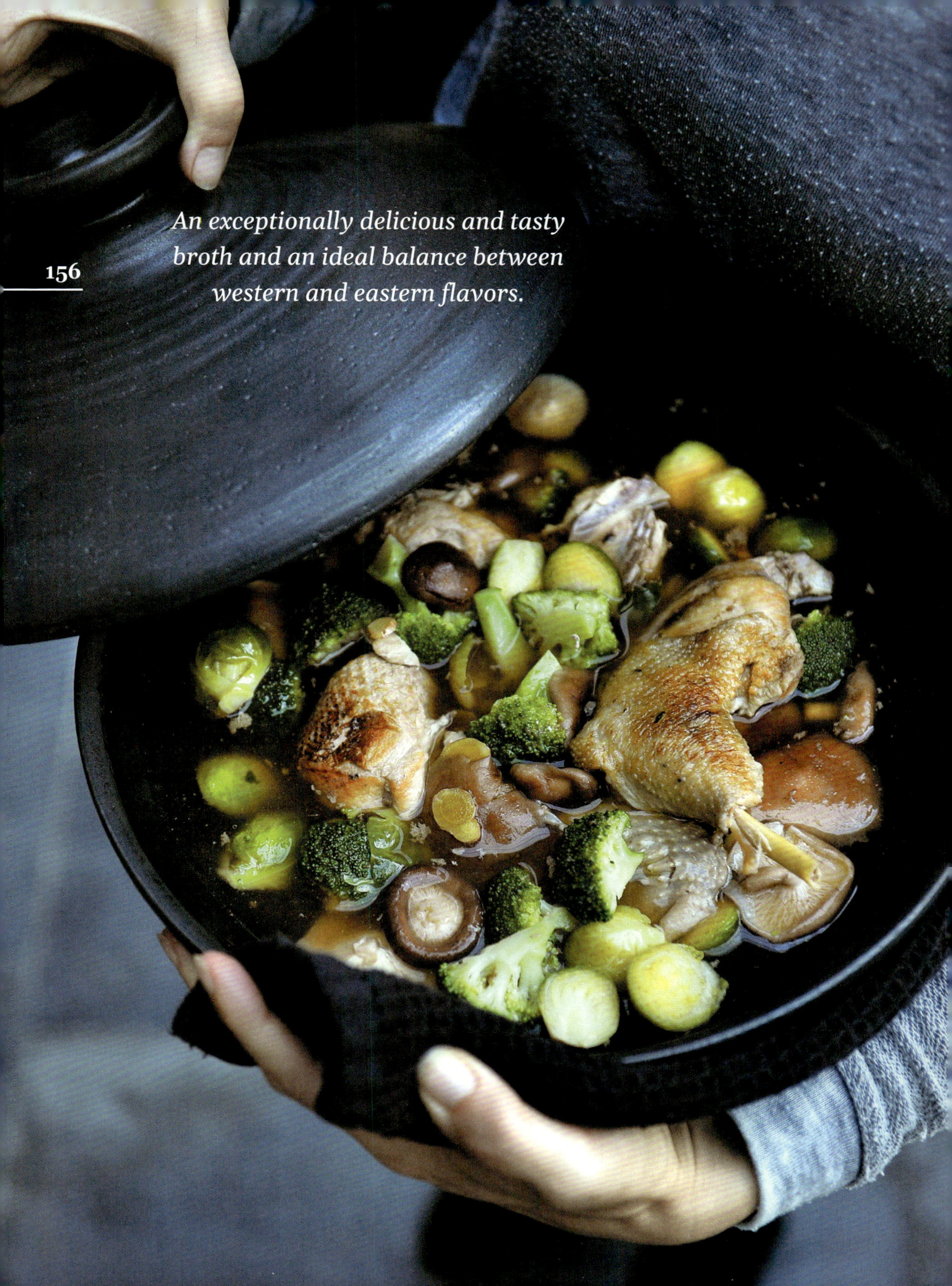

An exceptionally delicious and tasty
broth and an ideal balance between
western and eastern flavors.

Cooked chicken

WITH VEGETABLES

Preparation time: 15 minutes - cooking time: 1 hour and 20 minutes - serves 2

1 organic chicken (2 lbs/1 kg) - 9 oz (250 g) brown mushrooms
20 brussels sprouts (7 oz/200 g) – 1/2 head of broccoli (10 1/2 oz/300 g)
3 tablespoons light soy sauce (3/4 oz/20 g) - 2 cloves of garlic
1-inch (2 cm) piece of ginger root (3/4 oz/20 g) - 2 oz (60 g) butter

Chop the chicken into pieces (or have your butcher do it for you), brown the chicken pieces in the butter and then pour water over the pieces until the meat is just submerged. Simmer gently for about 45 minutes. Meanwhile, clean and trim the vegetables. Slice the broccoli into florets and halve the brussels sprouts. Finely chop the ginger and slice the garlic.
Once the chicken has cooked for 45 minutes, add the ginger and garlic. Season with salt, pepper and soy sauce. After 1 hour of cooking, add the mushrooms. After another 15 minutes of cooking, add the brussels sprouts (see tip) and the broccoli and let the vegetables cook for about 5 minutes. The chicken will have cooked for a total of 1 hour and 20 minutes.
Serve in deep dishes.

Tip: Brussels sprouts
I like my brussels sprouts *al dente*, in which case 5 minutes of cooking time should be enough. If you prefer softer brussels sprouts, cook them a little longer.

Tip: chicken broth
Who makes their own broth nowadays? I can tell you that it's a wonderfully satisfying experience. This is what cooking is all about. It brings out that instinctive, primitive wisdom in us, because we all know from the generations before us that broth made from bones can be highly restorative and nutritious. Broth strengthens our immune systems, heals our guts, digests easily and provides us with nutrients that are easy to absorb. Commercially produced bouillon cubes and powders are simply no match for home-brewed broth ...

Per serving: 49.9g P (32%) / 42.8g F (62%) / 8.5g NetC (6%)

DAY 14
DINNER

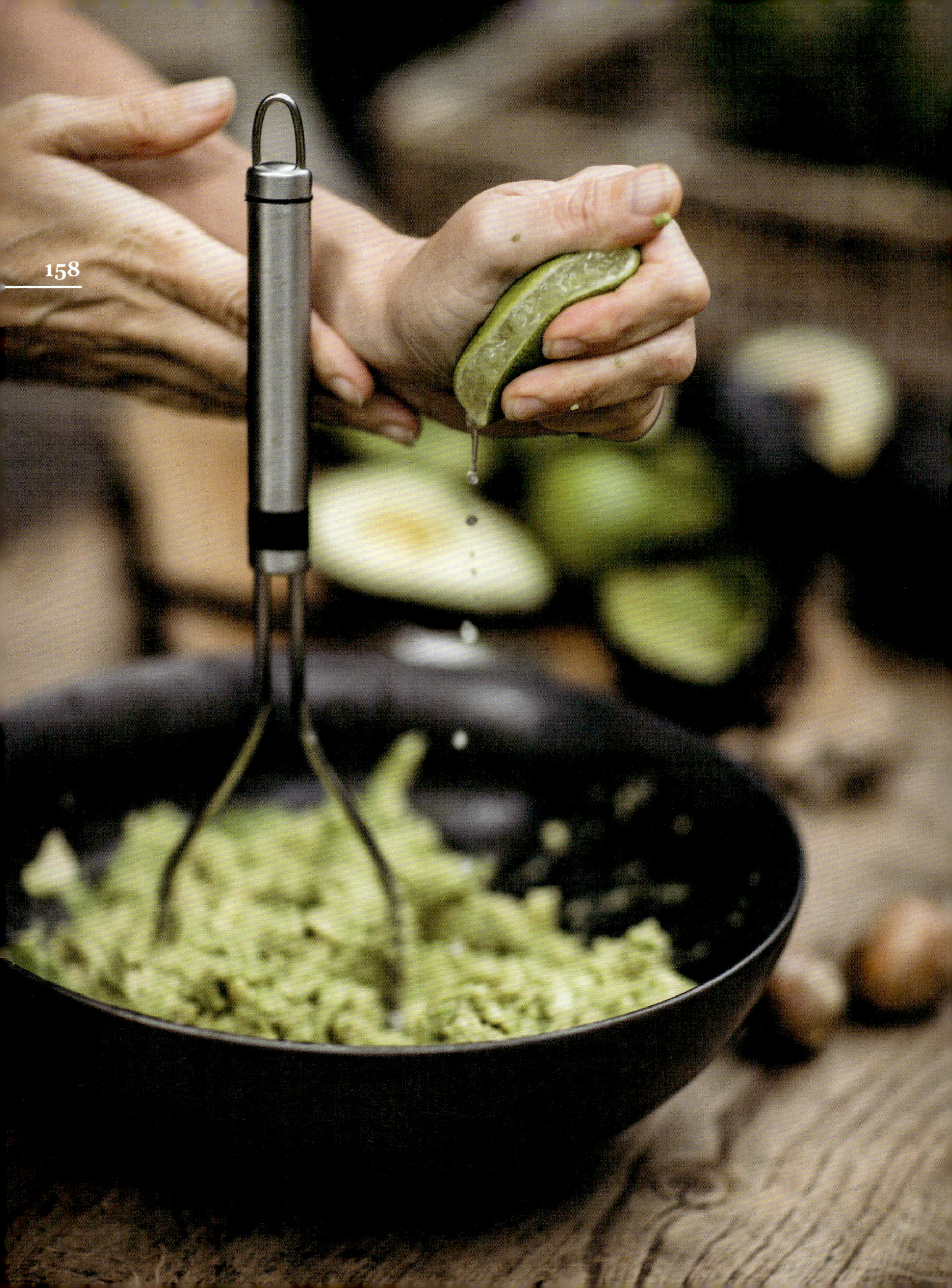

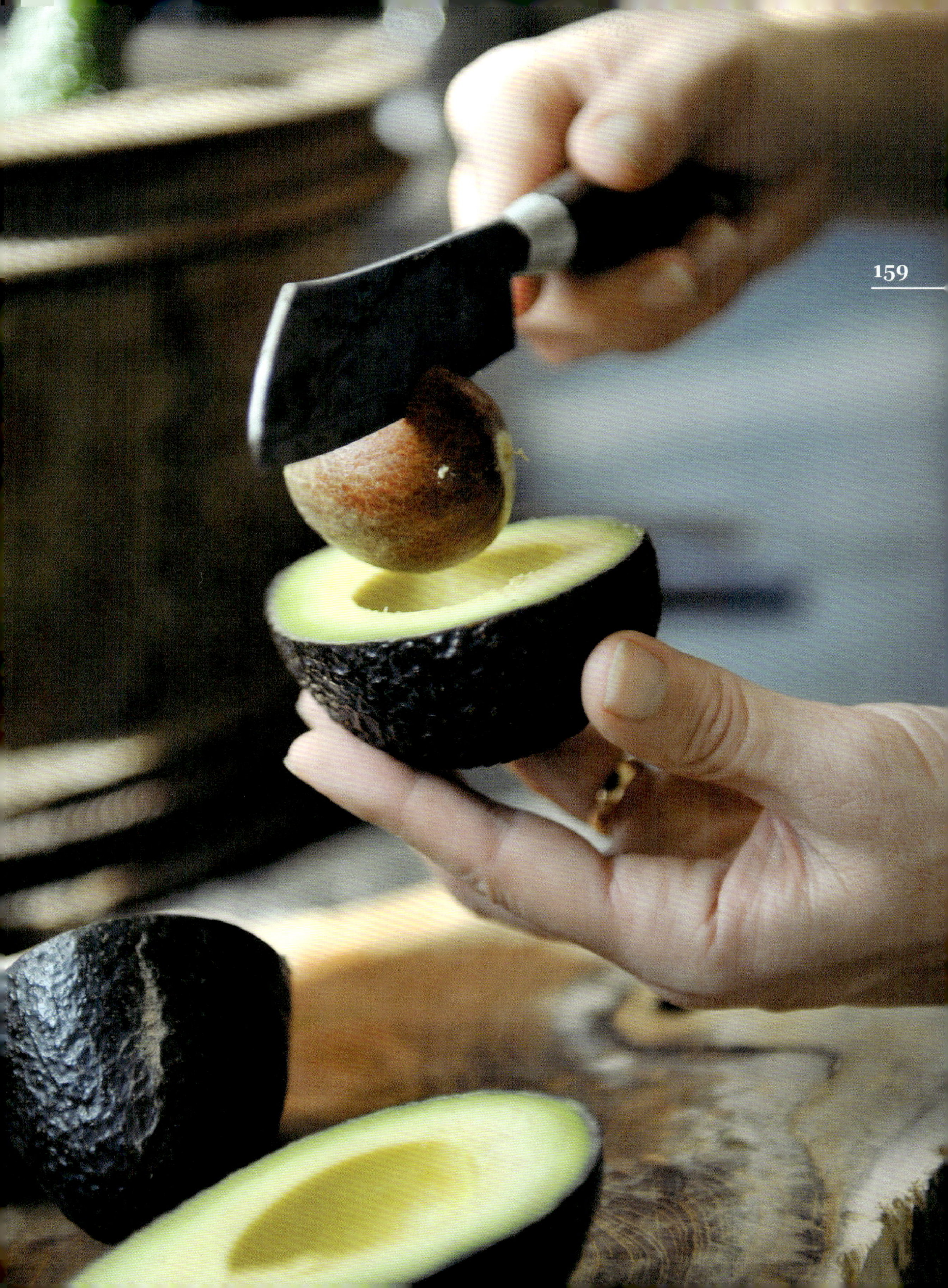

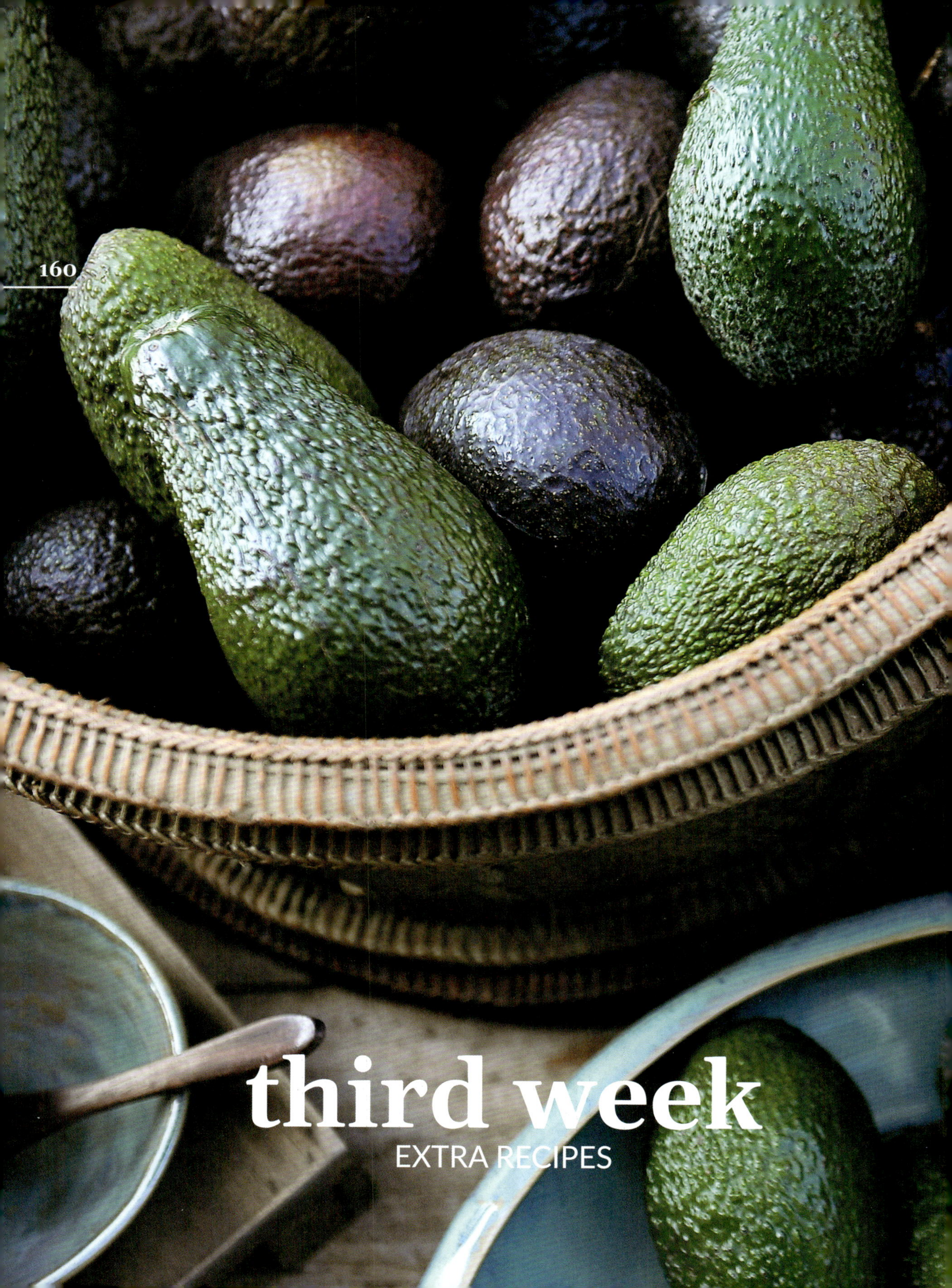

third week
EXTRA RECIPES

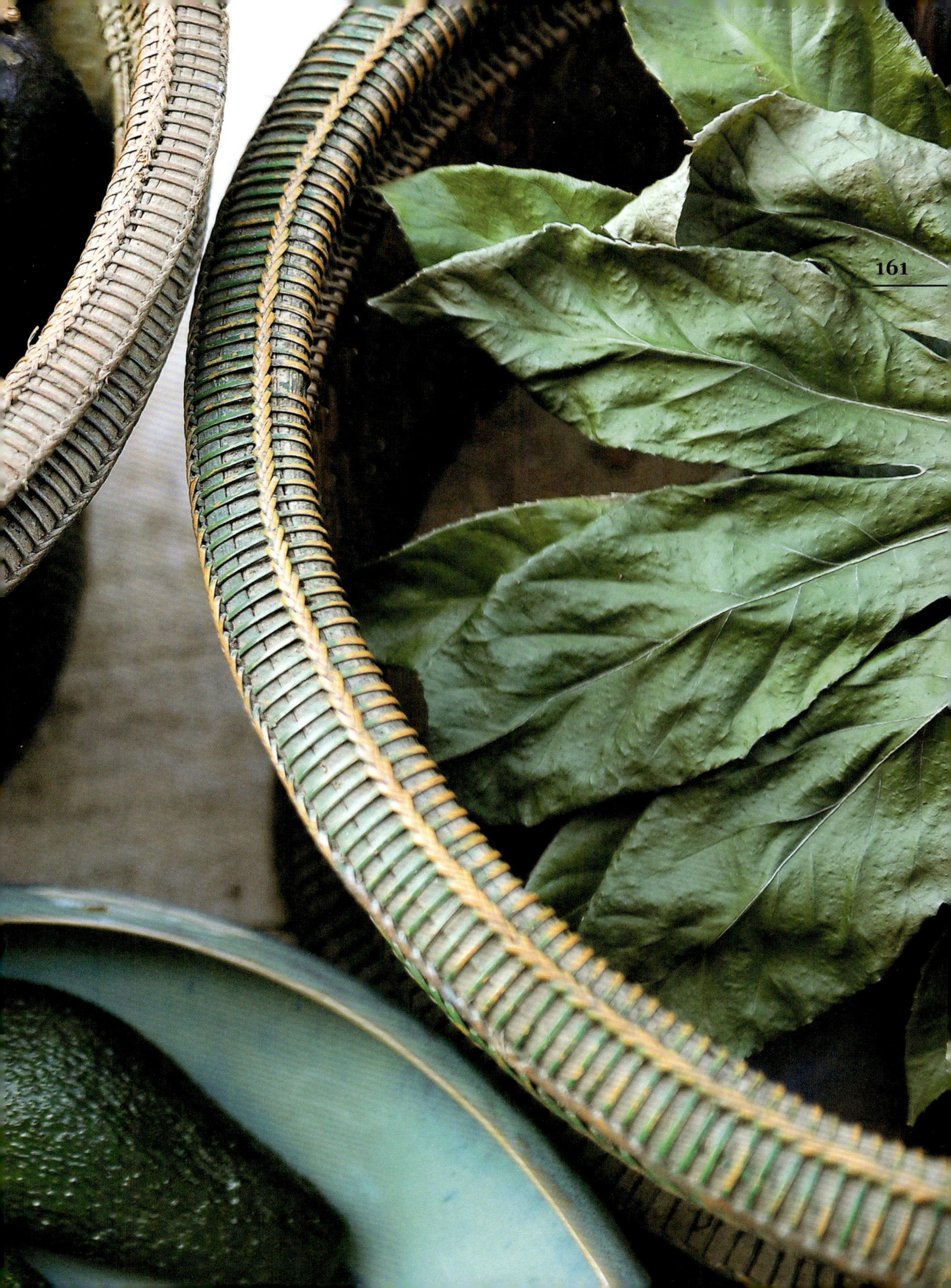

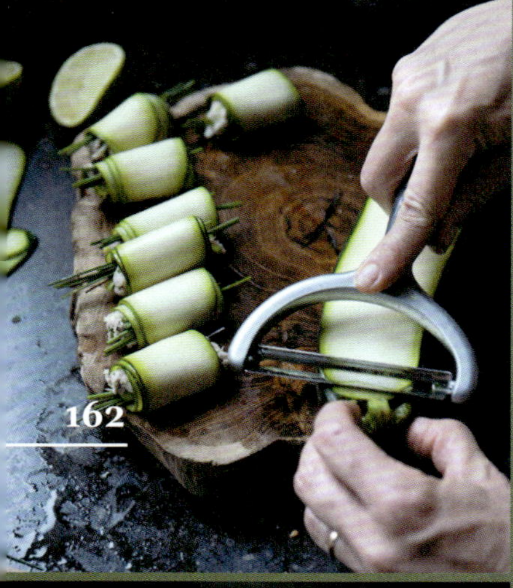

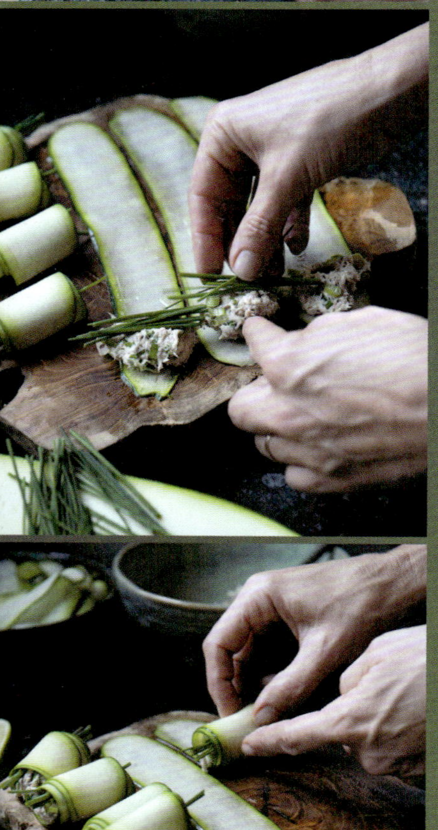

Zucchini roll-ups

WITH MACKEREL

Preparation time: 15 minutes - cooking time: none - makes 15 roll-ups

1 zucchini (9 oz/250 g)
5 oz (150 g) smoked or steamed mackerel
2 spring onions
1 jar of salmon roe
1 tablespoon mayonnaise
(optional, without added sugar)
1 lime
chives

With a vegetable peeler, slice 10 thin strips from the zucchini. Put them in a bowl and pour a generous splash of olive oil and the juice of half a lime over the top. Season with salt and pepper.
Mash the mackerel using a fork. Finely chop the spring onions and add them together with the mayonnaise and the salmon roe to the mackerel. Season to taste with salt and pepper. Divide the mackerel mixture over the zucchini slices, sprinkle some of the finely chopped chives over the top and roll the zucchini up. Serve on a stick or on a plate.

Per 3 1/2 oz (100g): 8.6g P (18%) / 16.7g F (80%) / 1g NetC (2%)
Per roll of 1 1/3 oz (38g): 3.2g P (18%) / 6.4g F (80%) / 0.4g NetC (2%)

EXTRA RECIPE
SNACK

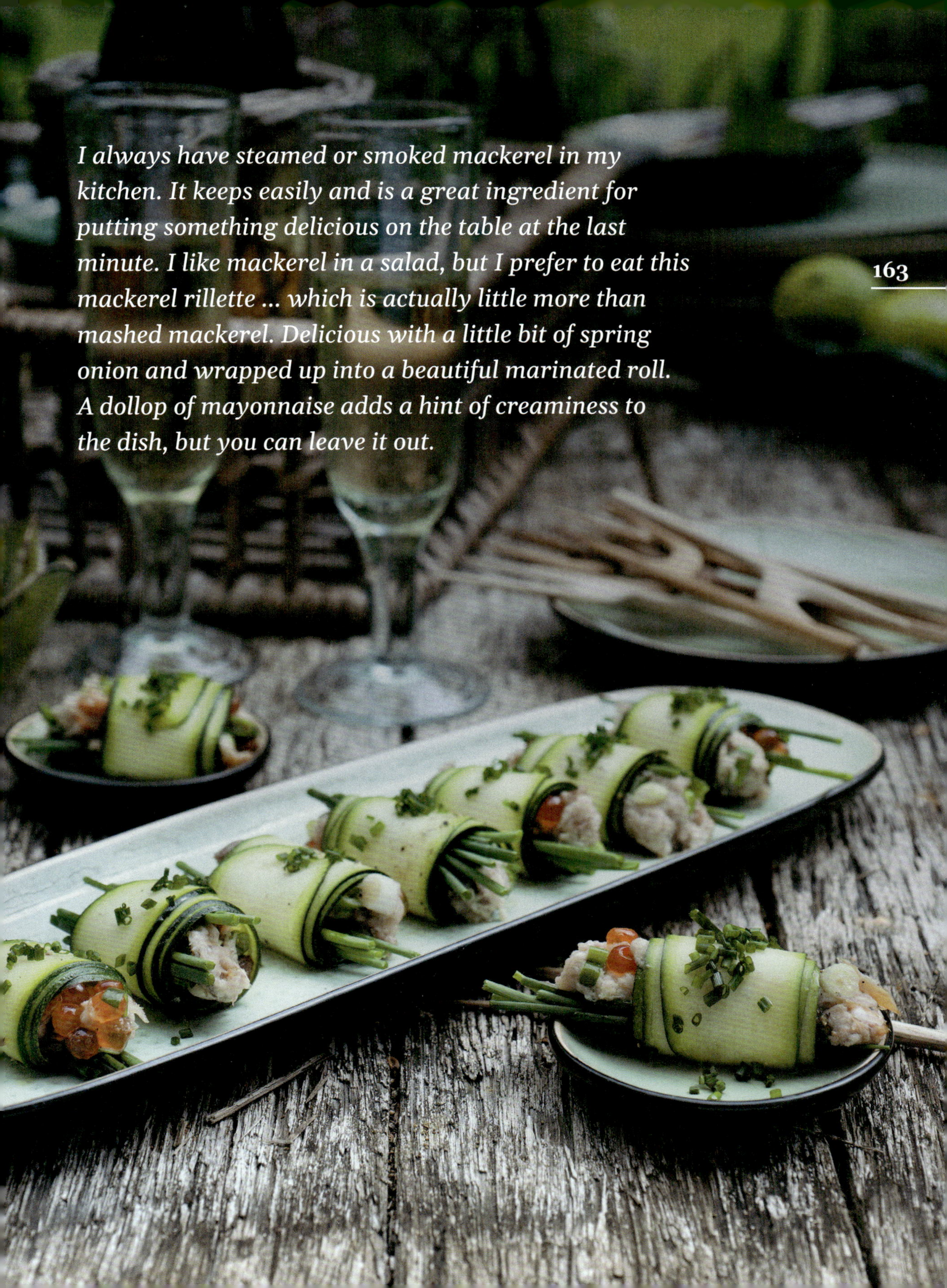

I always have steamed or smoked mackerel in my
kitchen. It keeps easily and is a great ingredient for
putting something delicious on the table at the last
minute. I like mackerel in a salad, but I prefer to eat this
mackerel rillette … which is actually little more than
mashed mackerel. Delicious with a little bit of spring
onion and wrapped up into a beautiful marinated roll.
A dollop of mayonnaise adds a hint of creaminess to
the dish, but you can leave it out.

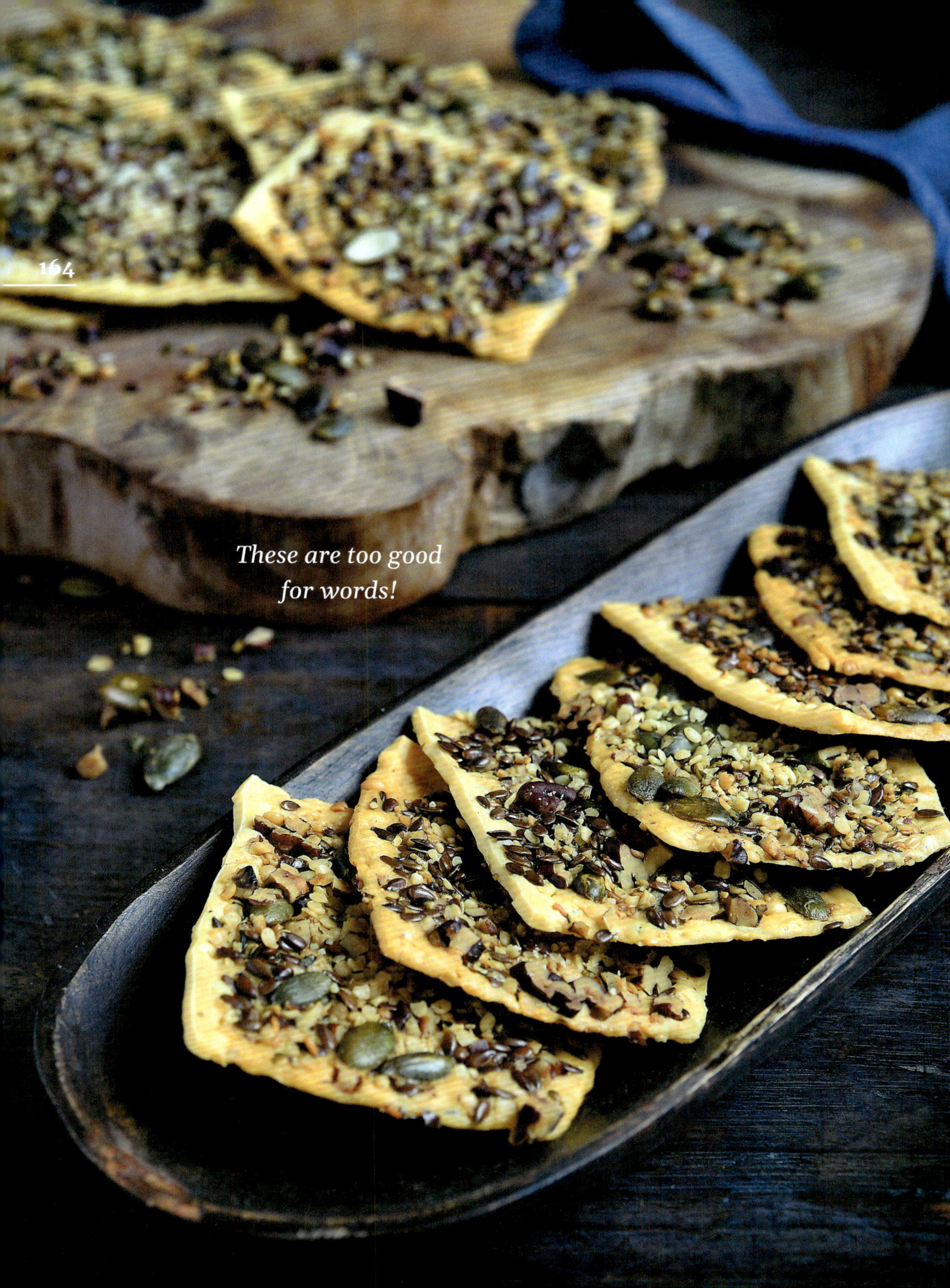

These are too good
for words!

Delicious keto cheese crackers

Ready in 20 minutes - makes about 20 crackers

3/4 oz (20 g) flaxseeds

3/4 oz (20 g) pumpkin seeds

3/4 oz (20 g) hemp seeds

3/4 oz (20 g) pecans

6 oz (170 g) mature cheese, for example Old Amsterdam

or mature Cheddar cheese, sliced

Extra: baking parchment

Coarsely chop the pecans and combine them with the seeds. Slice the cheese slices into quarters to match the size of the crackers and place them on the parchment paper. Sprinkle the seed-nut mixture on top of the cheese slices. Press the nuts and seeds lightly into the cheese (see tip).
Bake in the oven for 13 to 15 minutes at 350 °F (180 °C) or until the cheese starts to brown slightly at the edges. Let the crackers cool.

Tip: cheese in the oven
Check regularly, because every oven is different, and the cheese and seeds should definitely not burn. It is important to let them cool off completely; as soon as the crackers are cold, they become hard and crispy. If the cheese is still soft in the middle, then they haven't been in the oven for long enough. Use mature cheese that hardens after baking, as opposed to young cheese that remains soft.

Tip: egg whites
You can mix the nuts and seeds with an egg white if you prefer, so they stick easily to the cheese.

For 3 1/2 oz (100 g): 28.5g P (30%) / 29.7g F (69%) / 1.2g NetC (1%)

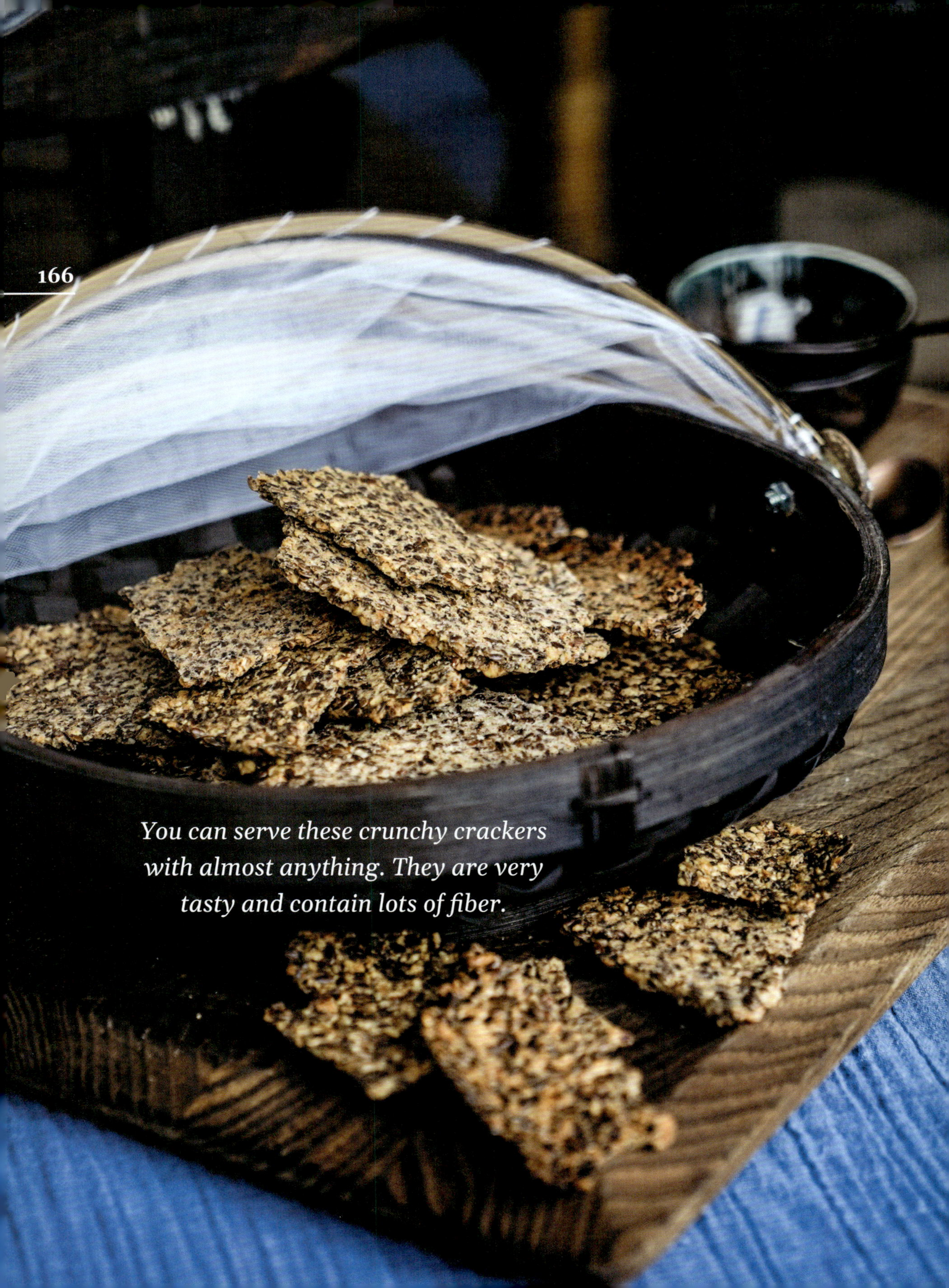

You can serve these crunchy crackers
with almost anything. They are very
tasty and contain lots of fiber.

Keto nut and seed crackers

Preparation time: 15 minutes - for a sheet of 20x30 cm

5 oz (150 g) pecans

5 oz (150 g) flaxseeds

3 egg whites

2 tablespoons olive oil

Extra: baking parchment

Preheat the oven to 350 °F (180 °C).

Mix the nuts and the seeds in a blender. Blend into a coarse flour. Stir the egg whites and olive oil into the mixture.

Place a sheet of parchment paper on a flat work surface. Spread a layer of the nut and seed mixture thinly out over the parchment paper. Place a second sheet of parchment paper on the mixture and flatten with a rolling pin or rub evenly over the paper using a dish towel until the dough is no more than 1/4 inch (1/2 cm) thick. Remove the top sheet of parchment paper. Transfer the dough to a baking sheet and put it in the oven.

Turn the crackers over after 10 minutes, remove the parchment paper, and cook for an additional 5 minutes. Note that every oven is different so keep checking regularly the first time you make these.

Tip: quantities
Use 1 egg white per 5 ounces (150 g) of mixed nuts and seeds. You can also add fresh herbs such as finely chopped garlic, rosemary or thyme.

Tip: how can I best store these crackers?
I keep them under a dishtowel in the kitchen so they'll stay crispy and keep for four or five days.

Per 3 1/2 oz (100g): 12.8g P (10%) / 48.7g F (87%) / 3.6g NetC (3%)

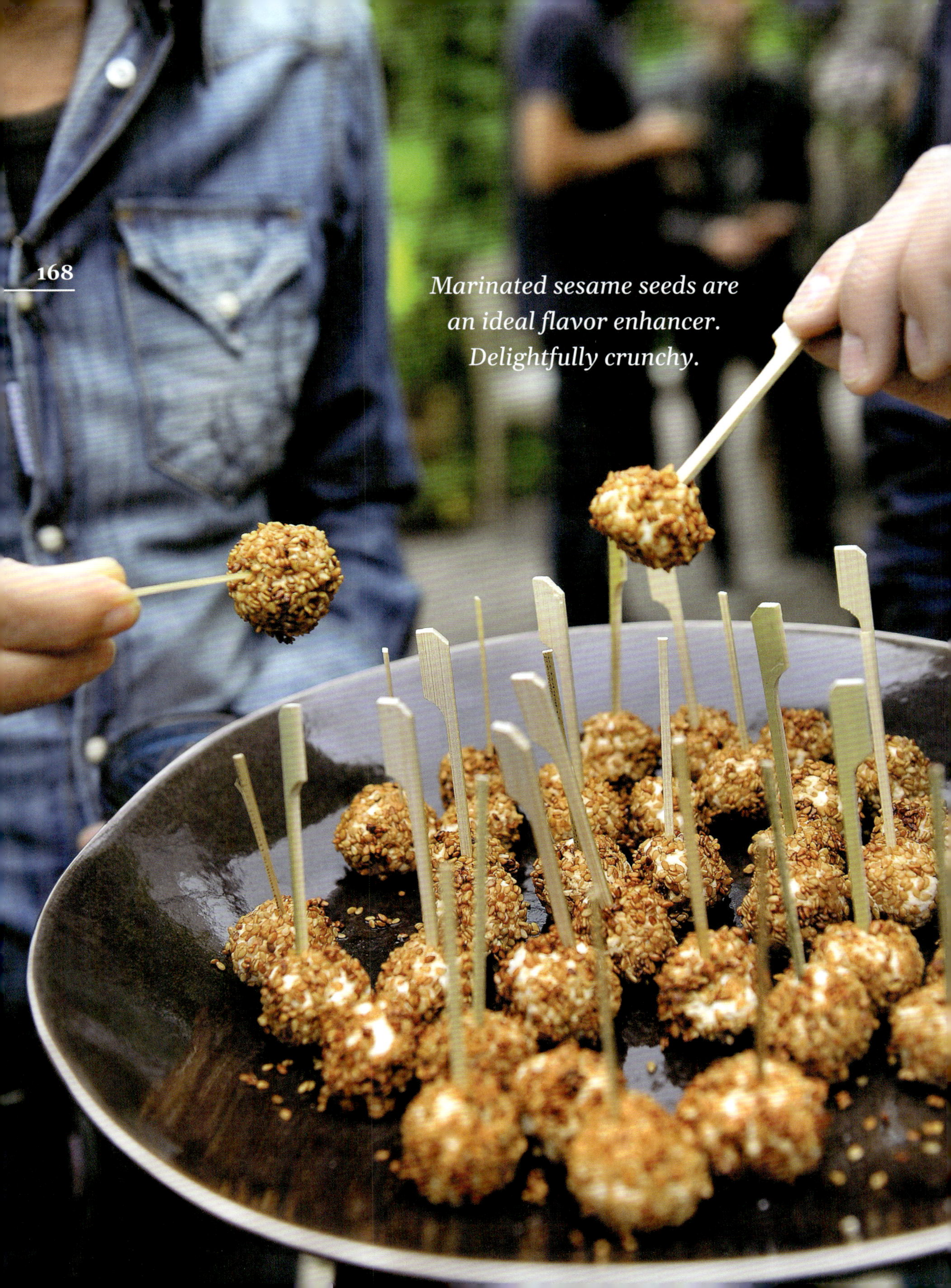

168
Marinated sesame seeds are
an ideal flavor enhancer.
Delightfully crunchy.

Goat cheese

WITH MARINATED SESAME SEEDS

Preparation time: 10 minutes - cooking time: 6 to 10 minutes - marinade time: at least 15 minutes - makes 6 to 10

7 oz (200 g) soft goat cheese

3 oz (75 g) roasted sesame seeds (see tip)

1 3/4 oz (50 g) soy sauce

Extra: baking parchment

Preheat the oven to 350 °F (180 °C).
Put the sesame seeds in a bowl and pour soy sauce over the top until the seeds are just submerged.
Let the seeds soak for at least 15 minutes.
Line a baking tray with baking parchment and spread out the still-wet sesame seeds.
Bake for 6 to 10 minutes in the preheated oven.
Roll the goat cheese into balls which are then rolled in the sesame seeds.

Tip: marinated sesame seeds
As far as marinades go, the following rule always applies: the longer, the better. I marinate the seeds the night before, even if I don't need them until the following evening. Moreover, I make more than I need. You can easily keep them for a few days (in a cool spot on paper towels) and use them in other dishes; they are an ideal flavoring. I use them in salads, but you can also simply put a bowl of seeds on the table to sprinkle over your vegetables or fish. If they're not as crunchy the next day, just pop them in the oven briefly.

Tip: sesame seeds in the oven
Keep checking the seeds regularly when they're in the oven to make sure they don't burn; stir occasionally so they dry evenly and become crispy on all sides. They should be light brown in color, definitely not dark brown. If necessary, lower the oven temperature and leave them in the oven a little longer.

Per 3 1/2 oz (100g): 16.8g P (23%) / 24g F (73%) / 3.5g NetC (4%)

EXTRA RECIPE
SNACK

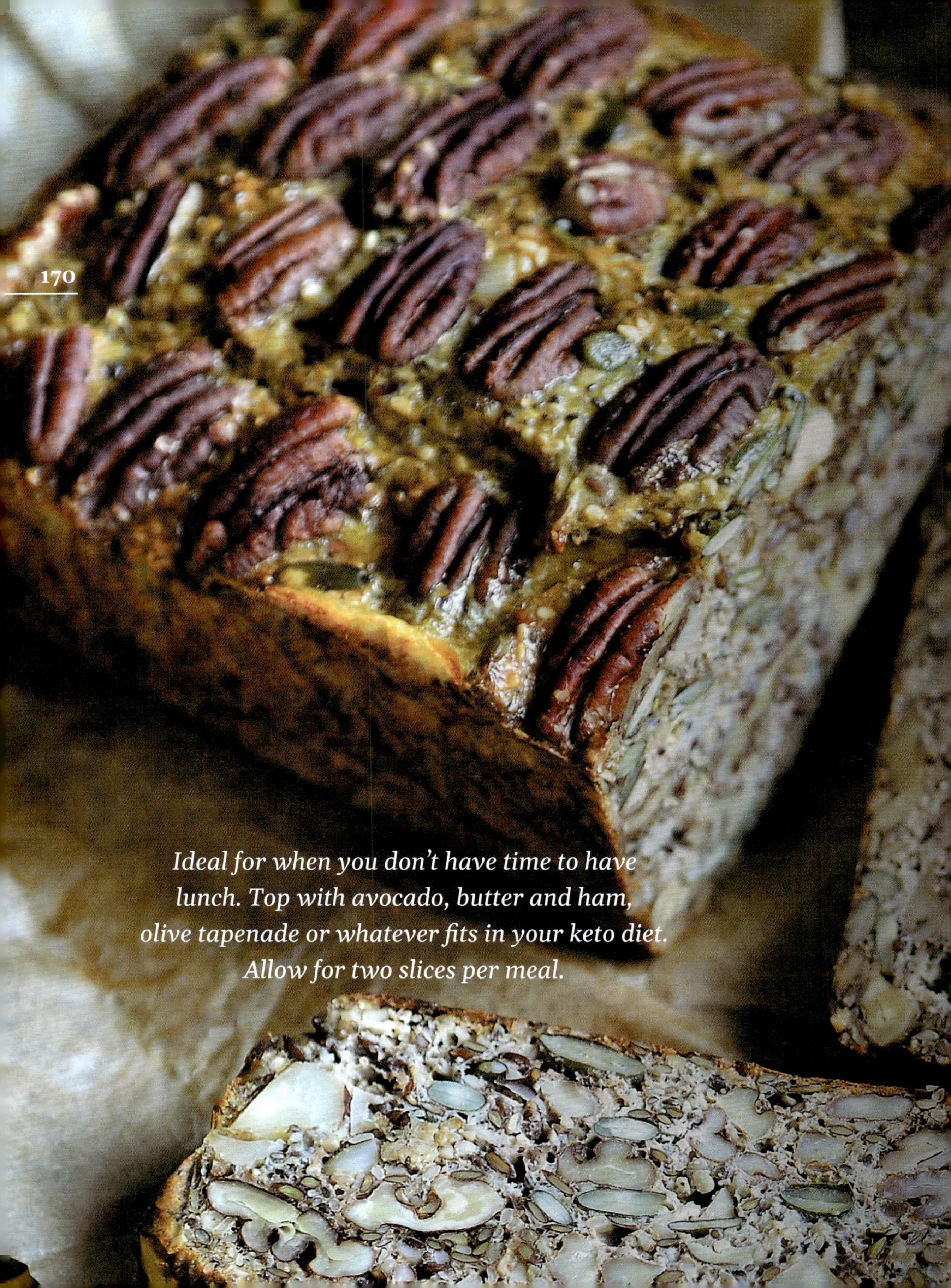

Ideal for when you don't have time to have
lunch. Top with avocado, butter and ham,
olive tapenade or whatever fits in your keto diet.
Allow for two slices per meal.

Nut bread

Preparation time: 15 minutes - cooking time: 40 minutes - makes 10 slices

3 1/2 oz (100 g) pecans - 2 oz (60 g) flaxseed - 2 oz (60 g) pumpkin seeds
2 oz (60 g) sesame seeds - 1 oz (30 g) chia seeds - 1 oz (30 g) hemp seeds
3 1/2 oz (100 g) Brazil nuts - 3 1/2 oz (100 g) walnuts - 5 (small) eggs
2 tablespoons ground cinnamon - 7 oz (200 ml) full-fat cream

Preheat the oven to 350 °F (180 °C).
You can chop the nuts, but you don't have to. Combine all the ingredients with a pinch of salt and pour the batter into a cake tin or small loaf pan lined with baking parchment.
Bake in the oven for 30 to 40 minutes.

Tip: toppings
Top the slices of bread with some avocado, olive tapenade, cheese, salmon, or slices of ham. Delicious and convenient every time.

Tip: no time?
I always have some variation of this nut bread stored in the freezer. For the low-carb version, I add dried fruit or berries and whatever nuts and seeds I feel like. I then freeze the slices separately so I always have something available for those times I need something at the last-minute.

Tip: herbs
Nut bread should have a relatively neutral flavor so you can top it with whatever you feel like. But you can always add some pepper, black olives, rosemary or cinnamon (for sweetness). Or even feta or another dry cheese.

Per 3 1/2 oz (100 g) with cream: 13.4g P (12%) / 41.8g F (85%) / 3.9g NetC (3%)

Nut bread variation
Replace the cream with 1 3/4 oz (50 g) coconut oil. This will make the bread taste even nuttier.

Per 3 1/2 oz (100 g) with coconut oil: 15.2g P (13%) / 45.7g F (84%) / 3.9g NetC (3%)

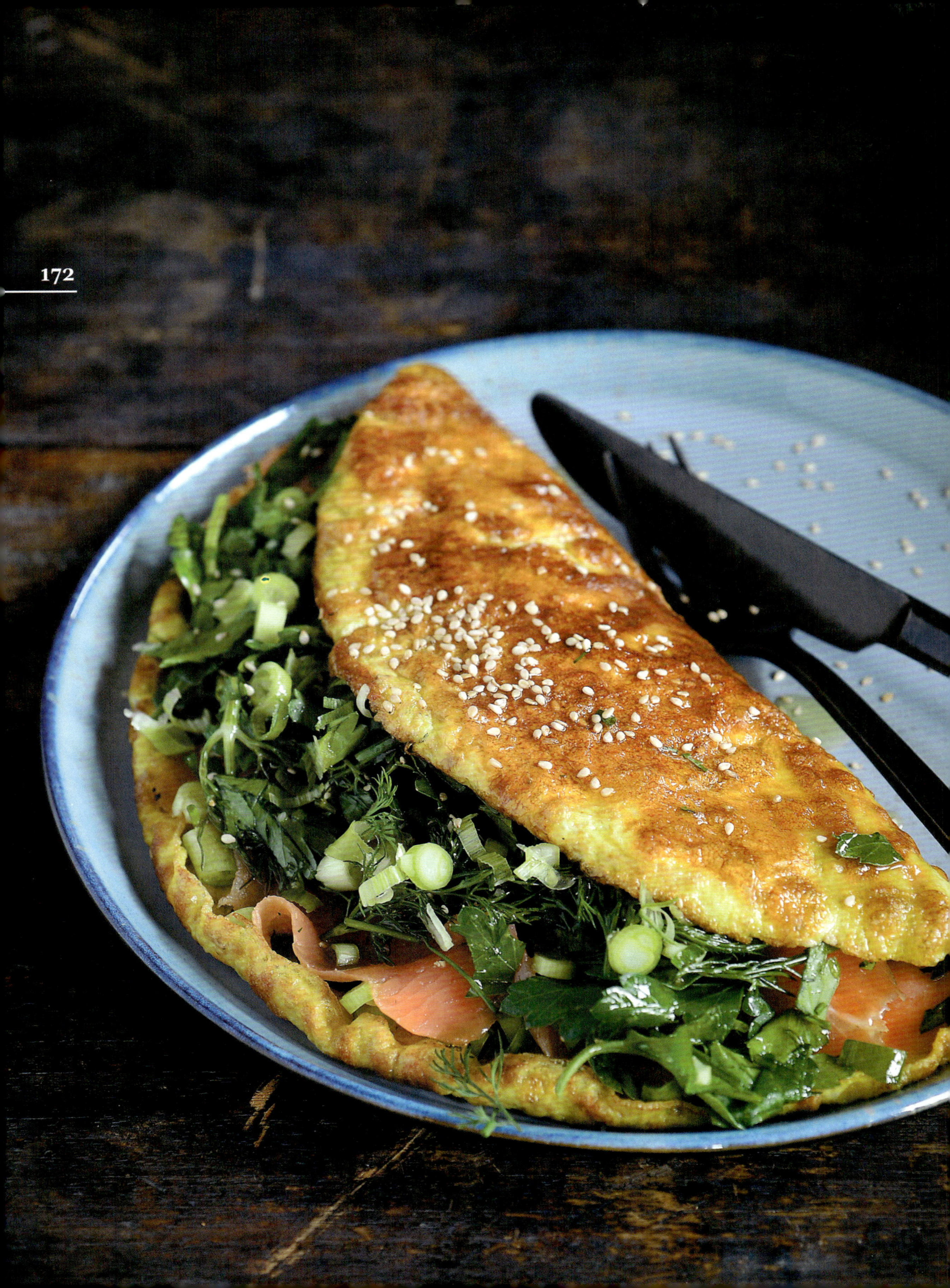

Delicious omelet

WITH SALMON AND FRESH HERBS

Ready in 20 minutes - serves 2

4 eggs

6 tablespoons cream (1 3/4 oz/50 g)

3/4 oz (20 g) sesame seeds

7 oz (200 g) smoked salmon

2 large bunches of fresh herbs (flat-leaf parsley, dill ...)

2 spring onions

Whisk the eggs together with the cream. Season with salt and pepper and add the sesame seeds. Drizzle a bit of olive oil in a pan and pour half the egg mixture into the pan. Cover. Keep cooking the omelet until the top is completely dry. Do the same with the second omelet.
Meanwhile, finely chop the spring onions and combine them with some olive oil and a pinch of salt and pepper. Put half the salmon slices on top of one half of the omelet and arrange half the herbs on top. Fold the omelet over. Garnish the second omelet in the same way. Sprinkle a few sesame seeds on top, if desired.

Per serving: 39g P (28%) / 44g F (71%) / 2g NetC (1%)

EXTRA RECIPE
BREAKFAST/LUNCH

Sautéed bok choy

WITH MUSHROOMS AND EGG

Ready in 20 minutes - serves 2

14 oz (400 g) bok choy (see tip)

2 oz (60 g) butter

7 oz (200 g) brown button mushrooms (cremini, baby bella)

1 oz (30 g) pecans

2 eggs

Trim the bottom inch (3 cm) from the bok choy. Melt half the butter in a pan, add the bok choy and pour a splash of water into the pan. Season with salt and black pepper. Cover the pan and cook for about 7 minutes. Check occasionally.
Coarsely chop the mushrooms and sauté them in the other half of the butter. Season with salt and pepper. Remove the lid from the pan and continue to cook until all the water has evaporated.
Place the bok choy along the edges of a deep dish and spoon the mushrooms into the middle. Make a well in the mushrooms with a spoon. Crack the eggs, separate the whites from the yolks, and place the egg yolk in the middle of the mushrooms. Season with salt and pepper and garnish with coarsely chopped pecans.

Tip: bok choy
Bok choy is a cabbage with Asian origins, but it is now also grown in many other places. It is lighter than traditional cabbage and the flavor is reminiscent of spinach. Bok choy is a versatile vegetable: you can steam, bake or stir-fry it. If you cook it briefly, the bok choy remains crunchy, making it ideal for salads. But in this dish, I want the leaves and the white stem to be very soft, which is why I cook them for at least 15 minutes.

Tip: feeling snacky or feeling hungry?
You can serve this as breakfast, lunch, or dinner. If you're not particularly hungry, use only one egg yolk. If you're really hungry, use two egg yolks. This will add some extra fat and protein to the dish.

Per serving with 2 egg yolks: 16g P (13%) / 46g F (84%) / 3g NetC (3%)

EXTRA RECIPE
BREAKFAST/LUNCH/DINNER

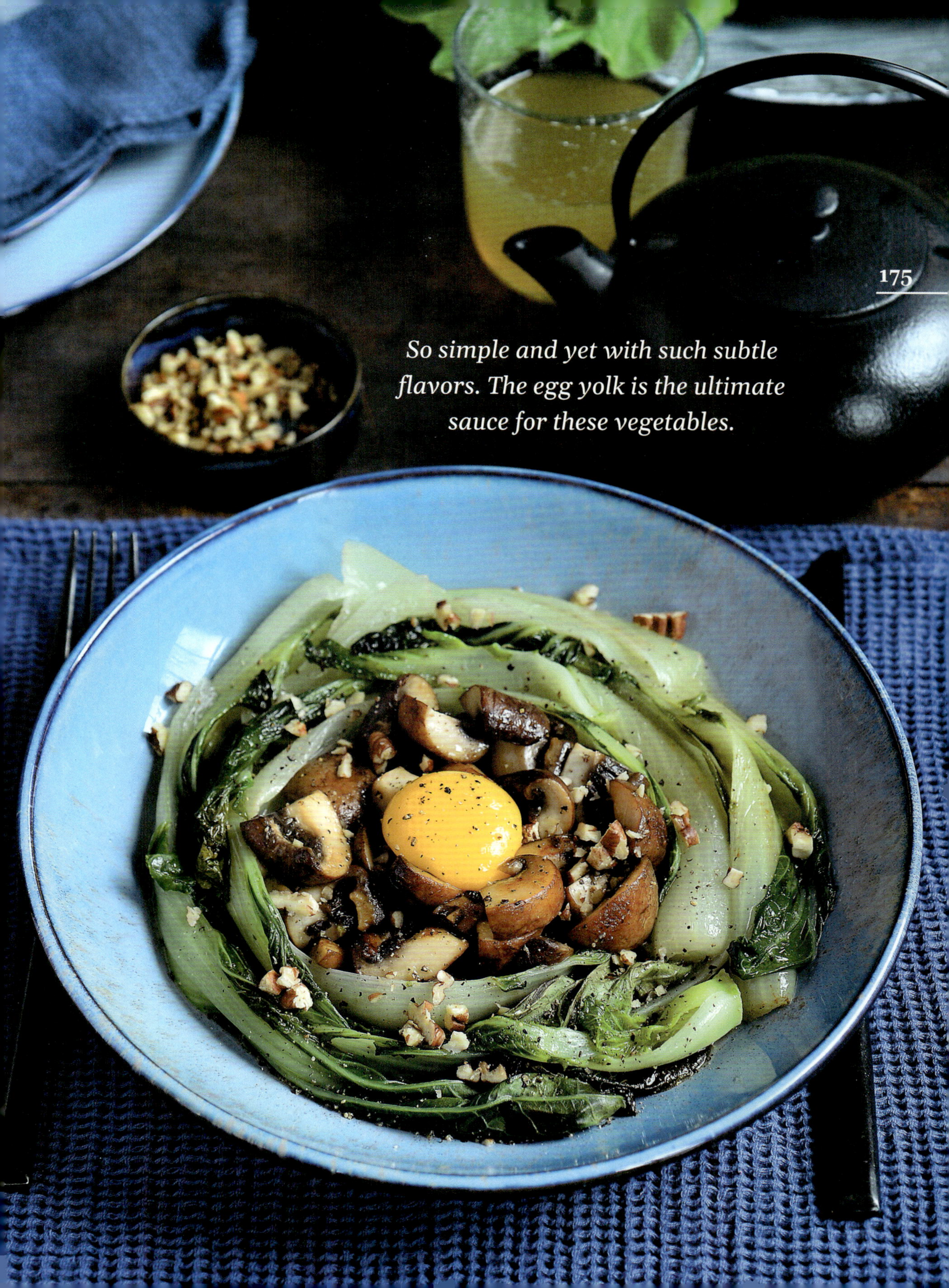

So simple and yet with such subtle flavors. The egg yolk is the ultimate sauce for these vegetables.

Avocado

WITH CRAB AND LUMPFISH EGGS

Preparation time: 15 minutes - cooking time: none - makes 4 small or 2 large servings

1 ripe avocado

1 shallot

wasabi (Japanese horseradish)

juice of 1 lime

1 can crab meat (7 oz/200 g)

1 jar lumpfish eggs

chives

Extra: cooking ring

Mash the avocado to a pulp and mix in some lemon juice to prevent discoloration. Finely chop the shallot and mix together with a teaspoon (or however much you want) of wasabi into the mashed avocado. Season the crab meat with some olive oil, salt and pepper. Press some of the crab meat into the bottom of a cooking ring, spoon the avocado mixture over the top and finish with some lumpfish eggs and chives.

Tip: no cooking ring?
This dish looks wonderful without a cooking ring as well. Start first by spreading out the avocado on the bottom, placing the crab meat on top and garnishing with a spoonful of lumpfish eggs and the chives.

Per serving: 28.6g P (25%) / 36.5g F (72%) / 4.2g NetC (3%)

EXTRA RECIPE
APPETIZER/FIRST COURSE

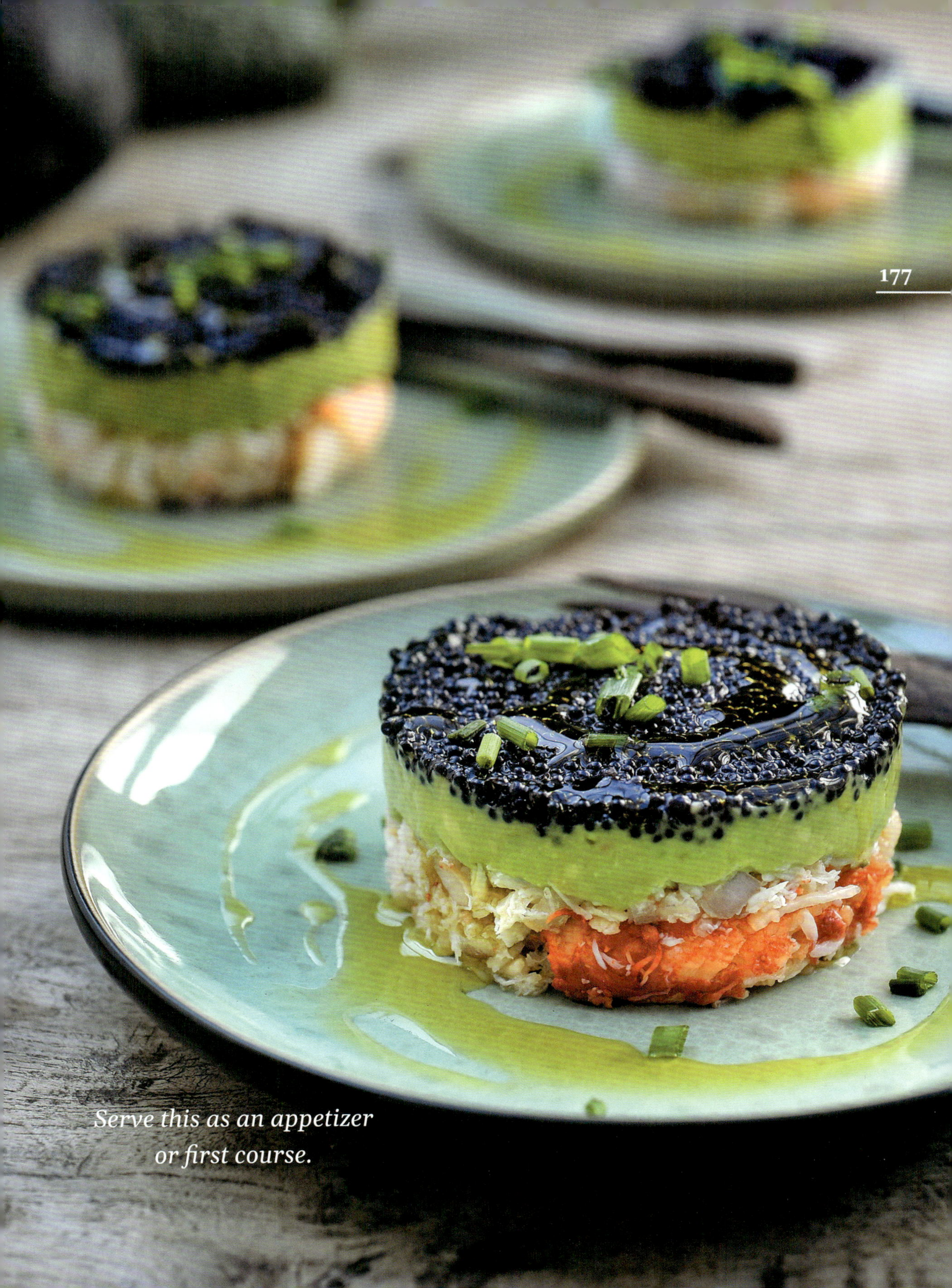
Serve this as an appetizer
or first course.

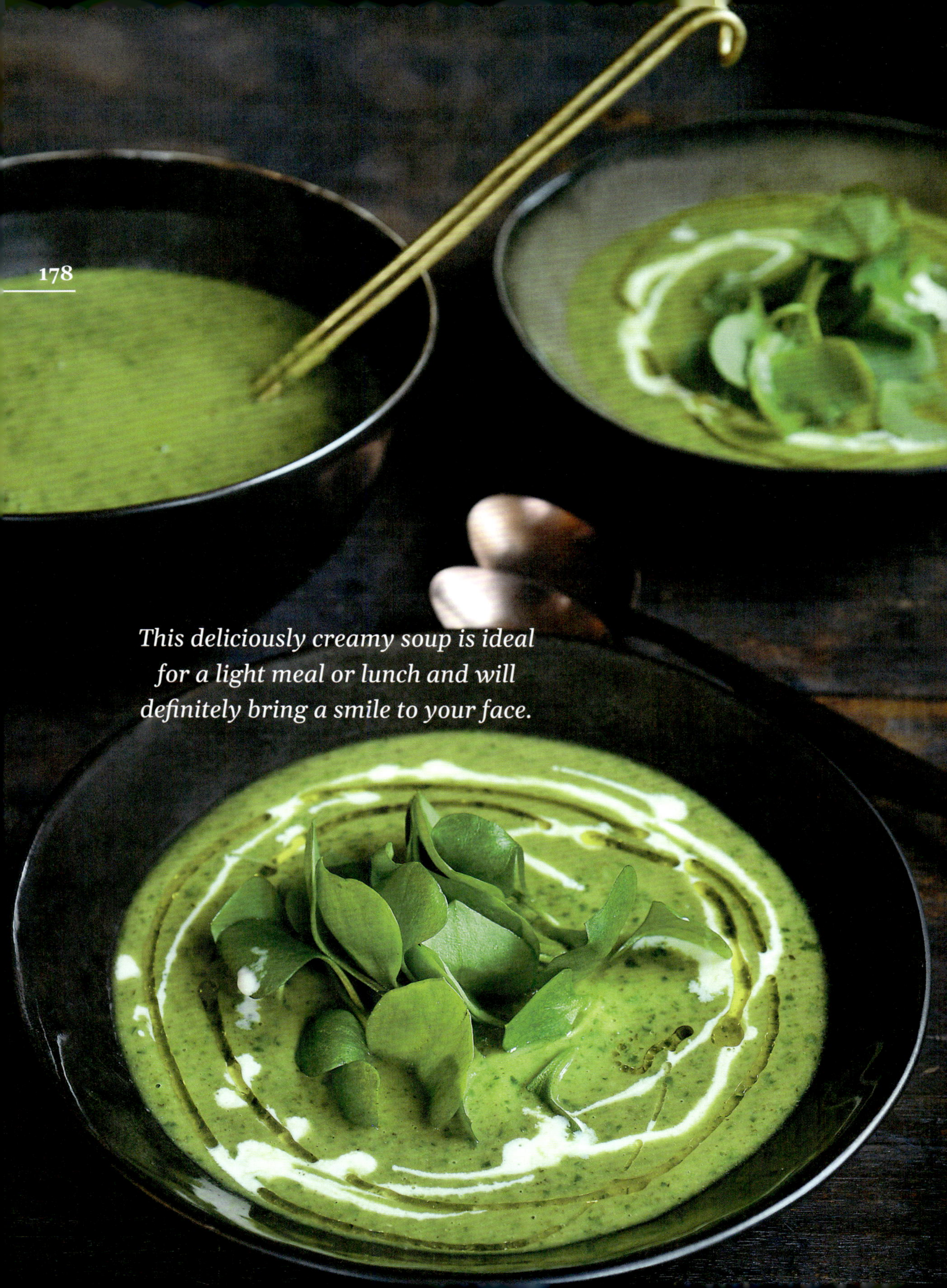

This deliciously creamy soup is ideal
for a light meal or lunch and will
definitely bring a smile to your face.

Green vegetable soup

Ready in 20 minutes - serves 2

1 zucchini (7 oz/200 g)

10 1/2 oz (300 g) broccoli

7 oz (200 g) spinach

2 tablespoons green curry paste
(1 1/2 oz/40 g)

1 3/4 oz (50 g) purslane

7 fl oz (200 ml) coconut milk

Chop the zucchini and broccoli into large chunks and put them in a large cooking pot. Add 1 1/2 quarts (1 1/2 liters) water to the vegetables. Season with salt and black pepper and bring to the boil. Let the vegetables cook for about 7 minutes. Remove the pot from the heat, add the fresh spinach, green curry paste, and coconut milk and blend to form a thick soup. Put the pot back on the heat, but don't let the mixture come to a boil. Check the seasoning. Spoon the soup into wide, shallow soup dishes and garnish with the purslane and a dollop of coconut milk and olive oil.

Per portion: 8.5g P (10%) / 31.4g F (82%) / 6.7g NetC (8%)

EXTRA RECIPE
SNACK/LUNCH

Raw salmon

WITH AVOCADO AND TOMATO IN A LOVELY CREAM SAUCE

Ready in 15 minutes - serves 2

10 1/2 oz (300 g) fresh salmon

2 avocados

fresh herbs such as chives and cilantro (see tip)

1 3/4 oz (50 g) full-fat sour cream

6 tablespoons full-fat cream (1 3/4 oz/50 g)

1 tomato

1 tablespoon sesame seeds (1/3 oz/10 g)

Extra: cooking ring

Dice the salmon, avocados and tomatoes, put everything in a bowl and add the sour cream. Sprinkle some finely chopped herbs into the bowl, season with salt and pepper and stir to combine.
Put the mixture into a cooking ring and place the ring on a plate. Spoon the full-fat cream around the salmon mixture and garnish with some additional fresh herbs and the sesame seeds.

Tip: Fresh herbs
I always have fresh herbs in my home. In the summer I plant them in my garden, and in the winter, I always bring some home with me whenever I go shopping. I use herbs such as chives, flat-leaf parsley, cilantro or dill. That way, I always have them on hand to add the finishing touch to a dish. Feel free to use any herbs you like.

Per serving: 34g P (16%) / 75g F (80%) / 7g NetC (4%)

EXTRA RECIPE
LUNCH/FIRST COURSE

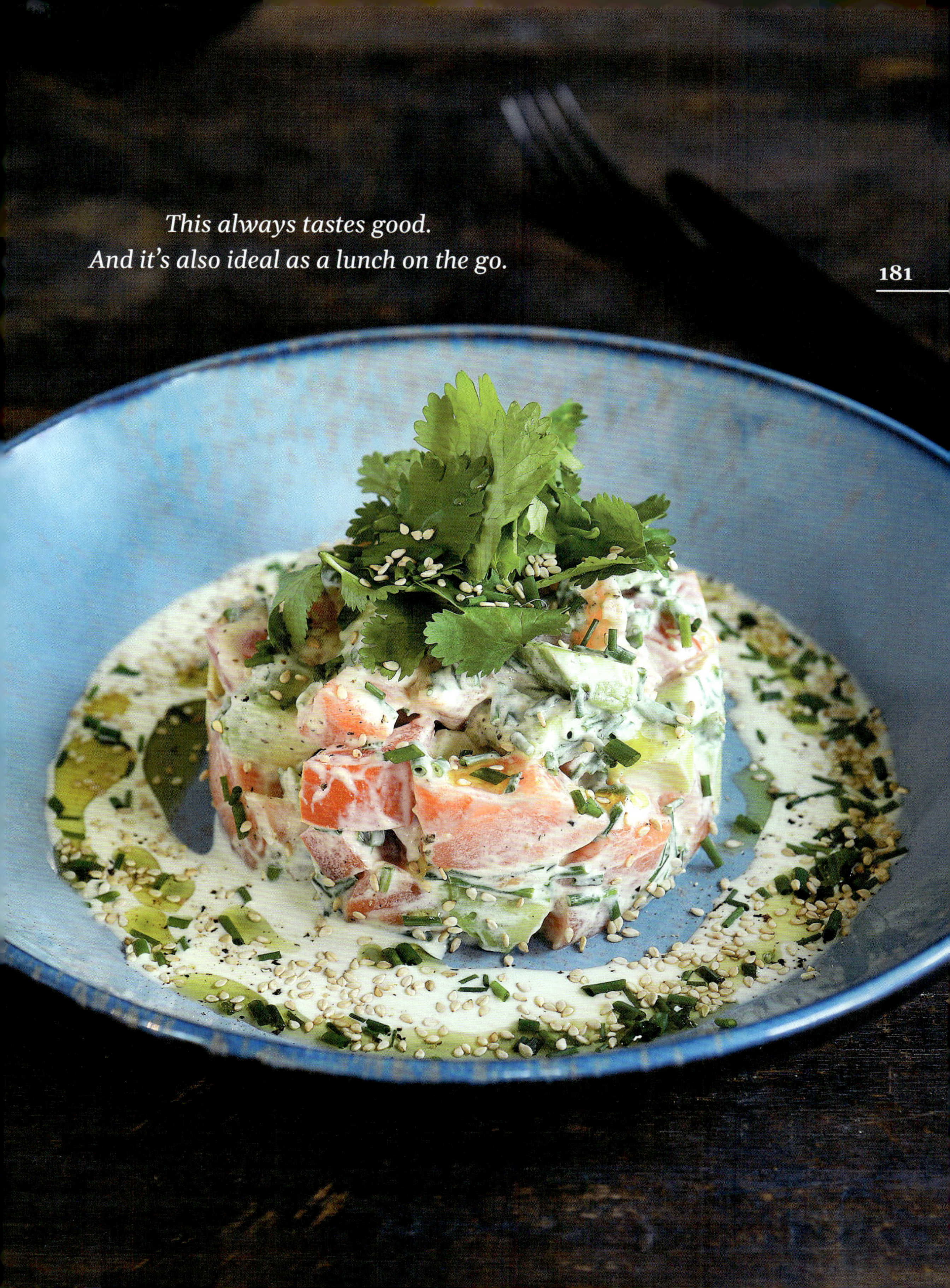

This always tastes good.
And it's also ideal as a lunch on the go.

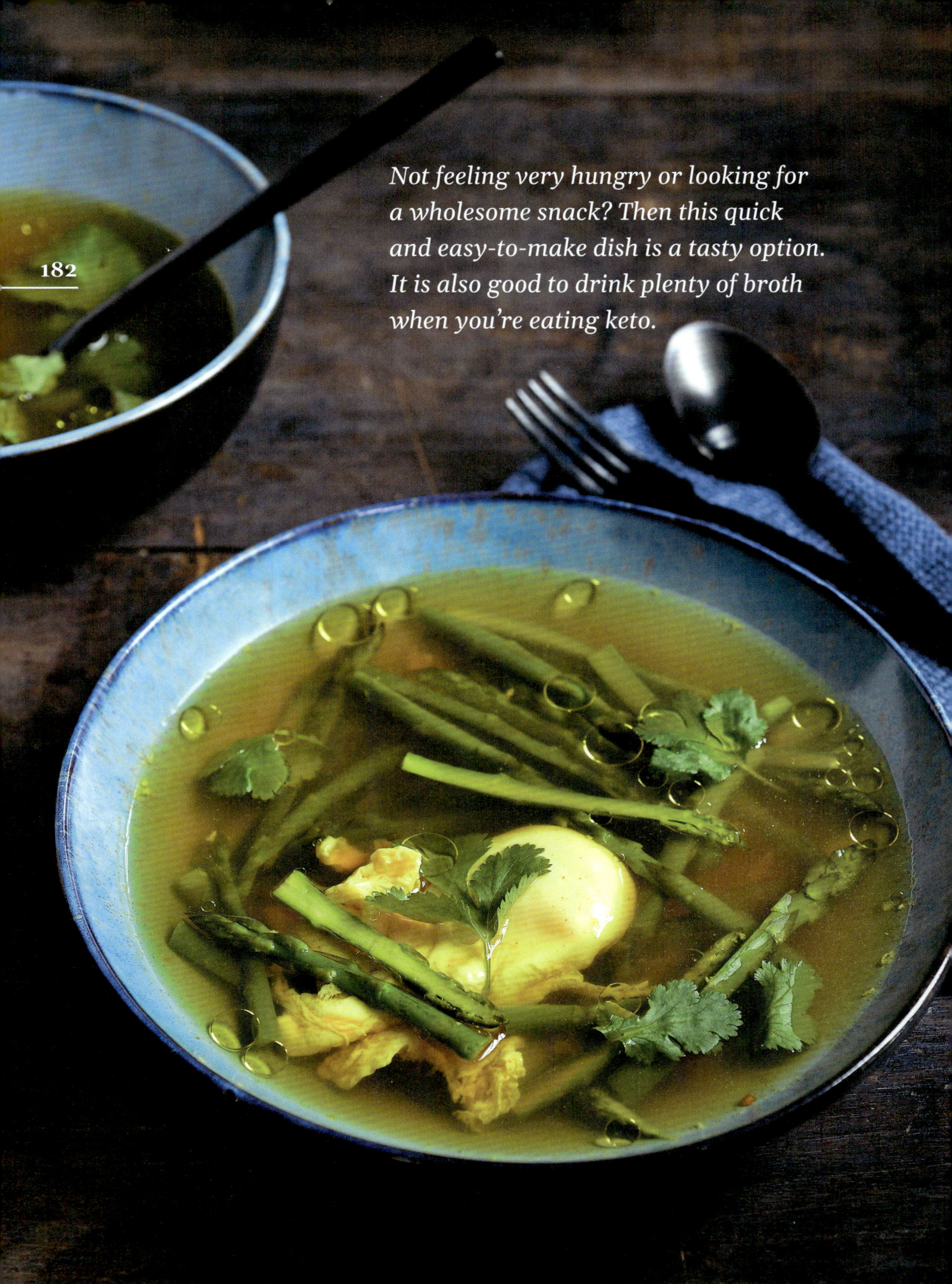

Not feeling very hungry or looking for a wholesome snack? Then this quick and easy-to-make dish is a tasty option. It is also good to drink plenty of broth when you're eating keto.

Quick broth

WITH POACHED EGG AND ASPARAGUS

Ready in 20 minutes - serves 2

1/2 quart (500 ml) chicken broth - 1/2 quart (500 ml) water
2 fresh eggs - 14 oz (400 g) asparagus - 2 tablespoons ras-el-hanout
4 tablespoons apple cider vinegar - cilantro leaves to garnish
1 1/2 oz (40 g) olive oil

Bring a large pot with water to the boil for poaching the eggs. Break each egg separately into a small ramekin (see tip). Once the water is boiling, add the apple cider vinegar. Don't add salt or pepper. Turn the heat down until the water is just barely simmering. Stir the water in a clockwise direction to create a whirlpool, and slide an egg into the center of the whirlpool. Let the egg cook for 2 or 3 minutes at the most. Remove the egg from the water using a slotted spoon. Do the same with the second egg. Put the broth in a pot and add 1/2 quart (500 ml) water. Season with salt, black pepper and the ras-el-hanout. Slice the asparagus in half lengthwise and then into 2-inch (5-cm) long pieces. Add them to the broth. Add a splash of olive oil and bring to a boil. Divide the soup evenly into two bowls and add the poached eggs. Garnish with the cilantro leaves and a drizzle of olive oil.

Tip: broth
Either make your own broth or buy organic broth, but don't use cubes. These often contain flavor enhancers, sugars and hydrogenated fats. Store-bought broth is almost always without fat. That's why I always add some extra fat to the broth to give it some flavor.

Tip: poached egg
If you don't want your poached eggs to have many strands, use ultra-fresh eggs. Another tip is to strain your eggs first. Break the egg over a small, fine-mesh strainer before pouring it into the ramekin. Any extra liquid from the egg (that's where you get those strands from) will drain out of the egg white. Don't be put off by the idea of making poached eggs. You'll see, poaching eggs is fun!

Per serving: 10g P (14%) / 26g F (81%) / 4g NetC (5%)

EXTRA RECIPE
SNACK/LUNCH

This dish is ready in no time. I serve it with a herbed salad when my girlfriends come over. But it's also an inspiring dish for when you're on the go. You can make countless variations using different ingredients: tomatoes, carrots, zucchini ... Throw them together or just use the one vegetable, either way you can't go wrong with this dish. Another handy tip: line the dish with baking paper so you can easily remove the quiche.

Savory broccoli quiche

Preparation time: 15 minutes - cooking time: 25 minutes - serves 2

1 head of broccoli (1 1/2 lbs/700 g)

9 oz (250 g) goat cheese

8 eggs

2 large bunches of basil (1 1/2 oz/40 g)

Blend the eggs with the basil in a blender until you have a green eggy mixture. Season with salt and pepper. Sauté the broccoli florets 3 to 4 minutes until al dente (or softer, if you prefer) in some olive oil with a splash of water.
Pour the egg mixture into a baking dish and arrange the broccoli over the mixture. Slice the goat cheese and arrange the slices among the broccoli florets. Bake the quiche in the oven at 350 °F (180 °C) for about 20 minutes.

Per serving: 72g P (35%) / 57g F (62%) / 6g NetC (3%)

EXTRA RECIPE
LUNCH

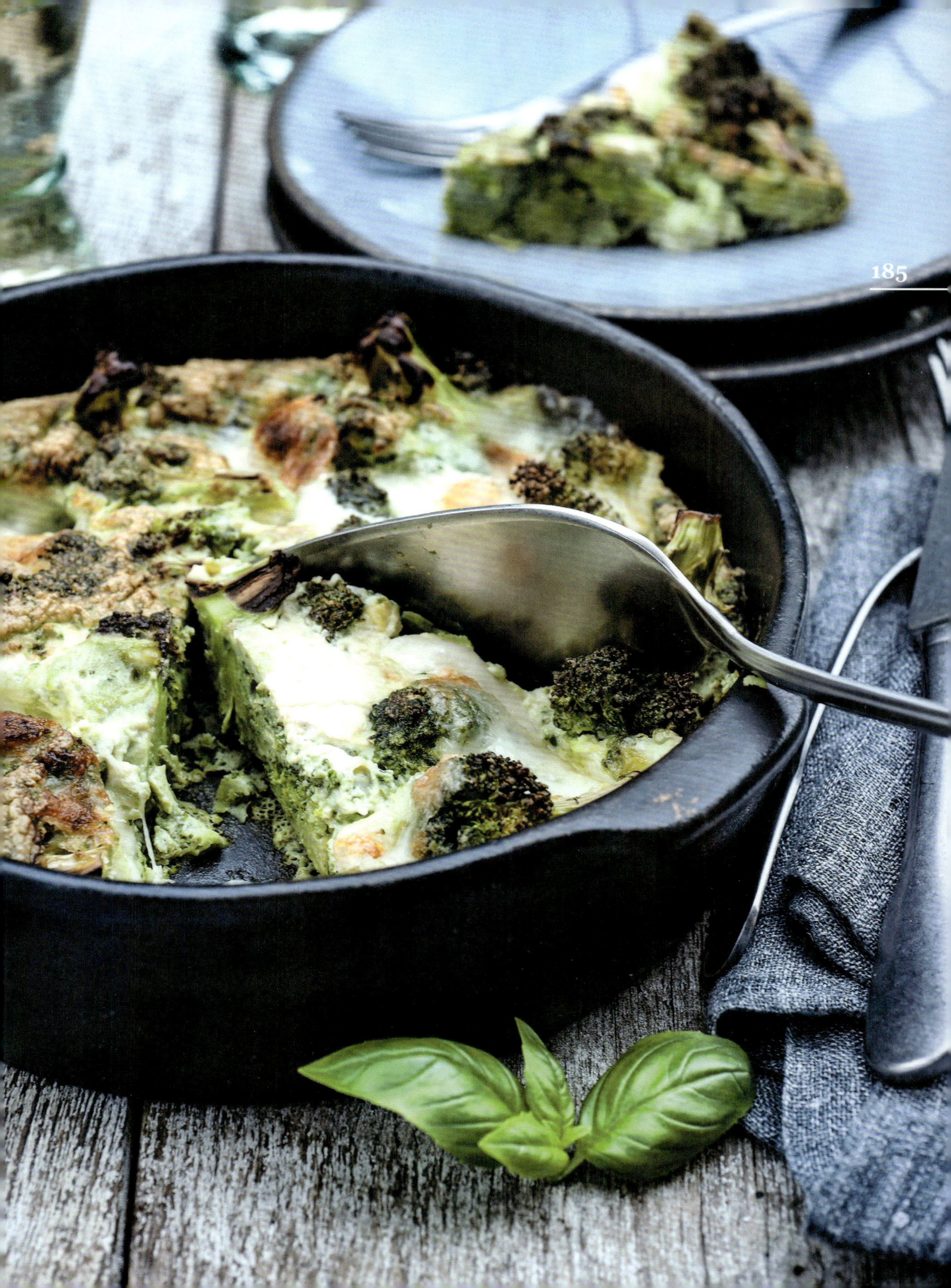

Flatbread wraps

Ready in 25 minutes - makes 4 wraps

5 oz (140 g) ground almonds - 1 oz (30 g) psyllium (see tip)

2 tablespoons olive oil - 5 fl oz (140 ml) water

For the filling:

Lettuce - 1 avocado - 12 slices ham

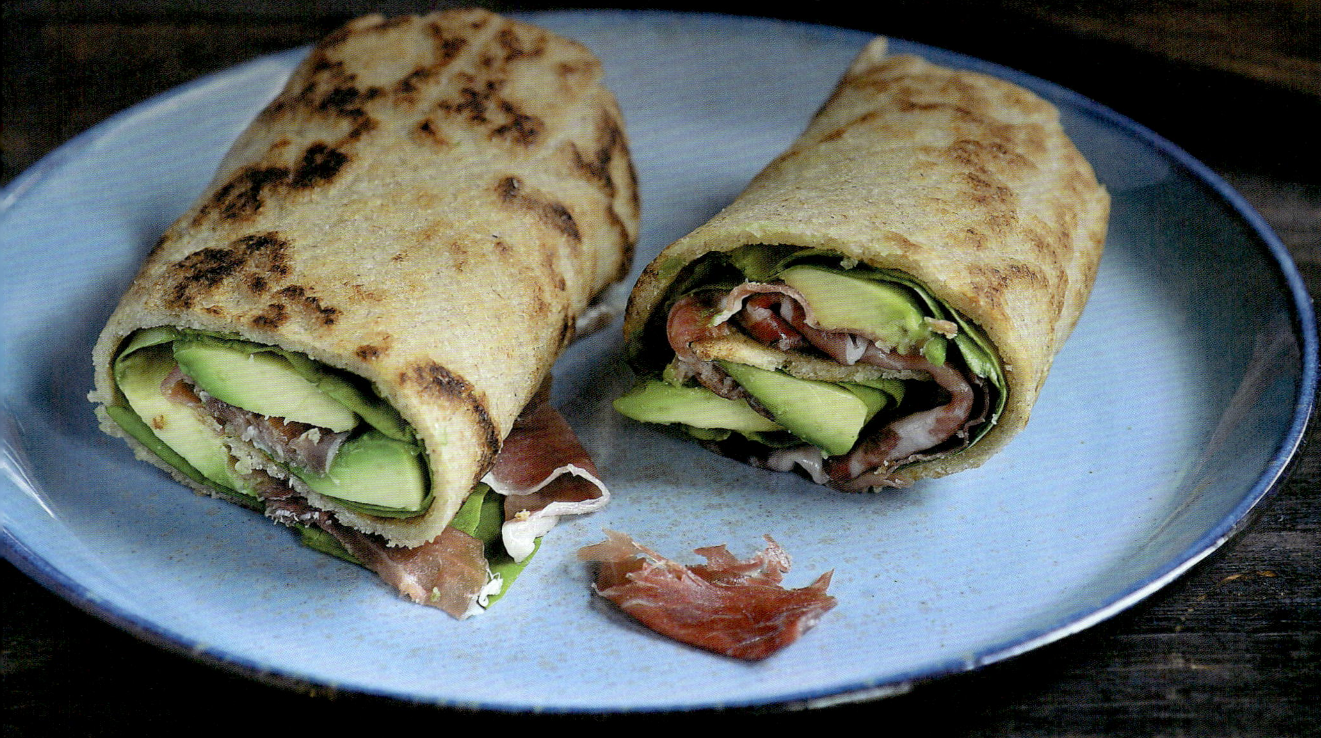

Combine the ground almonds with the psyllium, a little salt and the olive oil.

Bring the water to a boil and stir it into the almond mixture. You should now have a dough that you can knead without it sticking to your hands (see tip).

Let the dough rest for 10 minutes, giving the ingredients time to settle. Cut the dough into four pieces and roll them out between two sheets of baking paper. Carefully pull the baking paper away from the dough. Be careful as the dough may tear easily. Did you mess up? Roll the dough out once more and try again. Practice makes perfect!

In a frying pan with a little olive oil, fry the flatbreads for 3 minutes on one side, and 2 minutes on the other side. Don't fry them until they're crunchy, otherwise they'll break when you roll them up. If you cooked them for too long, use them as crackers, because they still taste great. Divide the lettuce, avocado and ham evenly across the four pieces of bread and roll them up. Bon appétit!

Tip: finely ground almonds

It is important that the almonds are finely ground, otherwise the flatbreads will not be firm enough. Your best option is to use store-bought finely-ground almonds.

Tip: dough

If the dough is too soggy, add some extra psyllium. And if it's too dry, add a couple of extra drops of water.

Tip: what is psyllium?

Psyllium are seed husks, in other words: fiber. In this recipe, they are effectively the glue keeping the dough together. Psyllium soaks up a lot of moisture, so bear that in mind. You can also add psyllium to your breakfast or to other dishes to increase your fiber intake. Although if you have a fiber deficiency, it's better to eat more vegetables, nuts or seeds because the types of fiber you get from whole foods are much healthier.

Tip: freezing

You can easily store these flatbreads in the freezer. Separate them with a piece of baking paper so they don't stick together. That way, you'll always have last-minute flatbreads to make and take with you.

Per 2 flatbreads with toppings: 32g P (16%) / 69g F (79%) / 9g NetC (5%)

*They're not only very tasty,
but also really easy to take with you.
You can roll them up with whatever you like.*

EXTRA RECIPE
LUNCH

Raw salmon

WITH ZUCCHINI NOODLES

Preparation time: 10 minutes - cooking time: none - serves 2

a little over 1 lb (500 g) raw salmon, sliced thinly

1 1/4 lb (600 g) long, firm zucchini

1 bunch of parsley

juice of 1 lemon

2 oz (60 g) hazelnut oil

1 tablespoon dried pink peppercorns

Peel the zucchini down its entire length with a special julienne peeler or a spiralizer to make long, thin strands. Put the strands in a bowl.

Finely chop the parsley and add to the zucchini noodles.

To make the vinaigrette, combine the hazelnut oil, lemon juice, and some fleur de sel and pepper. Add half the vinaigrette to the zucchini noodles and set aside the other half for the salmon. Put the zucchini noodles in the refrigerator to marinate.

Divide the salmon evenly between the plates and arrange the zucchini noodles in the middle. Spoon some of the remaining vinaigrette over the salmon and sprinkle some of the dried pink peppercorns on top.

Per serving: 49.9g P (23%) / 71.4g F (75%) / 4.6g NetC (2%)

EXTRA RECIPE
LUNCH

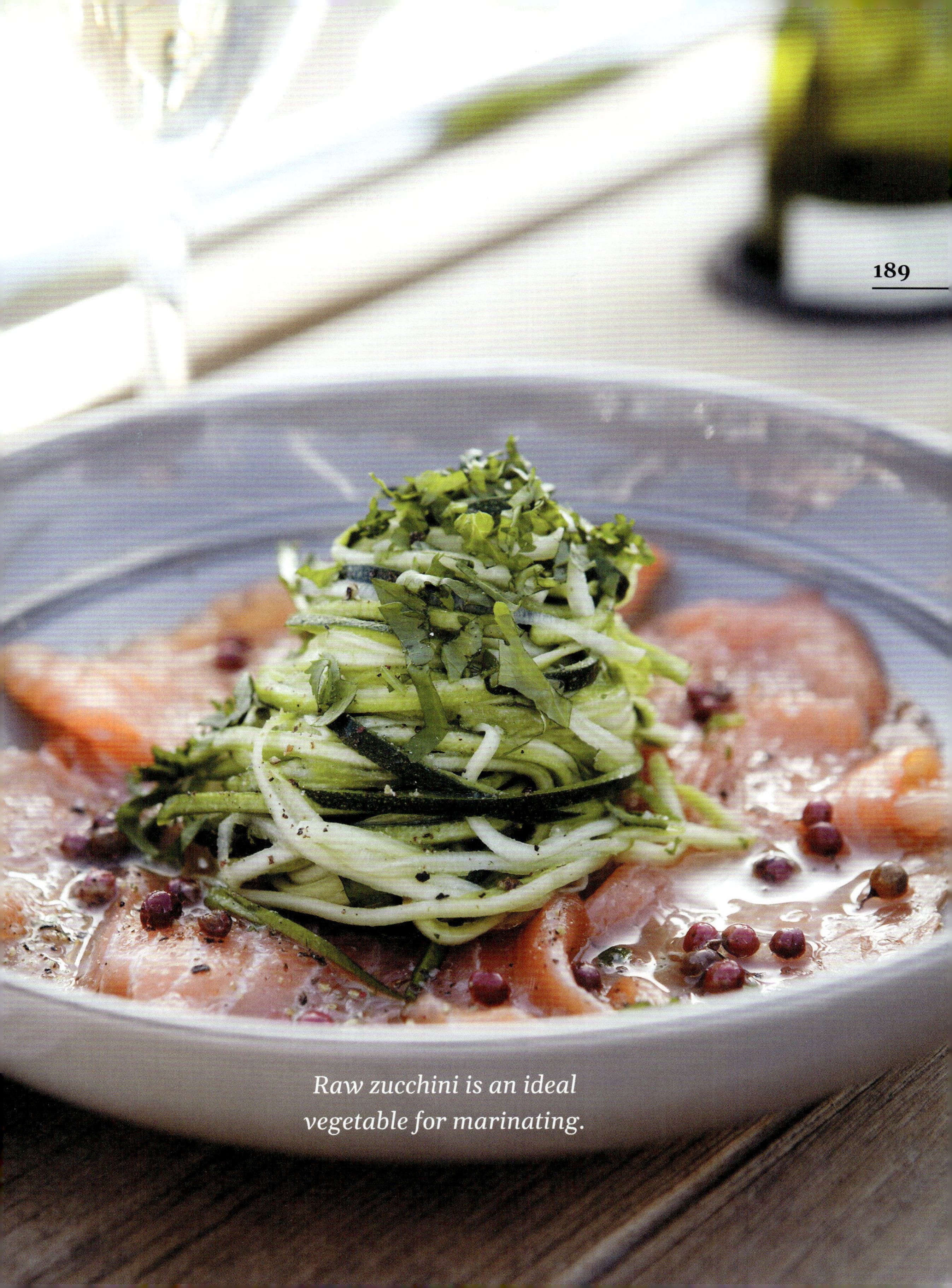

Raw zucchini is an ideal vegetable for marinating.

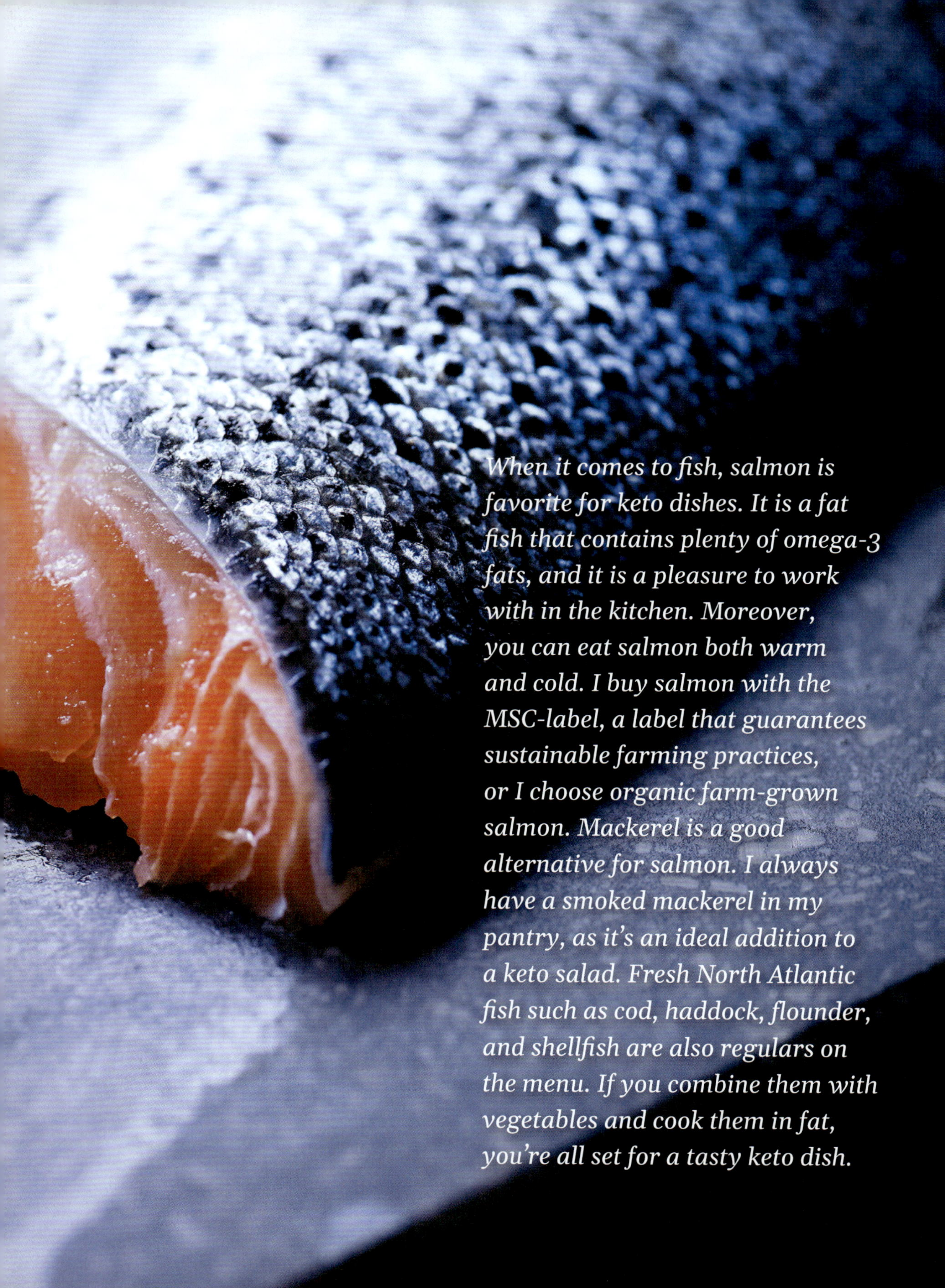

When it comes to fish, salmon is favorite for keto dishes. It is a fat fish that contains plenty of omega-3 fats, and it is a pleasure to work with in the kitchen. Moreover, you can eat salmon both warm and cold. I buy salmon with the MSC-label, a label that guarantees sustainable farming practices, or I choose organic farm-grown salmon. Mackerel is a good alternative for salmon. I always have a smoked mackerel in my pantry, as it's an ideal addition to a keto salad. Fresh North Atlantic fish such as cod, haddock, flounder, and shellfish are also regulars on the menu. If you combine them with vegetables and cook them in fat, you're all set for a tasty keto dish.

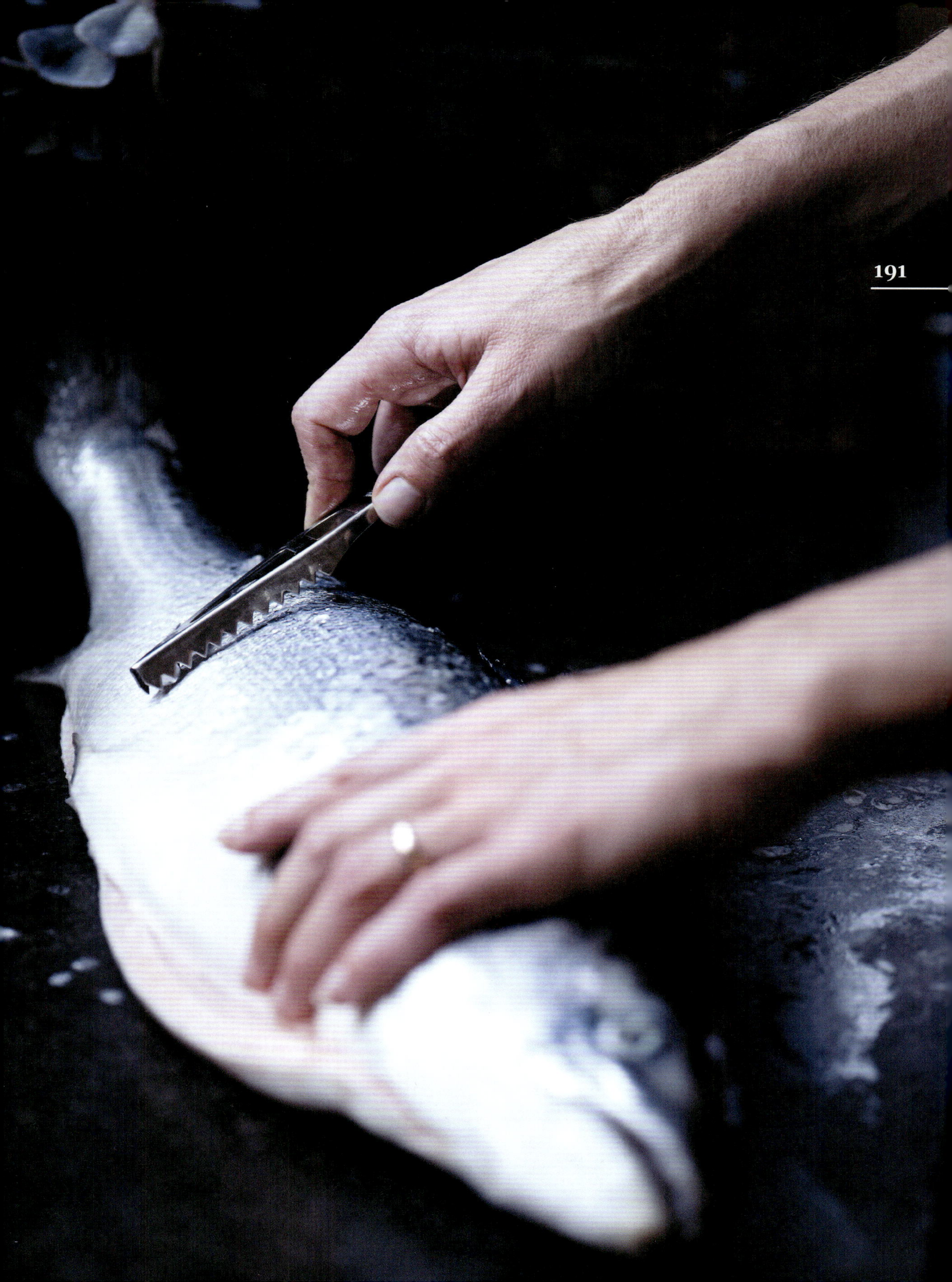

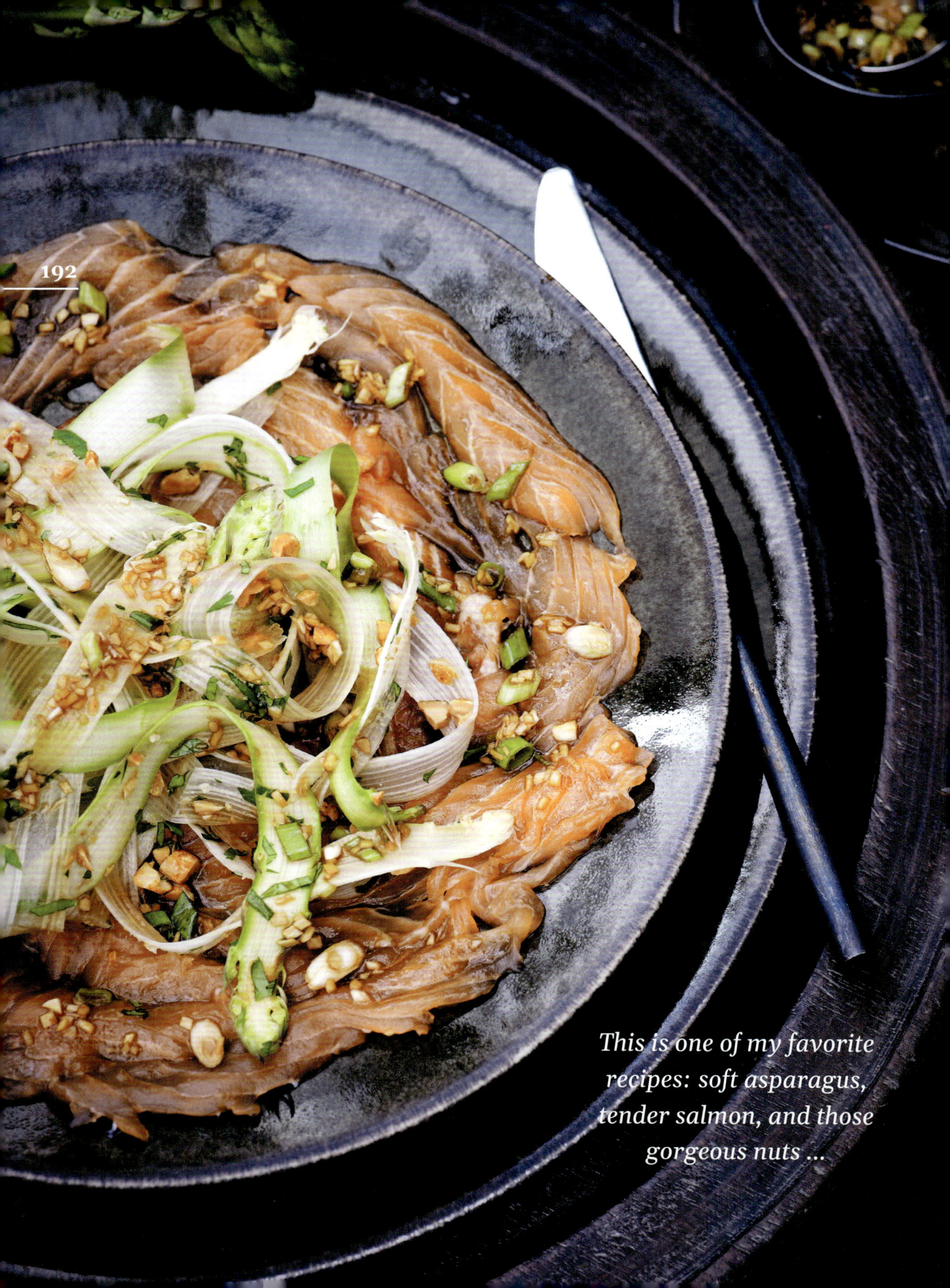
This is one of my favorite
recipes: soft asparagus,
tender salmon, and those
gorgeous nuts ...

Salmon carpaccio

WITH THINLY SLICED GREEN ASPARAGUS

Preparation time: 15 to 20 minutes - cooking time: none - serves 2

14 oz (400 g) green asparagus

10 1/2 oz (300 g) salmon carpaccio

For the sauce:

1 lime

2 tablespoons toasted sesame seed oil (3/4 oz/20 g)

4 tablespoons soy sauce

1 oz (30 g) roasted peanuts

1 3/4-inch (2-cm) piece of ginger (3/4 oz/20 g)

1 clove of garlic

1 spring onion

First, make the sauce. Coarsely chop the peanuts in a blender.
Put them in a bowl and add the sesame oil, soy sauce and juice of half a lime. Grate the ginger and garlic into the sauce and stir well to combine. Finely chop the spring onion and add to the sauce. Remove the woody ends from the asparagus stalks and peel the asparagus lengthwise with a vegetable peeler into long, thin strands. Arrange the salmon on the plates. Arrange the asparagus over the salmon. Drizzle the delicious sauce over the top.

Per serving: 36g P (27%) / 40g F (67%) / 8g NetC (6%)

EXTRA RECIPE
LUNCH/DINNER

These spinach nests are both a pleasure to eat and a feast for the eye. I often serve them as a side dish with a cheesy casserole or as a light lunch with a salad. They are also an ideal side dish for when you're dining with guests. Everyone loves them and you can make them beforehand. All you need to do is bake the nests in the oven. Use spinach with larger leaves and leave the stems on, this will make it easier to make the nests.

Spinach nests

WITH MOZZARELLA

Preparation time: 15 minutes - cooking time: 15 minutes - makes 4 nests

14 oz (400 g) fresh spinach

1 ball mozzarella cheese

handful of pine nuts (about 1 1/2 oz/40 g)

turmeric or sweet paprika powder to garnish

Sauté the spinach in plenty of olive oil until the spinach has wilted. Season with salt and pepper. Remove the pan from the heat and let the spinach cool slightly. Meanwhile, divide the mozzarella into four pieces.

Take a large fork and twirl the spinach around the fork (as you would do with spaghetti). Put the nest into an ungreased baking dish, tweak the spinach into shape with your fingers and press a well in the middle. Make four nests. Divide the mozzarella over the nests and sprinkle some turmeric or sweet paprika powder (for a bit of color) and pine nuts over the top. Bake in the oven at 350 °F (180 °C) for about 10 minutes or until the mozzarella has fully melted.

Per 5 1/2-ounce (150 g) nest: 10g P (16%) / 20g F (79%) / 3g NetC (5%)

EXTRA RECIPE
LUNCH/DINNER

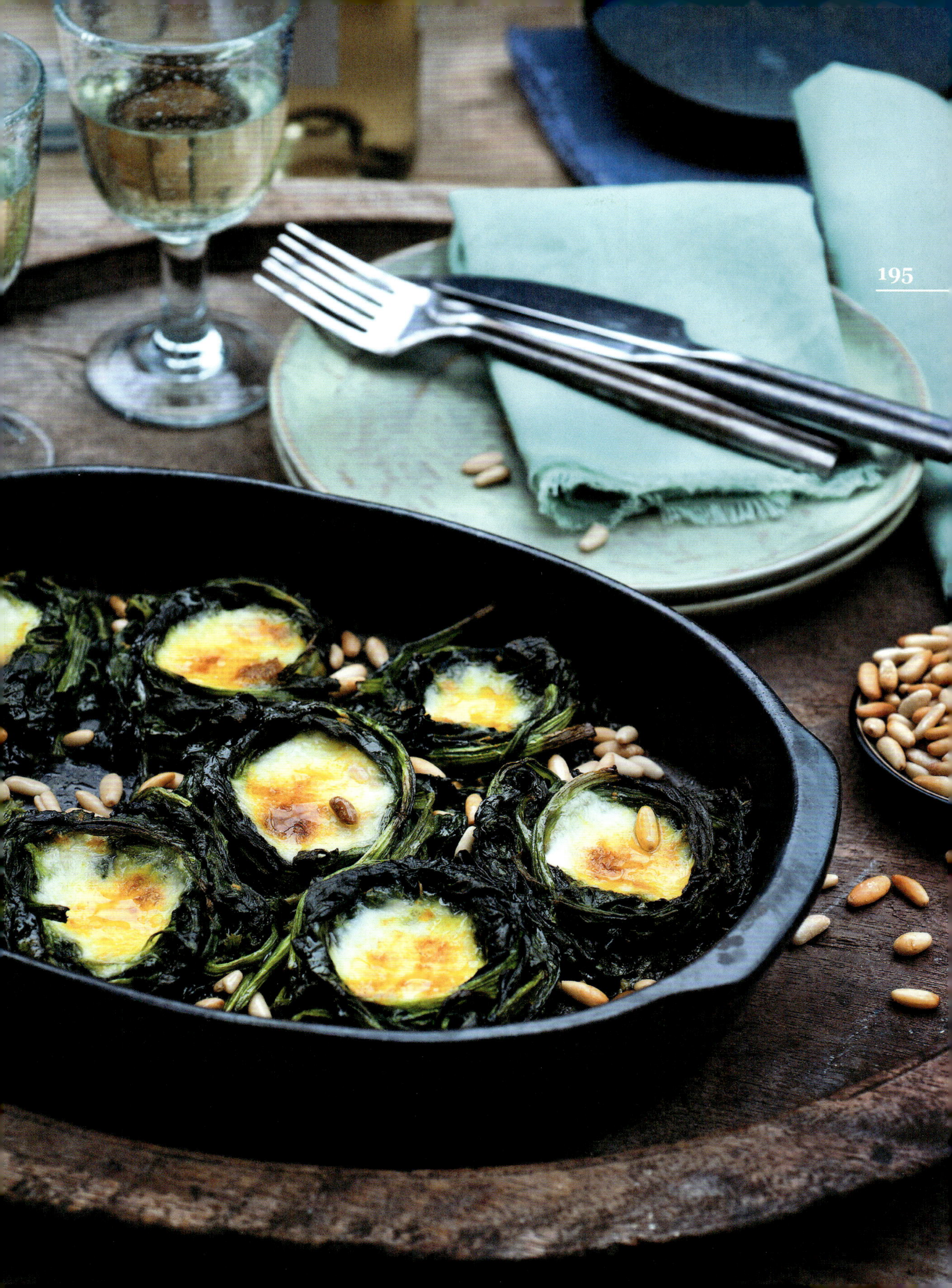

Baked cauliflower mash

WITH MUSHROOMS

Preparation time: 15 minutes - cooking time: 20 minutes - serves 2

1 small head of cauliflower (14 oz/ 400 g)

9 oz (250 g) brown button mushrooms (cremini, baby bella)

5 1/4 oz (150 g) pumpkin seeds

1 1/2 oz (40 g) olive oil

Scrape the outer 1/4 inch (1/2 cm) from the cauliflower, so you end up with tiny couscous-like grains. Rub the cauliflower between your fingers to crumble it into tiny pieces. Coarsely chop the inner part of the cauliflower and cook the pieces in lightly salted water.

Add a generous splash of olive oil to a pan and cook the pumpkin seeds over medium heat. Season with pepper and a little salt (see tip). Set the pumpkin seeds aside on paper towels once they have turned golden brown and have puffed up slightly.

Slice the mushrooms into thick slices and sauté them in the same pan with a generous splash of olive oil. Add the cauliflower couscous and stir-fry everything over medium heat. Add extra olive oil if needed. Season with pepper and a little salt.

Drain the water from the cauliflower pieces. Put the pot back over the heat and pour a generous splash of olive oil into the pot. Briefly fry the cooked cauliflower and then blend. Season with pepper and a little of salt. Spoon the cauliflower puree into the middle of the plate, spoon the fried cauliflower and mushroom mixture over the top and garnish with the pumpkin seeds.

Tip: cooking pumpkin seeds
You'll notice that the pumpkin seeds may pop out of the pan as they're being heated, so keep a lid on hand.

Per serving: 25.2g P (17%) / 54.3g F (78%) / 8.2g NetC (5%)

EXTRA RECIPE
DINNER

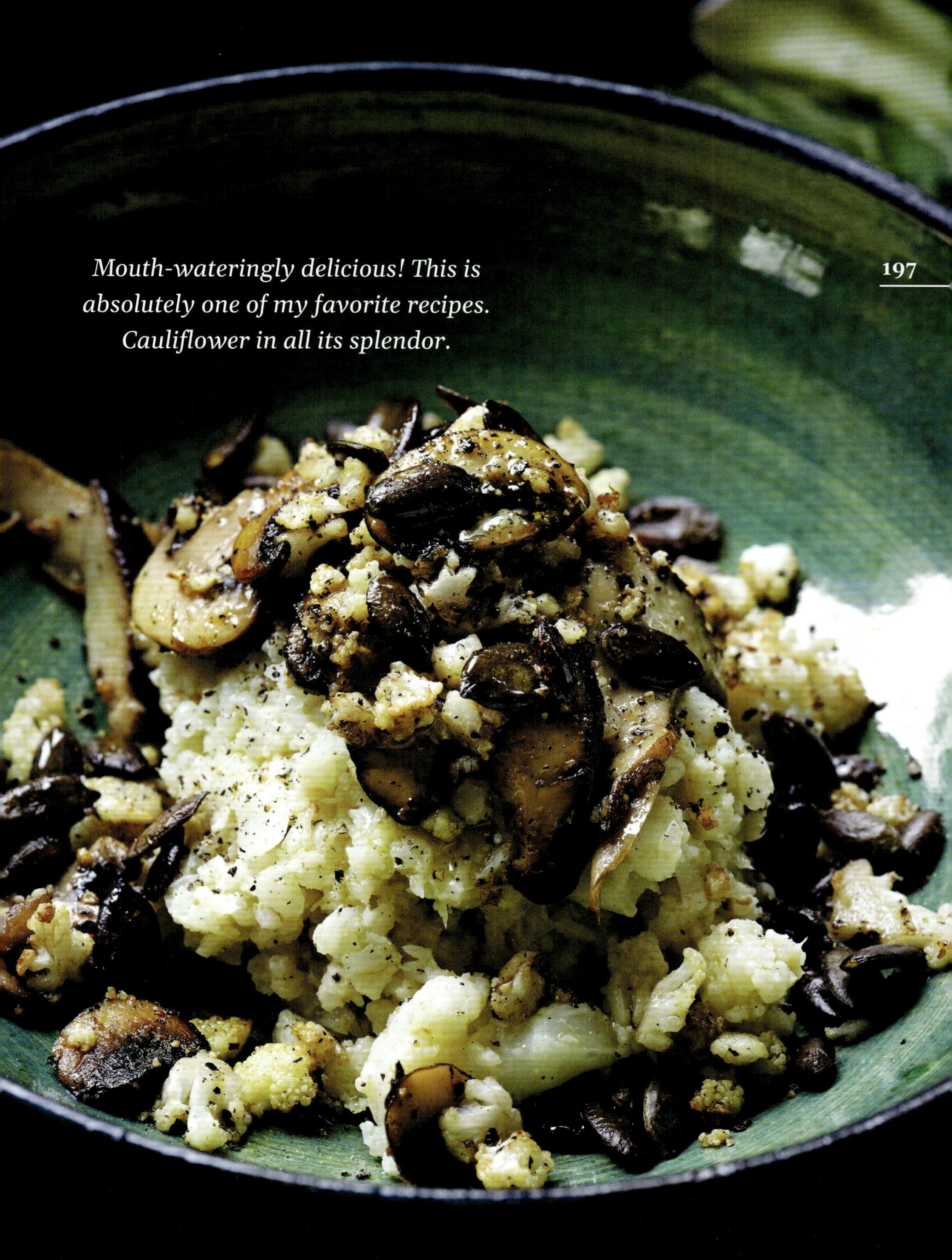

Mouth-wateringly delicious! This is absolutely one of my favorite recipes. Cauliflower in all its splendor.

Sautéed pointed cabbage

WITH CHICKEN MEATBALLS IN BUTTER SAUCE

Ready in 25 minutes - serves 2

14 oz (400 g) pointed cabbage

14 oz (400 g) ground chicken

3 oz (90 g) butter

2 teaspoons ras-el-hanout

Slice the pointed cabbage lengthwise into four pieces. Make sure you slice through the stalk so the leaves stay together. Melt 1 1/2 oz (50 g) of the butter in a pan and put the pointed cabbage pieces into the pan, cut side down. Pour a generous splash of water into the pan, season with salt and pepper and cover. Let the cabbage cook for about 7 minutes. Check regularly and turn the cabbage pieces over once to brown the other side as well.

Combine the ground chicken with the ras-el-hanout, salt and black pepper. Shape them into six meatballs and flatten them slightly, making them easier to cook. Cook the meatballs in some butter in a covered pan. Arrange the pointed cabbage and the meatballs on the plates. Pour the fat out of the pan but leave any leftover bits of meat that have stuck to the pan. Return the pan to the heat and add the remaining 1 1/2 oz (40 g) of butter. Let the butter melt, stirring to mix in the pan drippings. Spoon the sauce over the pointed cabbage and the meatballs.

Per serving: 40.3g P (27%) / 44.4g F (67%) / 8.2g NetC (6%)

EXTRA RECIPE
DINNER

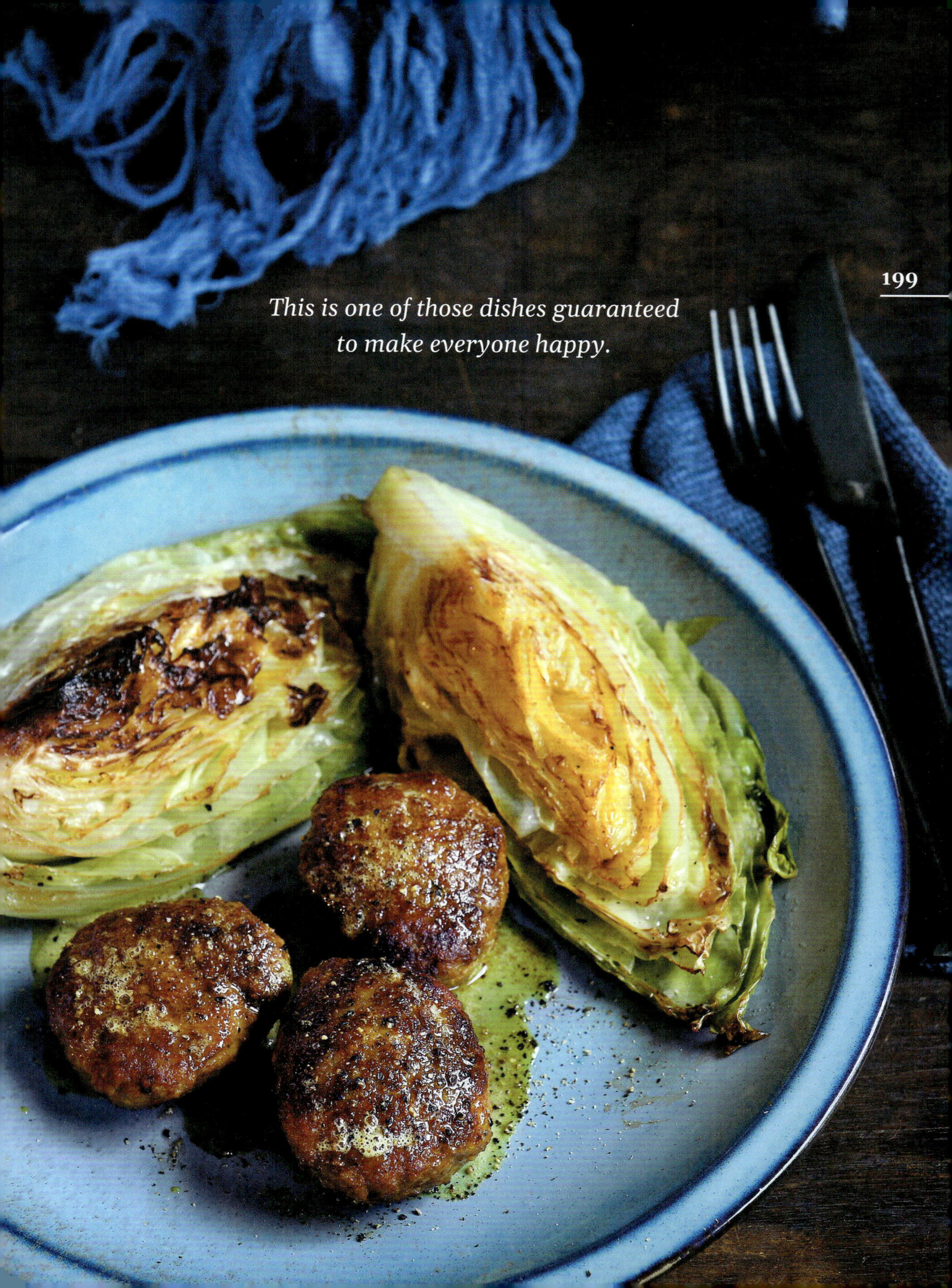

199
This is one of those dishes guaranteed
to make everyone happy.

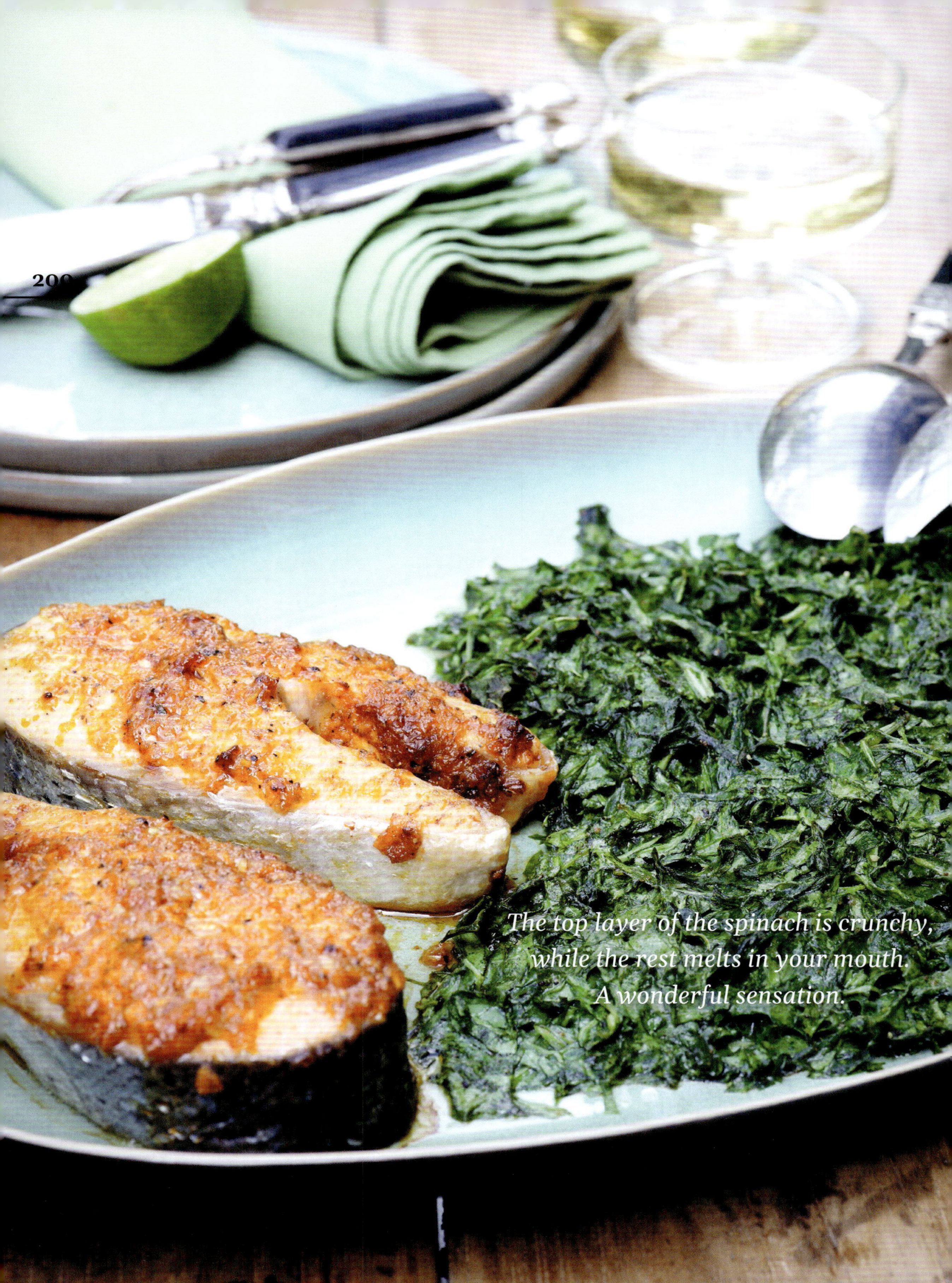
The top layer of the spinach is crunchy,
while the rest melts in your mouth.
A wonderful sensation.

Spicy salmon

WITH OVEN-BAKED SPINACH

Preparation time: 15 minutes - cooking time: 20 minutes - serves 2

2 pieces of salmon (12 oz/350 g)

1 lime

For the sauce:

3 garlic cloves

1 teaspoon harissa (5 g)

a little over 1 lb (500 g) fresh spinach

1 teaspoon ground nutmeg

1 1/2 oz (40 g) olive oil

Preheat the oven to 350 °F (180 °C).

Blend (or grind with a mortar and pestle) the garlic together with the harissa, salt, pepper and a splash of olive oil to a thick paste. Rub the paste into the salmon and place the salmon in a baking dish. Cut the lime in two and place it next to the fish. Bake in the oven for 20 minutes.

Wash the spinach and pat dry. Slice into thin strips. The easiest way to do this is by rolling up the spinach leaves first. Put the spinach in a bowl. Season with salt, pepper and nutmeg and add the olive oil. Toss well until all the spinach pieces are coated with olive oil. Add the spinach to the fish during the final 10 minutes of cooking.

Per serving: 36.7 g P (24%) /51.7g F (75%) / 2g NetC (1%)

EXTRA RECIPE
DINNER

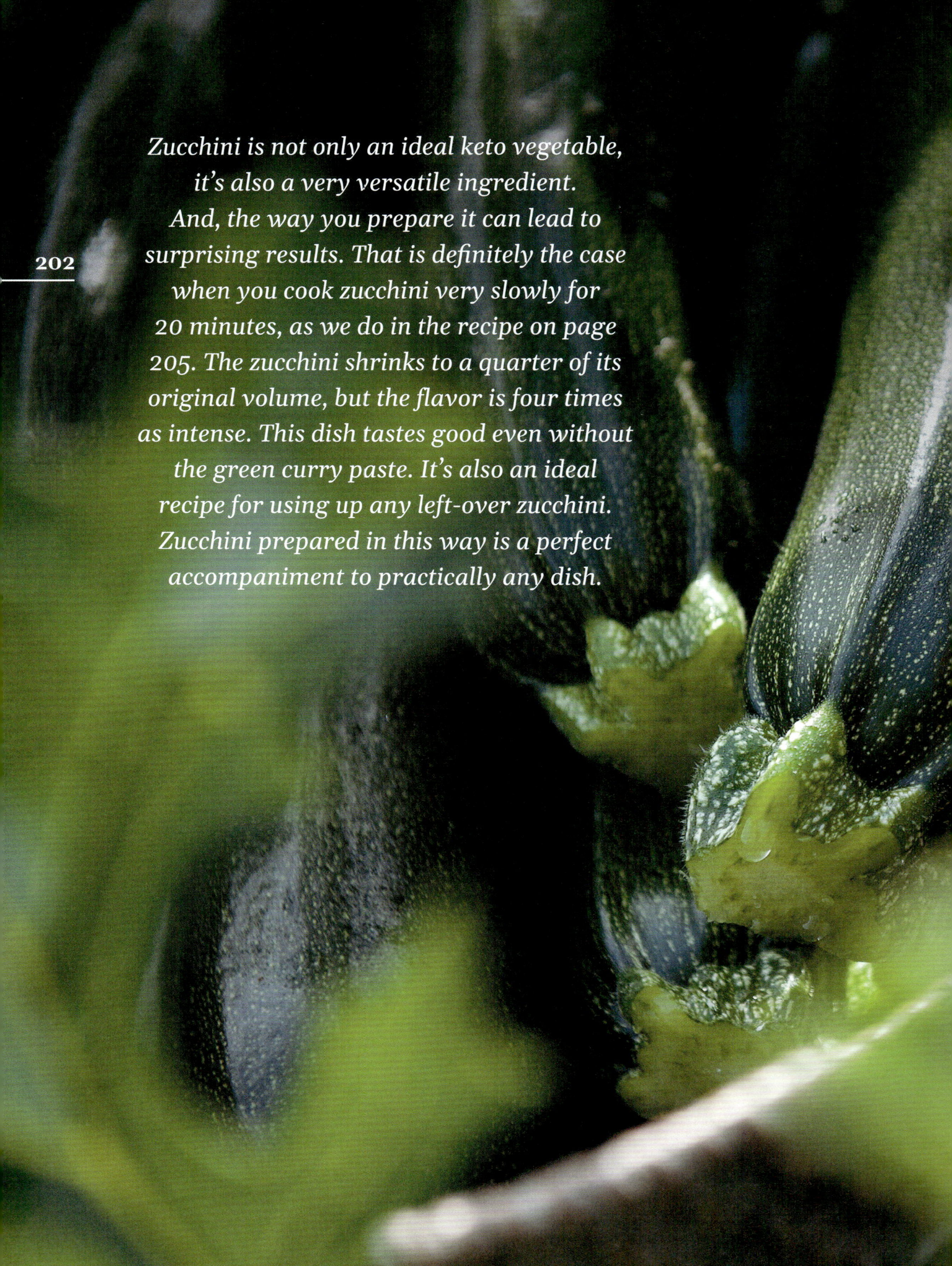

Zucchini is not only an ideal keto vegetable, it's also a very versatile ingredient. And, the way you prepare it can lead to surprising results. That is definitely the case when you cook zucchini very slowly for 20 minutes, as we do in the recipe on page 205. The zucchini shrinks to a quarter of its original volume, but the flavor is four times as intense. This dish tastes good even without the green curry paste. It's also an ideal recipe for using up any left-over zucchini. Zucchini prepared in this way is a perfect accompaniment to practically any dish.

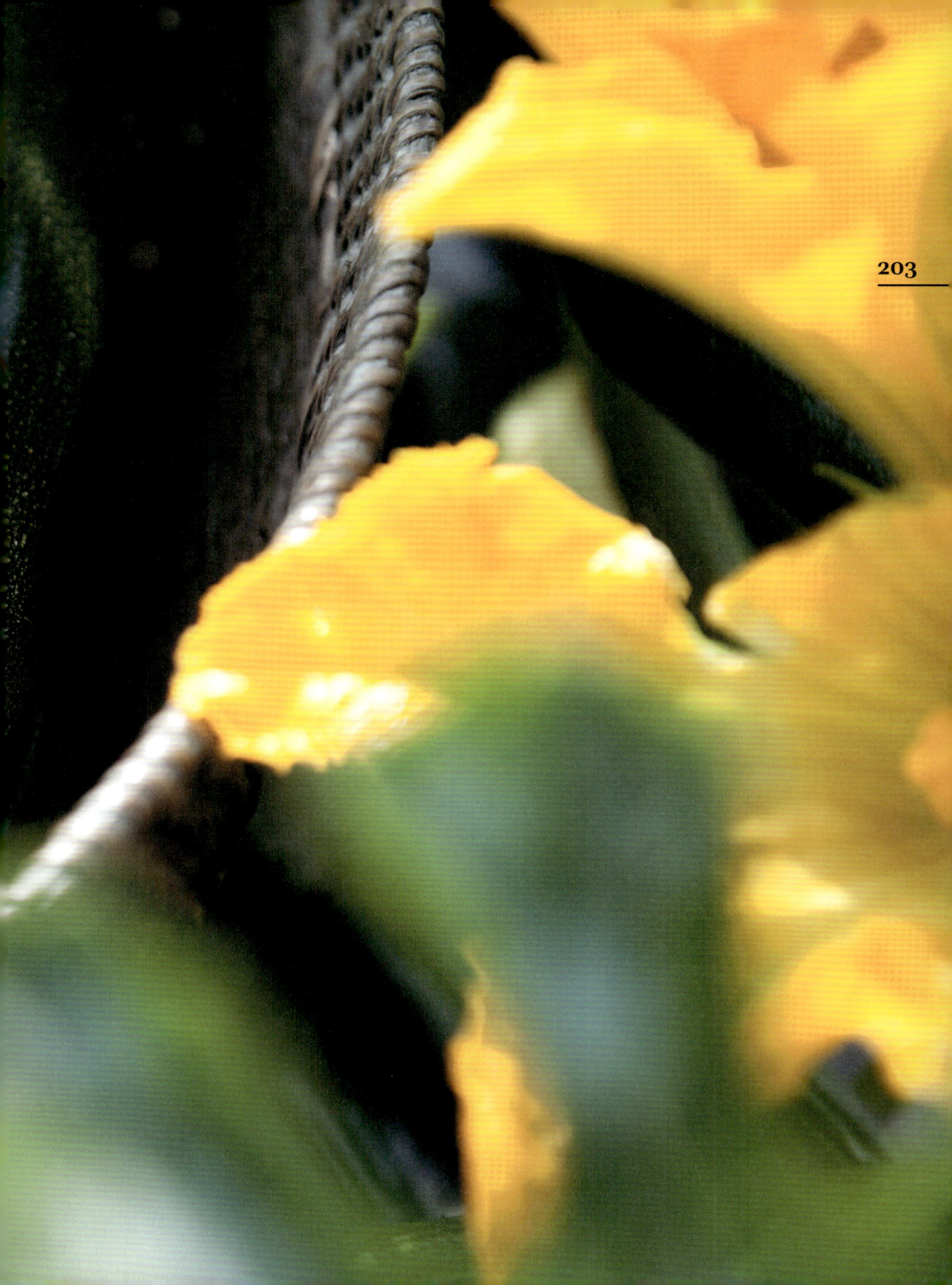

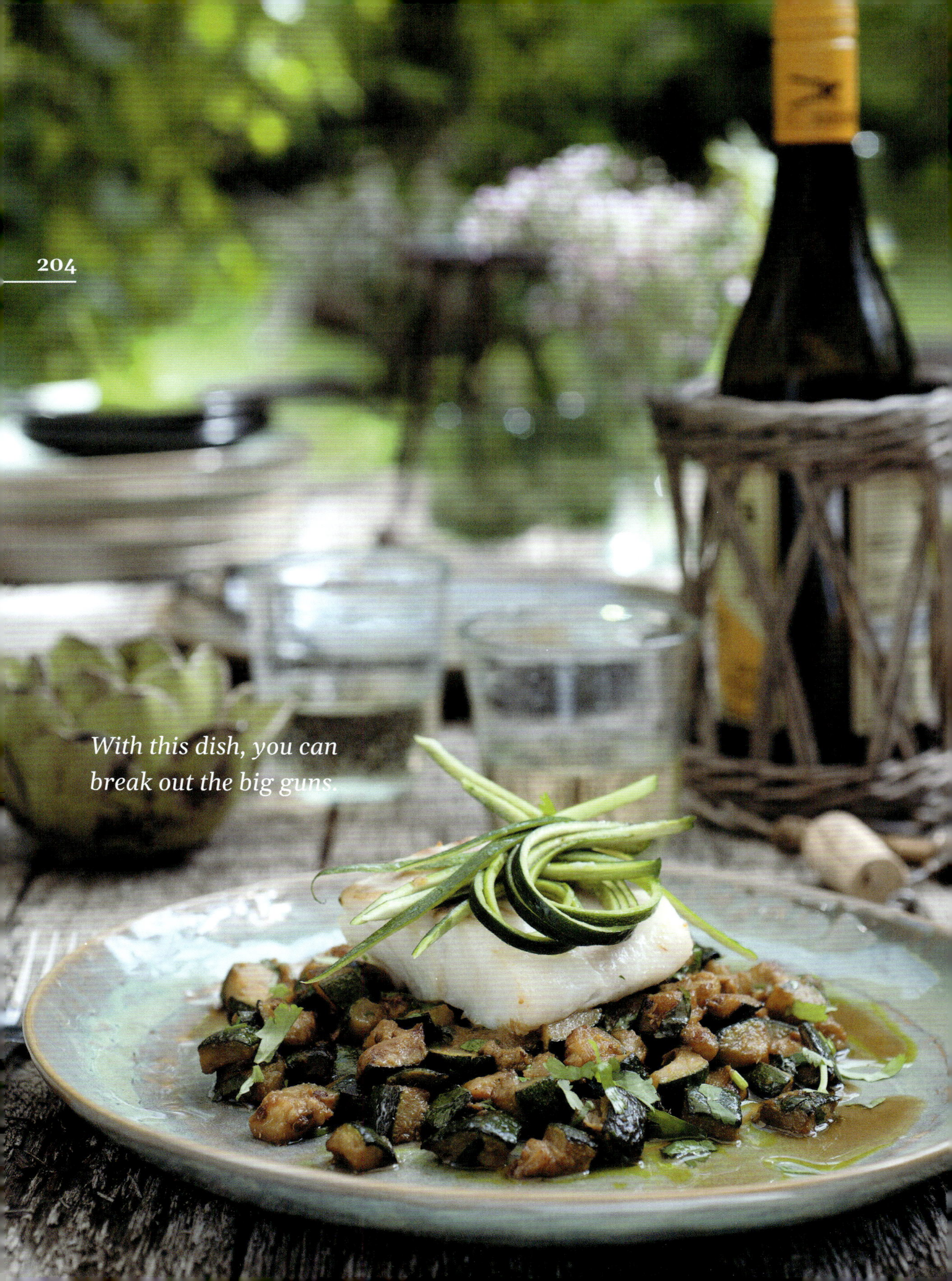

With this dish, you can
break out the big guns.

Spicy fried zucchini

WITH FISH

Preparation time: 15 minutes - cooking time: 20 minutes - serves 2

1 1/4 lb (600 g) zucchini

12 1/2 oz (350 g) whitefish fillet (sea bass, cod ...)

1 tablespoon green curry paste (1 oz/30 g)

a handful fresh cilantro (or parsley) (1 1/2 oz/40 g)

1 3/4 oz (50 g) olive oil

1 3/4 oz (50 g) coconut oil

First slice a couple of thin strands from the zucchini with a vegetable peeler. You will need this for the garnish later. Dice the rest of the zucchini and cook over low heat in the olive oil and coconut oil. Cook gently for about 20 minutes, stirring regularly. Don't panic: you will be left with about a quarter of the original volume. Mix in the curry paste 5 minutes before the end of the cooking time.
Bake the fish in the oven at 350 °F (180 °C) for 10 to 15 minutes while the zucchini is gently cooking.
Season the fish with just a little salt and pepper and pour a drizzle of olive oil over the top.
Finely chop the cilantro and add it to the zucchini just before serving. Place the vegetables on a plate, arrange the fish on top and garnish with the zucchini slices.

Per serving: 45.8g P (26%) / 57g F (71%) / 6.2g NetC (3%)

EXTRA RECIPE
DINNER

Curried spinach

WITH JUMBO SHRIMP

Preparation time: 15 minutes - cooking time: 15 to 20 minutes - serves 2

14 oz (400 g) fresh spinach
12 jumbo shrimp (14 oz/400 g)
14 fl oz (400 ml) coconut cream
1 1/2 oz (40 g) green curry paste (see tip)
1 tablespoon ras-el-hanout
1 1/2 oz (40 g) olive oil

Preheat the oven to 350 °F (180 °C).
Mix the curry paste together with half of the olive oil, then
combine it with the coconut cream. Take a large bowl and
toss the fresh spinach with the curried coconut mixture.
Season with some salt and pepper and spoon the mixture into
a baking dish. Put the dish in the oven for 15 to 20 minutes.
Put the jumbo shrimp in a bowl and toss them with the
remaining olive oil and the ras-el-hanout. Combine thoroughly
until everything is a warm yellow color. Add the jumbo shrimp
to the spinach 10 minutes before the end of the cooking time.

Tip: green curry paste
Be careful with curry paste. Some brands are really spicy,
while others are very mild. Add the paste one spoonful at a
time, and make sure to keep tasting.

Per serving: 31.7g P (20%) / 53.6g F (76%) / 6.6g NetC (4%)

EXTRA RECIPE
DINNER

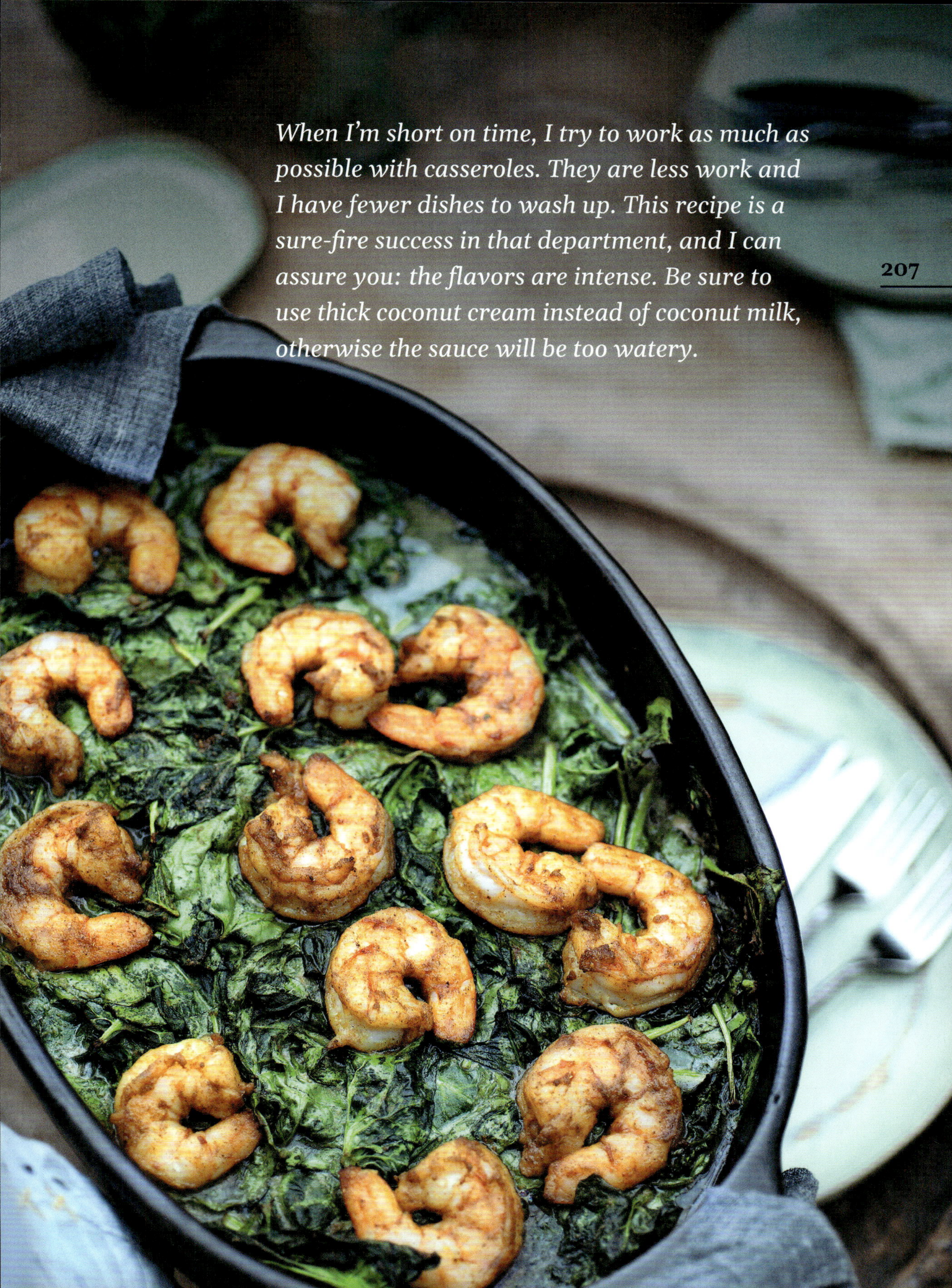

When I'm short on time, I try to work as much as possible with casseroles. They are less work and I have fewer dishes to wash up. This recipe is a sure-fire success in that department, and I can assure you: the flavors are intense. Be sure to use thick coconut cream instead of coconut milk, otherwise the sauce will be too watery.

Sole

WITH BROCCOLI PUREE

Preparation time: 25 minutes - cooking time: 20 minutes - serves 2

2 sole, skin and bony fin ridges removed

a little over 1 lb (500 g) broccoli

For the sauce:

2 oz (60 g) butter

12 small tomatoes

4 anchovy fillets

1/3 oz (10 g) parsley

1 tablespoon sliced almonds

Slice the broccoli into florets. Remove the outer layer from the stalk and slice the stalk. Cook the broccoli florets and slices in some water with a generous splash of olive oil, salt and pepper until tender. Cover the pan. Drain off the water, return the pan to the heat and add another generous splash of olive oil to the broccoli. Briefly stir-fry the broccoli before mashing it into a thick pulp.
Bake the sole for about 4 minutes on each side in butter with some salt and pepper.
Now, make the sauce: Halve the tomatoes, chop the anchovies into tiny pieces and finely chop the parsley. Heat up plenty of butter in a small pan over low heat. Add the tomatoes, parsley, anchovies and the sliced almonds. Cook for a few minutes so the ingredients release their flavors; make sure the butter doesn't turn brown. You can add pepper, but you don't need to add any salt - the anchovies are salty enough. Spoon the broccoli puree onto the plates, arrange the fish over the top and garnish with the delicious sauce.

Per serving: 47.2g P (26%) / 57.6g F (72%) / 3.9g NetC (2%)

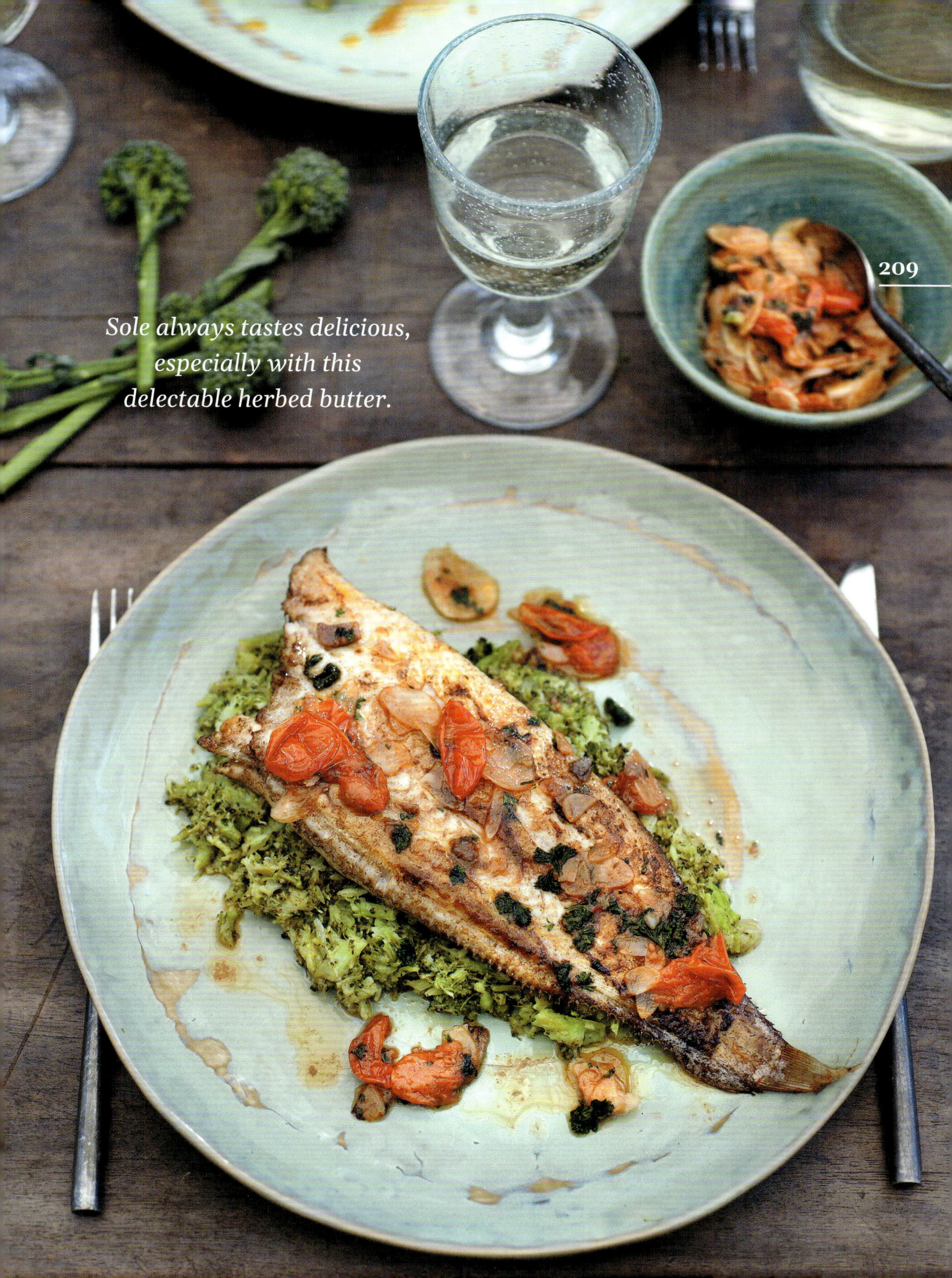

Sole always tastes delicious, especially with this delectable herbed butter.

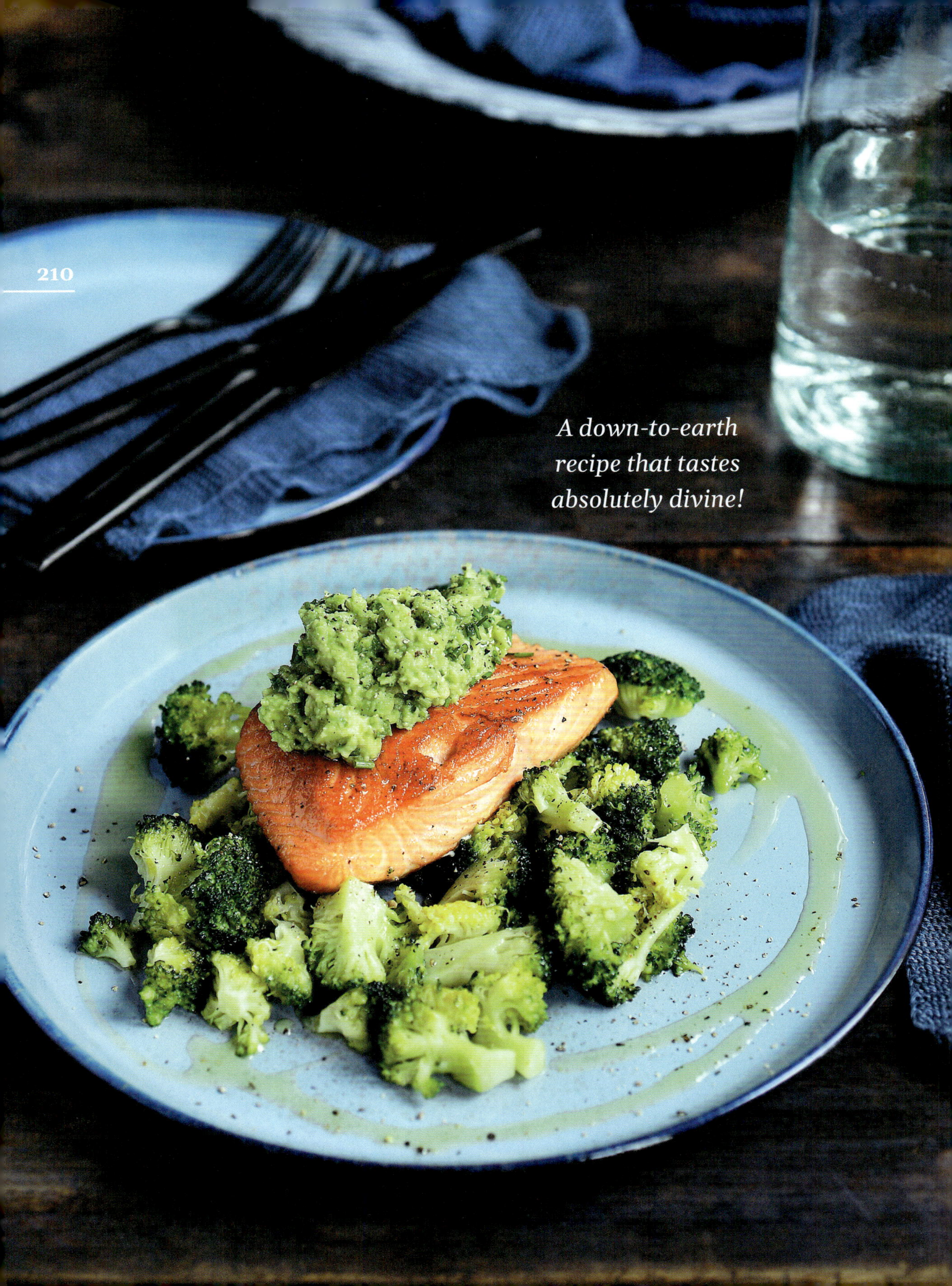

A down-to-earth
recipe that tastes
absolutely divine!

Salmon

WITH GUACAMOLE AND SAUTEED BROCCOLI

Ready in 25 minutes - serves 2

1 head of broccoli (14 oz/400 g)

2 salmon fillets (14 oz/400 g)

1 avocado

juice of 1/2 lime

2 oz (60 g) butter

handful of fresh herbs (1 oz/ 25 g)

Slice the broccoli into florets and sauté in 1 1/2 oz (40 g) butter (or coconut oil) with a splash of water.

Cover the pan. Stir regularly.

Mash the avocado flesh with the lime juice and finely chopped fresh herbs.

Season with salt and black pepper.

Sear the salmon fillets over a high heat in the remaining butter (or olive oil).

Place the broccoli on a plate and arrange the salmon with the guacamole over the top.

Garnish with olive oil and black pepper.

Per serving: 45g P (23%) / 64g F (75%) / 4g NetC (2%)

EXTRA RECIPE
DINNER

Chocolate cake

Preparation time: 15 minutes - cooking time: 15 minutes - serves 2

1 1/2 oz (40 g) dark chocolate (at least 85% cocoa)

1 3/4 oz (50 g) nut flour (hazelnut or walnut)

1 oz (25 g) cocoa powder

1 egg

2 oz (60 g) butter

ground cinnamon

Extra: baking parchment

Preheat the oven to 350 °F (180 °C).

Melt the chocolate together with the butter (see tip). Keep some of the cocoa powder aside to garnish. Combine the nut flour with the cocoa powder and the egg. Stir in the melted butter and chocolate. Pour the batter into a cake tin lined with baking parchment. Sprinkle some cocoa powder over the top and bake in the oven for about 15 minutes.

Tip: melting chocolate

I put the chocolate and butter in a bowl and place it in the oven at 175 °F (70 °C). The mixture is completely melted after about 7 minutes. It's a lot less work than using a water bath.

Tip: cake tin

I'm often asked this question: which cake tin? Just have a look and see which cake tins or baking dishes you have in your cupboard. I like to use my small baking dishes for this cake, they are 15 cm (about 6") in diameter.

Tip: sugar substitute

You can also find this dessert in my book *Nog Eenvoudiger 2*. I use sugar in that recipe, but that doesn't fit into a keto diet. Dark chocolate lovers will love these cakes without sugar. If you prefer your cakes a little sweeter, you can add some xylitol (see p. 64 for more information on sugar substitutes).

Per serving: 6g P (8%) / 29g F (88%) / 3g NetC (4%)

EXTRA RECIPE
DESSERT

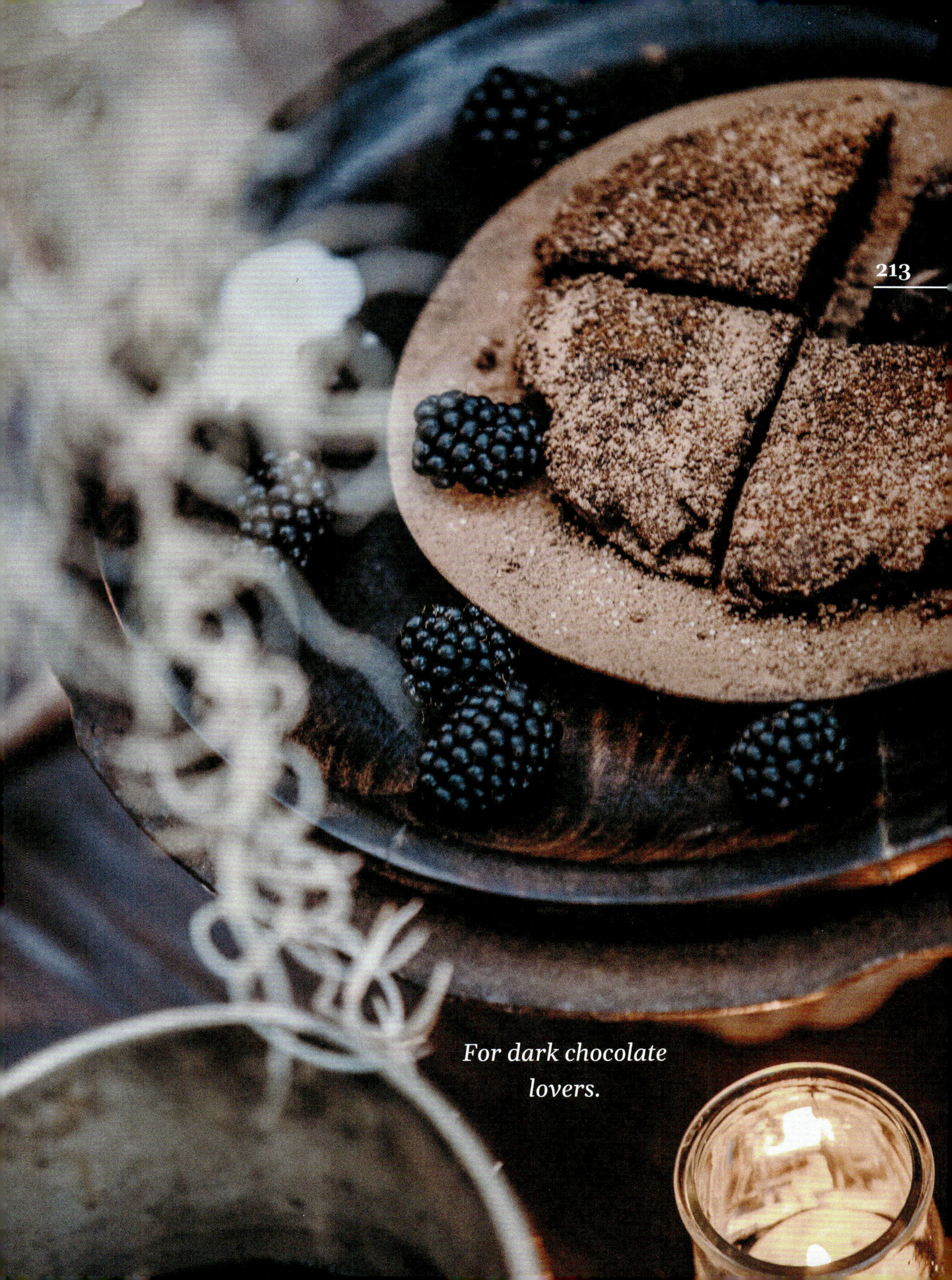

For dark chocolate lovers.

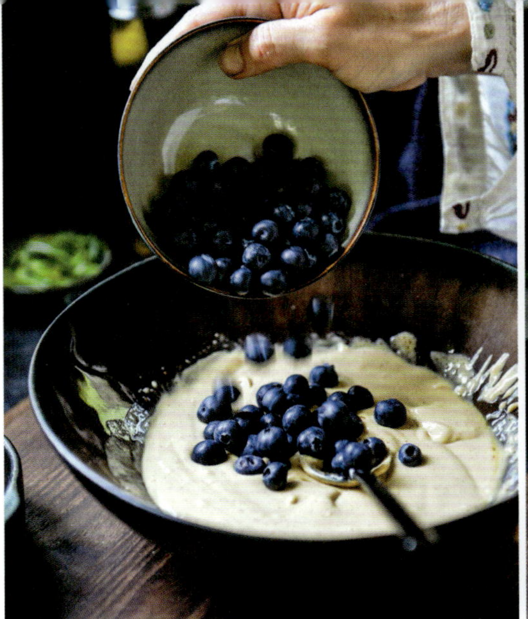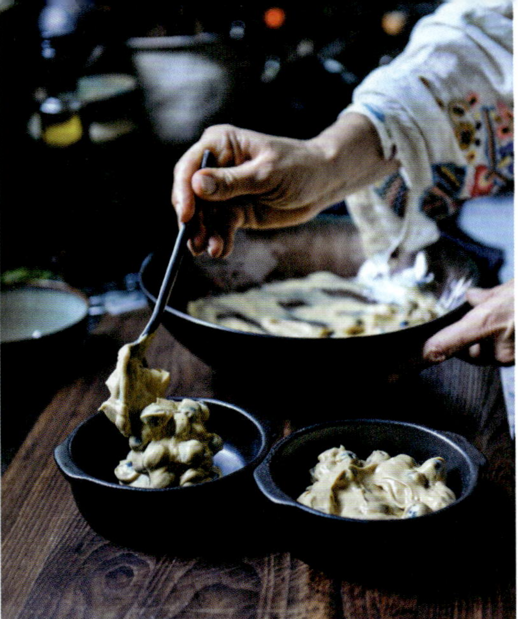

Delicious dessert

WITH MASCARPONE AND BLUEBERRIES

Preparation time: 4 minutes - cooking time: 15 minutes - serves 2

7 oz (200 g) mascarpone

3 1/2 oz (100 g) blueberries

2 eggs

Preheat the oven to 350 °F (180 °C).

Separate the eggs into yolks and whites. We only need the yolks. You can save the whites for another recipe if you wish.

Mix the egg yolks with the mascarpone and stir in the blueberries.

Spoon into ramekins or small ovenproof bowls and place them in the oven for 13-14 minutes.

Tip: sugar substitute

If you prefer your dessert a little sweeter, you can add xylitol or erythritol, but before you do, read more about sugar substitutes on page 64.

Per serving: 9.5g P (7%) / 49.9g F (87%) / 7.3g NetC (6%)

EXTRA RECIPE
DESSERT

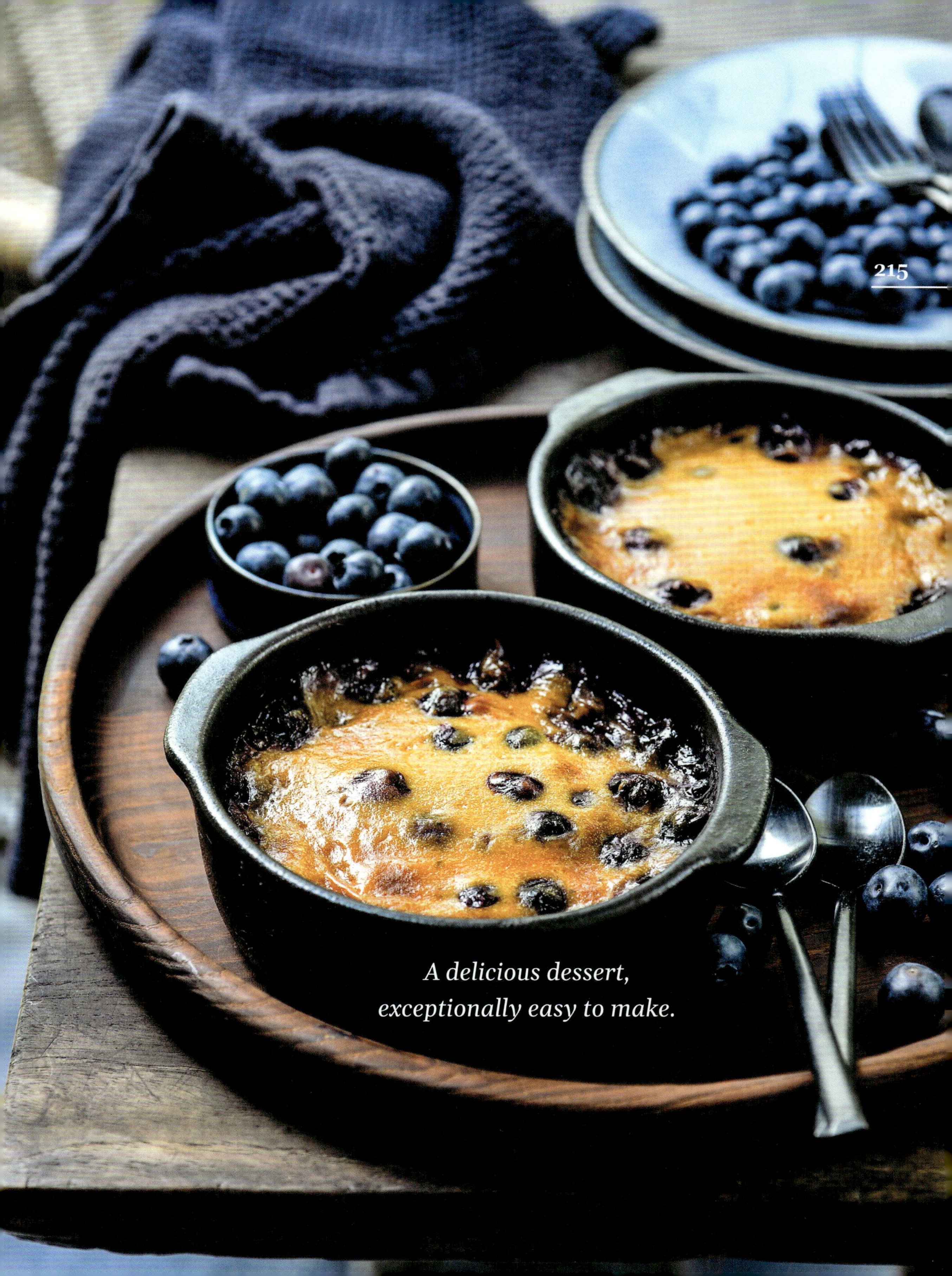

A delicious dessert,
exceptionally easy to make.

Keto chocolate mousse

Preparation time: 10 minutes - setting time: 5 minutes - serves 2

7 fl oz (200 ml) coconut cream

2 oz (60 g) nut butter

1 oz (30 g) cocoa powder

1/2 oz (15 g) cocoa nibs to garnish

A few blueberries to garnish

Thoroughly combine the coconut milk, the nut butter and the cocoa powder. Let the mixture briefly set in the refrigerator or for a couple of minutes in the freezer. Garnish with the cocoa nibs and the blueberries.

Tip: coconut cream
For this dessert, you really do need coconut cream instead of coconut milk. If you can't find coconut cream, use only the top creamy layer of coconut milk from the can or carton.

Per serving: 10.6g P (11%) / 36g F (82%) / 7.4g NetC (7 %)

EXTRA RECIPE
DESSERT

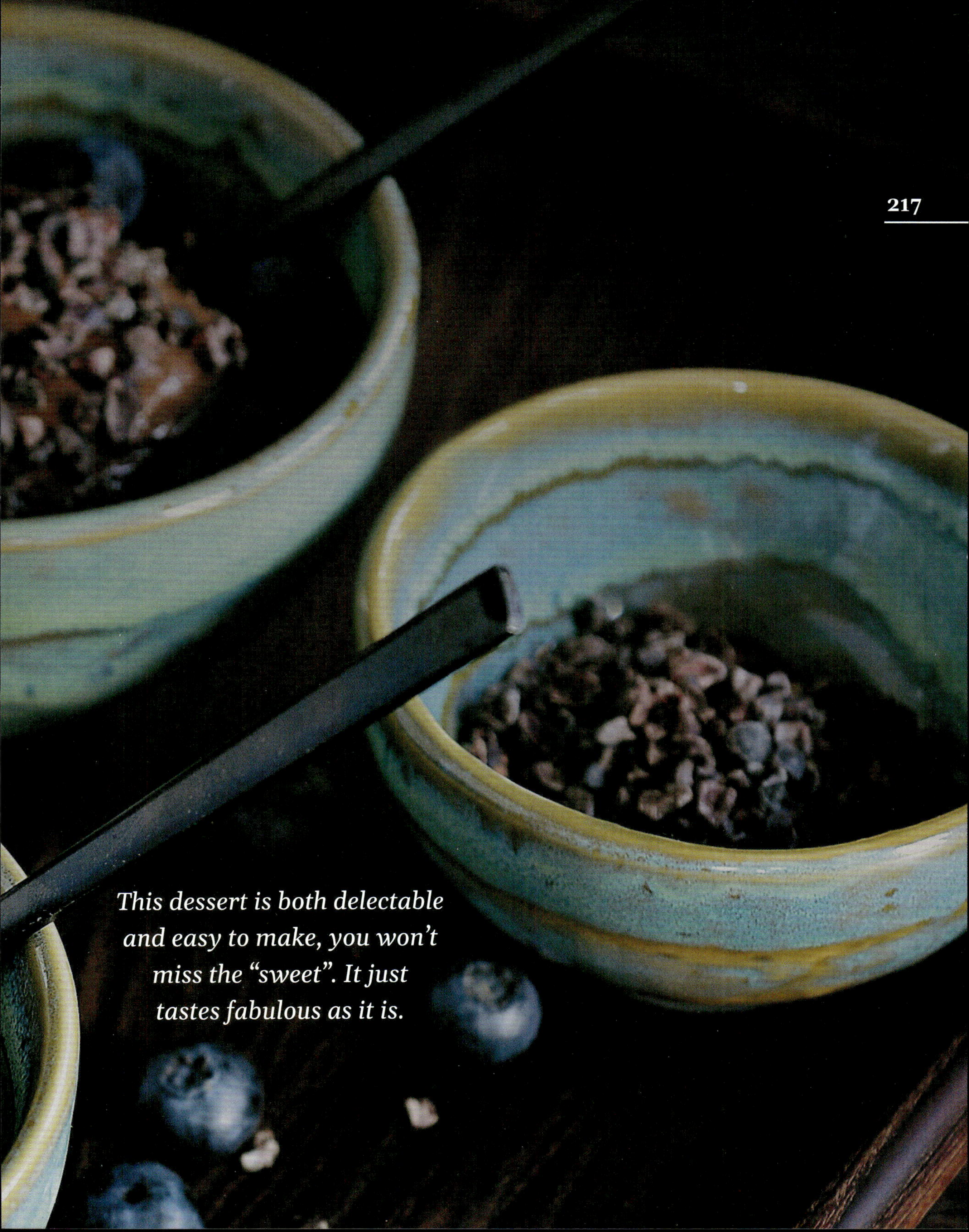

This dessert is both delectable and easy to make, you won't miss the "sweet". It just tastes fabulous as it is.

How the ketogenic diet originated

The keto diet has its origins in the 1920s and 1930s. It was developed by the Mayo Clinic (US) as a feasible alternative for the fasting diet recommended at the time for people with epilepsy. In 1921, endocrinologist Rollin Woodyatt discovered that fasting changes the body's metabolism. When the body is deprived of carbs (sugars), the liver starts burning body fats instead, producing ketones which are then used as a source of energy. The brain cannot use fatty acids as a source of energy because they cannot pass through the blood-brain barrier. Ketones (like glucose) can pass through this barrier, which was beneficial for patients with epilepsy. But people cannot fast forever, and as soon as the patients started to eat again, the seizures returned in many cases. Researchers started looking for a feasible diet that simulated the effects of fasting. Dr. Russell Wilder from the Mayo Clinic, who worked with diabetic patients, developed this research further and was the first to coin the term 'ketogenic diet'. He discovered that when you follow a diet high in fat and low in carbs, you can achieve the same effect as fasting. This diet also stimulates the development of ketones in the body, but it is much easier to achieve and maintain.

In the 1970s, Dr. Robert Atkins also experimented with the ketogenic diet. His low-carb diet started with a strict ketogenic diet in the first few weeks.

In the seventies, Professor Peter R. Huttenlocher introduced the MCT-diet (MCT = medium-chain triglycerides). These fatty acids are more easily converted into ketones and allowed epilepsy patients to eat slightly more carbohydrates while remaining in ketosis (see also page 28 about MCT oils).

Ketones look very promising and have become big business in recent years. In the sports world, extensive research is being conducted into exogenous ketones. We have known for some time that our bodies are not the only ketone producers: researchers can also produce artificial ketones, also known as exogenous ketones. They were introduced in 2003 to give American soldiers extra energy and keep them strong mentally. Today, one of the world's largest ketone manufacturers, H.V.M.N. in Silicon Valley, supplies exogenous ketones to practically all world-class professional cyclists.

In Belgium too, there is a large market for exogenous ketones and that, of course, has everything to do with the research conducted by Belgian professor Peter Hespel at KU Leuven, the results of which showed that endurance athletes performed up to 15 percent better when they took exogenous ketones during their recovery period. Ketones are the body's back-up fuel source. When the body has run out of all other sources of fuel, ketones come to the rescue of cells low on energy. Although this hardly compares to the nutritional ketosis discussed in this book, it does show that ketones show promise in many different fields.

Let's be clear: the ketogenic diet and the discovery of ketones are nothing new. The ketogenic diet has existed for more than a century and research has grown exponentially in this field from all corners of the scientific and medical world, from sports nutrition to diabetes and obesity research and from cancer research to neurology. It's no coincidence that this comes paired with the rise and increased popularity of the ketogenic diet with the general public. The studies conducted by cutting-edge researchers in particular point to the health benefits of the ketogenic diet, making the public enthusiastic about the possibilities.

While writing this book, I followed a keto diet and reached ketosis for an extended period of time. It was an exceptionally valuable experience that gave me new insight into nutrition. Physically, however, I noticed very little difference, perhaps because I have been eating moderately low-carb for years. I also didn't notice a difference in my energy levels, and I haven't lost weight (which was never my intention). What I did feel was great, just as always.

I would love to find out how you experienced going keto. Definitely let me know. Visit www.purepascale.com and send me a message via the "contact" page. You can read more stories under "testimonials". United we stand :-)

Index

Delicious dessert with
  mascarpone and blueberries 214
Mini-quiche with ham 122

marrow bones
Beef broth with savoy cabbage
  and marrow bones 127

mozzarella
Spinach nests with mozzarella 194

nuts
Sautéed bok choy with
  mushrooms and egg 174
Vegetables with hazelnuts 144
Delicious keto cheese crackers 165
Cod with spinach, tomato,
  eggplant and pistachio pesto 140
Keto nut and seed crackers 167
Eggplant noodles 129
Nut bread 171
Overnight chocolate mousse
  with macadamia nuts 102
Warm feta with vegetables
  and pecans 78
Seeds and nuts with full-fat
sour cream 89

olives
Chicken with olives
  and mushrooms 118
Pointed cabbage spaghetti
  with tomatoes and olives 151

bok choy
Sautéed bok choy with
  mushrooms and egg 174

bell peppers
Stuffed avocado with crawfish 117

pesto
Burrata with tomatoes,
  cream and pesto 98

snow peas
Avocado with bacon
  and snow peas 104

purslane
Smoked salmon with
  avocado and purslane 77
Green vegetable soup 179

green beans
Lamb chops with cauliflower,
  cream and sautéed green beans 94

crawfish
Stuffed avocado with crawfish 117

cream
Beef broth with tomato and cream 131
Burrata with tomato, cream
  and pesto 98
Raw salmon with avocado and
  tomato in a lovely cream sauce 180

savoy cabbage
Beef broth with savoy cabbage
  and marrow bones 127

jumbo shrimp
Curried spinach with jumbo shrimp 206

celery
Vegetables with hazelnuts 144

meat scraps
Beef broth with savoy cabbage
  and marrow bones 127

bacon
Avocado with bacon
  and snow peas 104

spinach
Green vegetable soup 179
Instant cold spinach soup 90
Cod with green curry 112
Cod with spinach, tomato,
  eggplant and pistachio pesto 140
Chicken broth with spinach 80
Spinach omelet roll-up with
  mushrooms and cheese 115
Spicy salmon with
  oven-baked spinach 201
Spinach soup with sliced
  almonds and a boiled egg 142
Curried spinach with
  jumbo shrimp 206
Spinach with tomato,
  turmeric and feta 149
Spinach nests with mozzarella 194
Spiced fish with coconut milk,
  lime and tomatoes 101

pointed cabbage
Sautéed pointed cabbage
  with chicken meatballs 198
Pointed cabbage spaghetti
  with tomatoes and olives 151

brussels sprouts
Cooked chicken with vegetables 157

tomatoes
Beef broth with tomato 131
Burrata with tomatoes,
  cream and pesto 98
Zucchini with smoked salmon,
  soy sauce and capers 137
Cod with green curry 112
Cod with spinach, tomato,
  eggplant and pistachio pesto 140
Raw salmon with avocado and
  tomato in a lovely cream sauce 180
Pointed cabbage spaghetti
  with tomatoes and olives 151
Spinach with tomato,
  turmeric and feta 149
Sole with broccoli puree 208
Creamy cheese with roast
  tomatoes and fresh herbs 133

Spiced fish with coconut milk,
lime and tomatoes

sole
Sole with broccoli puree

lamb's lettuce
Avocado with bacon
  and snow peas

fish
Spicy fried zucchini with fish
Spiced fish with coconut milk,
  lime and tomatoes

fish eggs
Avocado with crab
  and lumpfish eggs
Zucchini roll-ups with mackerel
Smoked salmon with
  mascarpone and fish eggs

white cabbage
White cabbage with shrimp

seeds
Roasted nuts and seeds
  with full-fat sour cream
Goat cheese with
  marinated sesame seeds
Greek yogurt with berries
  and seeds
Delicious keto cheese crackers
Keto nut and seed crackers
Nut bread
Seeds and nuts with full-fat
  sour cream

salmon
Zucchini with smoked salmon,
  soy sauce and capers
Smoked salmon with avocado
Smoked salmon with
  mascarpone and fish eggs
Delicious omelet with salmon
Spicy salmon with
  oven-baked spinach
Raw salmon with avocado and
  tomato in a lovely cream sauce
Raw salmon with zucchini noodles
Salmon with guacamole
  and broccoli

sour cream
Salmon carpaccio with thinly
  sliced green asparagus
Roasted nuts and seeds with
  full-fat sour cream
Raw salmon with avocado and
  tomato in a lovely cream sauce
Seeds and nuts with full-fat
  sour cream

Endnotes

1   The Ketogenic Diet: Evidence for Optimism but High-Quality Research Needed, David S Ludwig New Balance Foundation Obesity Prevention Center, Boston Children's Hospital and Harvard Medical School, Boston, MA, USA

2   A ketogenic diet may restore fertility in women with polycystic ovary syndrome: a case series, Ula Abed Alwahab, MD1; Kevin M. Pantalone, DO1; Bartolome Burguera, MD, PhD1,2

3   Cortvriendt W., Kankervrij, Uitgeverij Lucht, Amsterdam, 2020.

4   Klement R., Beneficial Effects of Ketogenic Diets for Cancer Patients - A Realist Review with Focus on Evidence and Confirmation. Med Oncol. 2017; 34: 132.
    Lv M., Zhu X., Wang H. et al., Roles of caloric restriction, ketogenic diet and intermittent fasting during initiation, progression and metastasis of cancer in animal models: a systematic review and meta-analysis. PLoS ONE. 2014; 9: e115147.
    Klement R., Champ C., Otto C. et al., Anti-tumor effects of Ketogenic diets in Mice: a meta-analysis. PLoS ONE. 2016: 11: e0155050.

5   Weiser M., Cabanillas M., Konopleva M. et al., Relation between the duration of remission and hyperglycemia during induction chemotherapy for acute lymphocytic leukemia with a hyperfractionated cyclophosphamide, vincristine, doxorubicin, and dexamethasone/ methotrexate-cytarabine regimen. Cancer. 2004; 100: 1179-1185.
    McGirt M., Chaichana K., Gathinj M. et al., Persistent outpatient hyperglycemia is independently associated with decreased survival after primary resection of malignant brain astrocytomas. Neurosurgery. 2008; 63: 286-291.
    Derr R., Ye X., Islas M. et al. Association between hyperglycemia and survival in patients with newly diagnosed glioblastoma. J Clin Oncol. 2009; 27: 1082-1086.
    Lamkin D., Spitz D., Shahzad M. et al., Glucose as a prognostic factor in Ovarian Carcinoma. Cancer. 2009; 115: 1021- 1027.
    Erickson K., Patterson R., Flatt S. et al., Clinically defined type 2 diabetes mellitus and prognosis in early-stage breast cancer. J Clin Oncol. 2011; 29: 54-60.
    Villarreal-Garza C., Shaw-Dulin R., Lara-Medina F. et al., Impact of diabetes and Hyperglycemia on survival in advanced breast cancer patients. Exp Diabetes Res. 2012; 2012: 732027.
    Minicozzi P., Berrino F., Sebastiani F. et al., High fasting blood glucose and obesity significantly and independently increase risk of breast cancer death in hormone receptor-positive disease. Eur J Cancer. 2013; 49: 3881-3888.
    Mayer A., Vaupel P., Struss H. et al., Strong adverse prognostic impact of hyperglycemic episodes during adjuvant chemoradiotherapy of glioblastoma multiforme. Strahlenther Onkol. 2014; 190: 933-938.
    Tieu M., Lovblom L., McNamara M. et al., Impact of glycemia on survival of glioblastoma patients treated with radiation and temozolomide. J Neurooncol. 2015; 124: 119-26.
    Monzavi-Karbassi B., Gentry R., Kaur V. et al., Pre-diagnosis blood glucose and prognosis in women with breast cancer. Cancer Metab. 2016; 4: 7.38.
    Adeberg S., Bernhardt D., Foerster R. et al., The influence of hyperglycemia during radiotherapy on survival in patients with primary glioblastoma. Acta Oncol (Madr). 2016; 55: 201-207.

6   Brünings W., Beiträge zum Krebsproblem. 1. Mitteilung: Über eine diätetisch-hormonale Beeinflussung des Krebses. (Contributions to the cancer problem. 1st communication: About a dietary hormonal influence on cancer.) Münch Med Wschr. 1941; 88: 117-123.
    Brünings W., Beiträge zum Krebsproblem. 2. Mitteilung: Klinische Anwendungen der diätetisch-hormonalen Krebsbeeinflussung ("Entzuckerungsmethode"). (Contributions to the cancer problem. 2nd communication: Clinical applications of dietary hormonal influence on cancer ("Desugarization method"). Münch Med Wschr. 1942; 89: 71-76.

7   Tan-Shalaby J., Carrick J., Edinger K. et al., Modified Atkins diet in advanced malignancies: final results of a safety and feasibility trial within the Veterans Affairs Pittsburgh Healthcare System. Nutr Metab. 2016; 13: 52.
    Nebeling L., Miraldi F., Shurin S., Lerner E., Effects of a ketogenic diet on tumor metabolism and nutritional status in pediatric oncology patients: two case reports. J Am Coll Nutr. 1995; 14: 202-208.

8 Fine E., Segal-isaacson C., Feinman R. et al., Targeting insulin inhibition as a metabolic therapy in advanced cancer: a pilot safety and feasibility dietary trial in 10 patients. Nutrition. 2012; 28: 1028-1035.

9 Schroeder U., Himpe B., Pries R. et al., Decline of lactate in tumor tissue after ketogenic diet: in vivo microdialysis study in patients with head and neck cancer. Nutr Cancer. 2013; 65: 843-849.

10 Branca J., Pacini S., Ruggiero M., Effects of Pre-surgical vitamin D supplementation and ketogenic diet in a patient with recurrent breast cancer. Anticancer Res. 2015; 35: 5525-5532.

11 Tan-Shalaby J., Carrick J., Edinger K. et al., Modified Atkins diet in advanced malignancies: final results of a safety and feasibility trial within the Veterans Affairs Pittsburgh Healthcare System. Nutr Metab. 2016; 13: 52.
Nebeling L., Miraldi F., Shurin S. et al., Effects of a ketogenic diet on tumor metabolism and nutritional status in pediatric oncology patients: two case reports. J Am Coll Nutr. 1995; 14: 202-208.
Abdelbary M., Elsakka A., Salah H. et al., Does Metabolic management of gliomas using restricted Ketogenic diet combined with hyperbaric oxygen therapy (HBOT) improve clinical outcome and reduce epileptic risk? (poster presentation). Tampa: Metabolic Therapeutics Conference. 2017.

12 Abdelwahab M., Fenton K., Preul M. et al., The ketogenic diet is an effective adjuvant to radiation therapy for the treatment of malignant glioma. PLoS ONE. 2012; 7: e36197.
Allen B., Bhatia S., Buatti J., Ketogenic diets enhance oxidative stress and radio-chemotherapy responses in lung cancer Xenografts Ketogenic diets enhance oxidative stress and radio- chemo-therapy responses in lung cancer xenografts. Clin Cancer Res. 2013; 19: 3905- 3913.
Poff A., Ari C., Seyfried T. et al., The Ketogenic diet and hyperbaric oxygen therapy prolong survival in mice with systemic metastatic cancer. PLoS ONE. 2013; 8: e65522.

13 Klement R., Restricting carbohydrates to fight head and neck cancer - is this realistic? Cancer Biol Med. 2014; 11: 145-161.
Allen B., Bhatia S., Anderson C. et al. et al., Ketogenic diets as an adjuvant cancer therapy: history and potential mechanism. Redox Biol. 2014; 2C: 963-970.

14 Klement R., Champ C., Calories, carbohydrates, and cancer therapy with radiation: exploiting the five R's through dietary manipulation. Cancer Metasta Rev. 2014; 33: 217-229.
Allen B., Bhatia S., Buatti J., Ketogenic diets enhance oxidative stress and radio-chemotherapy responses in lung cancer Xenografts Ketogenic diets enhance oxidative stress and radio- chemo-therapy responses in lung cancer xenografts. Clin Cancer Res. 2013: 19: 3905- 3913.
Sherwin R., Hendler R., Felig P., Effect of ketone infusions on amino acid and nitrogen metabolism in man. J Clin Invest. 1975; 55: 1382-1390.
Zuccoli G., Marcello N., Pisanello A. et al., Metabolic management of glioblastoma multiforme using standard therapy together with a restricted ketogenic diet: case report. Nutr Metab. 2010; 7: 33.
Klement R., Sweeney R., Impact of a ketogenic diet intervention during radiotherapy on body composition: I. Initial clinical experience with six prospectively studied patients. BMC Res Notes. 2016; 9: 143.

15 Fearon K., Borland W., Preston T. et al., Cancer cachexia: influence of systemic ketosis on substrate levels and nitrogen metabolism. Am J Clin Nutr. 1988; 47: 42-48.

16 Dorff T., Groshen S., Garcia A. et al., Safety and feasibility of fasting in combination with platinum-based chemotherapy. BMC Cancer. 2016; 10(16): 360.
De Groot G., Vreeswijk M., Welters M. et al., The effects of short-term fasting on tolerance to (neo) adjuvant chemotherapy in HER2-negative breast cancer patients: a randomized pilot study. BMC Cancer. 2015; 15: 652.

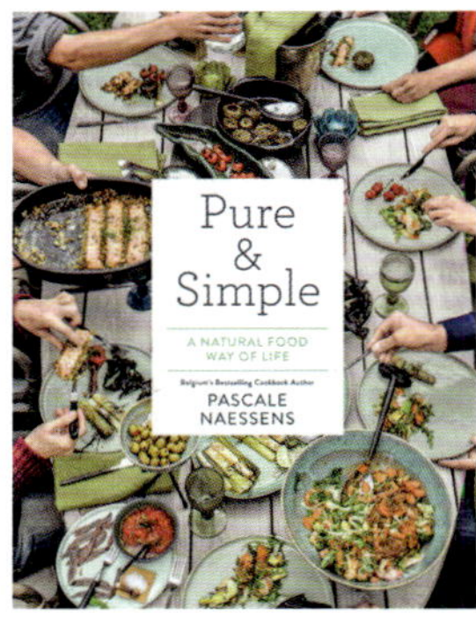

ISBN: 978 1 4197 2617 0

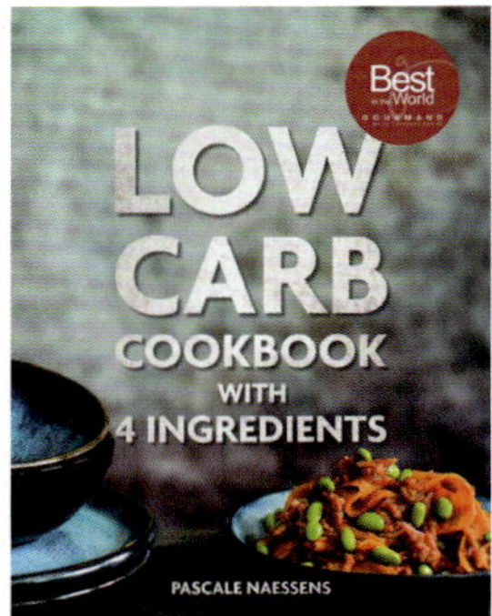

ISBN: 978 9 4014 6148 1

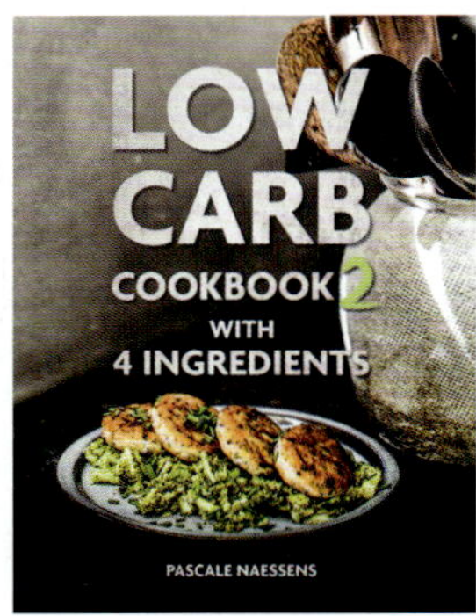

ISBN: 978 94 014 6841 1

www.purepascale.com
www.lannoo.com

I would like to thank my proofreaders, dieticians Hella Van Laer and Sabrina Mattens, keto-adept Katrijn Steenbeke and my assistant Tinneke Grietens. I would also like to thank my co-authors, Doctor William Cortvriendt and Professor Hanno Pijl, for their critical reading of my text and especially for their enthusiasm.

Have you had good experiences with this way of eating? We'd love to hear about it.
Visit the website mentioned above and send us a message via the "contact" page.
You can read more stories under "testimonials". United we stand!

RECIPES, STYLING AND CONCEPT: Pascale Naessens
TEXTS: Pascale Naessens, Hanno Pijl, William Cortvriendt
RECIPE MACRONUTRIENT CALCULATIONS: Dietician Sabrina Mattens
PHOTOGRAPHY: Roos Mestdagh, Diego Fransens, Wout Hendrickx
DESIGN: Kris Torfs - Gemex Publishing bvba
LAYOUT: Banananas.net
ENGLISH TRANSLATION: Textcase, Deventer

If you have any comments or questions, please do not hesitate to contact the publisher:
redactielifestyle@lannoo.be

© Pascale Naessens and Uitgeverij Lannoo nv, Tielt, 2021
D/2021/45/98 - NUR 440-441
ISBN: 978 94 014 7419 1

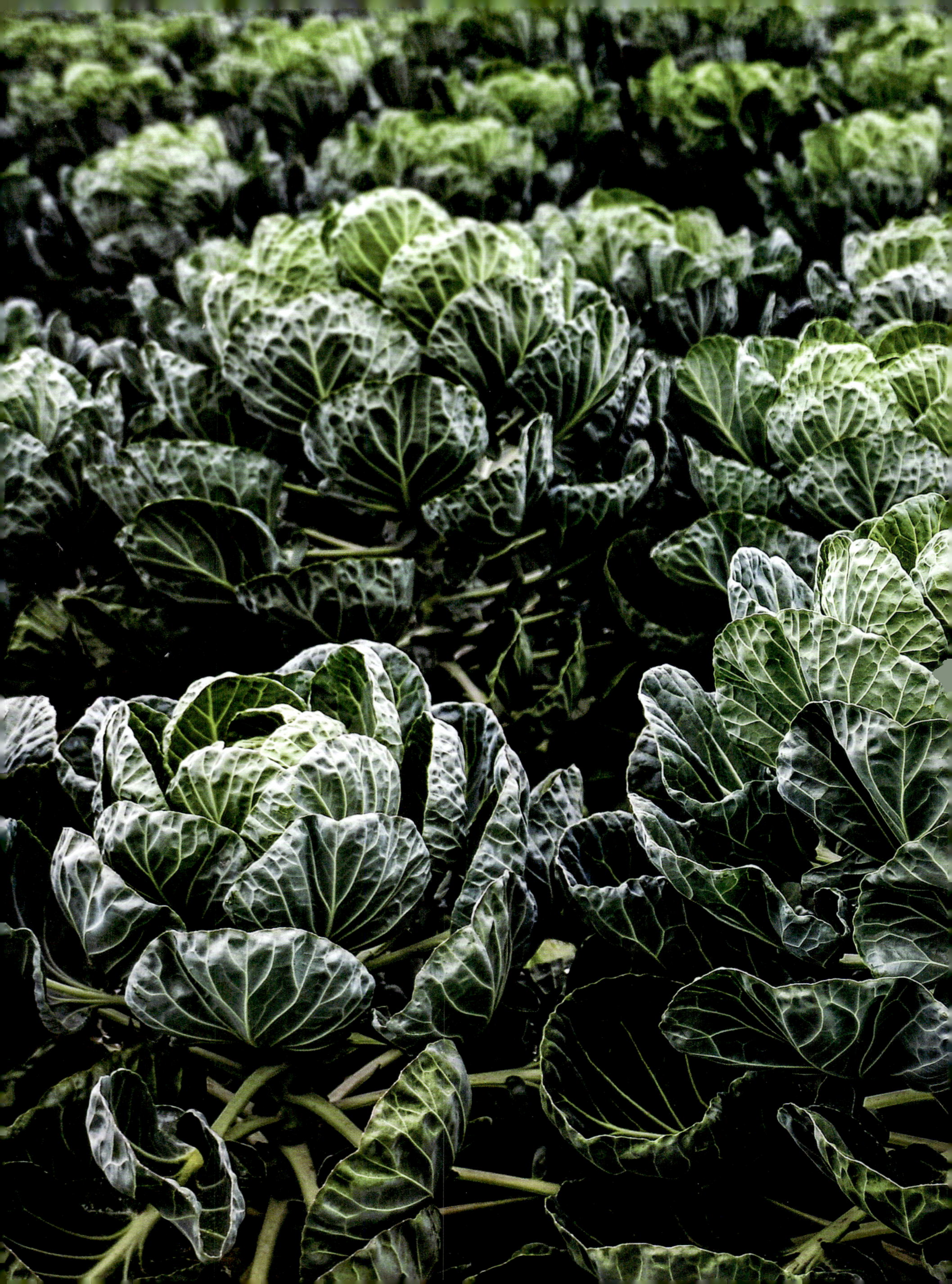